PENGUIN BOOKS

THE REAL LIFE NUTRITION BOOK

Susan Finn, Ph.D., R.D., is an ardent advocate for providing accurate nutrition information to the public. She is considered one of the nation's most articulate voices on nutrition services and practice, and is an internationally known lecturer, author, and practitioner.

Dr. Finn is president-elect of the 60,000-member American Dietetic Association (ADA), the nation's largest organization of nutrition professionals. She is also the director of nutrition services for Ross Laboratories, a leading research facility and manufacturer of scientifically formulated nutritional products. Dr. Finn holds a clinical professorship in the College of Medicine at Ohio State University.

Dr. Finn received her B.S. degree in nutrition from Bowling Green State University in Ohio. She earned her M.S. degree in public health nutrition from Case Western Reserve University in Cleveland, and her Ph.D. in nutrition science from Ohio State University.

She lives with her husband, Jim, in Columbus, Ohio.

Linda Stern Kass began working as a journalist, specializing in medical and health issues, in 1976. In the late 1970s, she wrote for various regional and national publications, including *Time, The Detroit Free Press, Monthly Detroit, Medical Tribune, Family Health, Ohio Magazine,* and *Columbus Monthly.* She received an honorable mention in the 1979 national Clarion awards competition. After spending seven years working in the telecommunications industry, she resumed her writing career with the preparation of *The Real Life Nutrition Book.*

Mrs. Kass received a Bachelor of Science degree in allied health medicine from the University of Pennsylvania in 1975 and a Master of Arts degree in journalism from Ohio State University in 1978.

She currently lives in Columbus, Ohio, with her husband, Frank, and son, Matthew.

The Real Life Nutrition Book

MAKING THE RIGHT FOOD CHOICES
WITHOUT CHANGING YOUR LIFE-STYLE

Susan Finn, Ph.D., R.D.
and
Linda Stern Kass

PENGUIN BOOKS

PENGUIN BOOKS
Published by the Penguin Group
Viking Penguin, a division of Penguin Books USA Inc.,
375 Hudson Street, New York, New York 10014, U.S.A.
Penguin Books Ltd, 27 Wrights Lane, London W8 5TZ, England
Penguin Books Australia Ltd, Ringwood, Victoria, Australia
Penguin Books Canada Ltd, 10 Alcorn Avenue, Suite 300,
Toronto, Ontario, Canada M4V 3B2
Penguin Books (N.Z.) Ltd, 182–190 Wairau Road,
Auckland 10, New Zealand

Penguin Books Ltd, Registered Offices:
Harmondsworth, Middlesex, England

First published in Penguin Books 1992

1 3 5 7 9 10 8 6 4 2

A NOTE TO THE READER
The ideas, procedures, and suggestions contained in this book are not intended
as a substitute for consulting with your physician. All matters regarding your
health require medical supervision.

LIBRARY OF CONGRESS CATALOGING IN PUBLICATION DATA
Finn, Susan Calvert.
The real life nutrition book / Susan Finn and Linda Stern Kass.
p.   cm.
Includes index.
ISBN 0 14 01.3174 4
1. Nutrition.   I. Kass, Linda Stern.   II. Title.
RA784.F54   1992
613.2—dc20   91-17467

Printed in the United States of America
Set in Baskerville and Bodoni Bold
Designed by Mary A. Wirth

Grateful acknowledgment is made for permission to use the following material:
Comparison of height-weight tables from *Principles of Geriatric Medicine and Gerontology,*
second edition, by R. Andres, et al. By permission of McGraw-Hill, Inc.
Nutritional charts by Linda J. Bethel. By permission of Linda J. Bethel.
Chart assessing blood lipids from *Controlling Cholesterol* by Kenneth H. Cooper, M.D.,
M.P.H. Copyright © 1988 by Kenneth H. Cooper. Used by permission of Bantam
Books, a division of Bantam Doubleday Dell Publishing Group, Inc.
FMI Supermarket Directory: Nutrition & Health Programs 1989 compiled by
FMI Consumer Affairs Department, Washington, D.C. By permission
of Food Marketing Institute.
Chart listing calorie expenditure from *Exercise Physiology: Energy, Nutrition
and Human Performance,* third edition, by W. D. McArdle, F. I. Katch,
and V. L. Katch. By permission of Lea & Febiger.
Metropolitan height and weight tables, courtesy of Metropolitan Life Insurance Co.

To the people who wish to
improve the quality of their
lives through good nutrition

Preface

My professional life as a nutritionist/dietitian began more than twenty years ago, and early on I learned a very important lesson. When I was graduated from Bowling Green University in 1966, I found myself working in the Hough neighborhood in Cleveland, where poverty and illiteracy were daily visitors. I was part of an outreach program from Cleveland Metropolitan General Hospital, and our mission was to reduce infant mortality by teaching mothers, some as young as twelve and thirteen, about nutrition.

We made home visits and talked about prenatal care, breast feeding, empty calories—the entire range of what goes into maternal infant care. But breast-feeding and talk of empty calories and a good breakfast were not especially popular among the poor young women who were my clients. In this troubled inner city, food stamps were higher on the priority list, and how to budget them to last a full month was a skill that needed to be taught. Additionally, alcohol and drugs were strong, persuasive enemies of family life and of the assistance we were trying to provide.

Yet, despite these frustrations, data from these programs demonstrated that they worked. Dietitians sent out into the community to teach changed lives for good. In this dramatic setting, I learned that new habits can be taught and that good nutrition can make a difference in people's lives. But few nutritional educational programs were available for the general public in those years. There was little interest in the medical schools, in the food industry, or among the general population.

In the intervening twenty-five years, we have undergone a revolution of interest and information. Eighty percent of all medical schools now offer at least an elective course in nutrition. Government funding is now allowing more research dollars to be allocated to investigate the role played by nutrition in the prevention and treatment of many diseases. But there are still wide gaps in the public's knowledge of nutrition in such areas as wise food choices.

I believe that one of the most vital roles of the dietitian today is to translate complex nutritional facts into language the general public can understand and to make that information readily accessible.

With that in mind, I envisioned this book as an opportunity to fill some of those gaps and to provide sound, comprehensible nutrition information in an interesting and readable format.

Susan Finn, Ph.D., R.D.
January 1992

Writing a book about nutrition was natural for me for several reasons. First, on a personal level, staying fit has been a part of my life since adolescence. I've always been curious about nutrition, and have been an avid reader of the subject over the years. As an undergraduate at the University of Pennsylvania, I majored in the allied health sciences, working in the field for several years before going on to get a master's degree in journalism at Ohio State University. On a professional level, I began writing about medical and health issues in 1976. I have written for various regional and national publications, including *Time,* where I reported on medicine and science for the magazine's Detroit bureau in the late seventies. From 1980 to 1987, I worked in the broadcasting and telecommunications industries and saw firsthand how health and nutrition became an integral part of broadcast programming.

Yet a reliable and credible nutrition book that took our increasingly mobile life-styles into account did not exist. Teaming up with an exceptionally knowledgeable expert like Susan Finn made such a book possible.

Many of the people I know have busy lives. They have children who need to be carpooled from one activity to another. They work. They make time to do volunteer work. They have trouble getting dinner on the table. They often can't fit regular exercise into their busy days. They don't understand labels, let alone have the time to read them during their rushed hour at the neighborhood grocery. They know some basic information about fats, cholesterol, sodium, and calories, but they don't know how to apply that information to making food choices at the supermarket or at a restaurant. They particularly don't wish to apply their information while traveling or entertaining. To many of the people I know, good nutrition seems like an unattainable goal.

These are the people I wanted to reach in a book about nutrition. When Susan Finn and I began discussing an angle for this book, we shared similar stories about people we knew. It became clear to us that we could make good nutrition a reality for people like yourself by approaching the subject in the context of your life—your real life.

We live in a society where medical technology is prolonging lives. We also live in a society offering the opportunity for diverse occupations and life-styles. Regardless of what "real life" is for you, there are nutritious alternatives at restaurants, at supermarkets, aboard airlines, and in your own home. We share them with you in this book.

Good nutrition doesn't have to conflict with social or business obligations. Society is adapting because real life demands it.

Linda Stern Kass
January 1992

Acknowledgments

The authors jointly would like to thank:

The six people who are featured as case studies in this book—Carole Gerber, Judy Markey, Burt Staniar, Jane Hartley, Barry Nash, and Herb Glimcher—for sharing their insights and experiences. Their comments will help make nutrition a "real life" subject for readers of this book.

Chefs Robert Briggs and Tracy Ritter for their expertise and creativity in making the challenge of cooking at home (Chapter 3) healthy and exciting.

Linda Bethel, R.D.; Margaret McWilliams, Ph.D., R.D.; and Virginia Vivian, Ph.D., R.D., for their valuable advice and guidance.

Susan Borra, R.D., Director of Consumer Affairs, Food Marketing Institute, for being so generous with both her time and knowledge.

Lori Lipsky, our editor at Penguin USA, for her enthusiastic support and flexibility, her assistant, Nicole Guisto, and everyone at Penguin USA who got behind this project from the outset and worked on it through all its phases.

Trish Todd (now an editor with Dell Publishing) and Sandra

Choron of March Tenth, Inc., who believed in the concept of "real life" nutrition. Thank you, Sandra, for bringing this project to the people who made it happen and for all your hard work and continued support.

Estelle Stern, who, as business manager of this project, deserves more appreciation than we could possibly express for more reasons than we could possibly list, and her assistant, Chris Carey, for handling many details with a smile.

Susan Finn would like to express her appreciation to:

"My husband Jim Finn and my son John for their patience and their willingness to be the subjects of so many dietetic and culinary experiences for so many years and for their never-swerving confidence in me and this project.

"My parents, Flora and Chalmers Davies, for the values and determination they instilled in me.

"Anita Owen, a friend and colleague of many years, who is the ultimate nutrition educator and the best role model I can think of for both new and experienced dietitians.

"My colleagues in the American Dietetic Association and the American Dietetic Association Foundation. Your dedication to the health and well-being of your society, your commitment to our profession, and your high level of expertise are a constant source of inspiration.

"The many, many registered dietitians I have been privileged to personally meet and work with, for continually coming up with new and creative ways to provide up-to-date and sound nutrition information to the public."

Linda Stern Kass would like to express her appreciation to:

"My best friend and husband, Frank Kass, who is an inspiration and a support to me always.

"My parents, Ernest and Aurelia Stern, who have never doubted my abilities, even when I did.

"My son, Matthew, and my stepsons, Jonathan and David, for tolerating all my nutritional 'advice.'

"Ron Johnson and his staff at Comdata Corporation for matching technology to creativity to keep the book on schedule.

"Those people who, over the years, shared their lifelong nutritional battles with me. Their challenges and pursuit of good nutrition convinced me of the universal interest in this topic and this book.

"All my devoted relatives and friends who were there to support me when personal tragedy interfered down the home stretch of this project and who continue to provide me with strength each day."

Contents

List of Charts

Introduction

In 1988, then–Surgeon General C. Everett Koop came out with a hard-hitting report on nutrition that shook the medical community. Too much fat, salt, and alcohol and not enough required nutrients are sending millions of Americans to early graves, he said. Diseases of dietary excess and imbalance, as he termed them, were among the leading causes of death in the United States in 1987. Nearly 1.5 million Americans, of the 2.1 million who died that year, succumbed to diseases associated with diet. "If you are among the two out of three Americans who do not smoke or drink excessively, your choice of diet can influence your long-term health prospects more than any other action you might take," Koop said.

Unfortunately, nearly five years later, the American public is confused and overwhelmed by seemingly contradictory reports about their diets. Too many people, in fact, get their nutrition education from the weekly tabloids at supermarket checkout stands rather than from reliable sources such as dietitians or medical doctors. Then there is the problem of the people who are nutritionally aware but are not acting on their information. A recent survey by the

Department of Agriculture found 78 percent of the respondents saying that there are so many recommendations related to diet, it's hard to know what to believe.

From a subculture of food faddists, we hear theories about the benefits of honey and sea salt and unrefined sugar. We read lists of foods that can be combined and foods that in combination can be harmful to our health. We're told that cholesterol levels higher than 200 milligrams can now be considered dangerous, but that shellfish (once thought to be forbidden for cholesterol watchers) can be eaten by some people on low-cholesterol diets since it is low in saturated fat. We hear that calcium supplements are important, but some articles warn that they can be hazardous because they block the absorption of trace minerals. We've heard so much about the benefits of fiber, yet we're now told that too much fiber can be harmful.

So first there's the problem of sifting through a lot of information and misinformation. You need basic nutritional principles, and you need them from reliable sources. Then there's the problem of maintaining good nutrition when your life-style involves many unpredictable situations and temptations—nonstop family activities and car pools, daily business lunches, frequent travel and entertainment, little time for cooking, and fast-food restaurants on every corner. The result is, you give up, you eat what's handy, you exercise if you can fit it into your already tightly scheduled day. Or, in other words, you eat potato chips for lunch, Lean Cuisine for dinner, and rationalize that you're watching your diet.

Whereas the "anything goes" attitude may be the easiest answer for today's hectic life-styles, it is also the most dangerous to your lifelong health. Furthermore, it is a black-and-white approach to nutrition. Who says good nutrition and general well-being can result only from strict calorie counting and limited food choices, supplemented by a rigid exercise program?

One fact is clear. Many of our lives cannot accommodate an inflexible nutritional regimen. That may explain why so many new diet books are published each year. Each one makes promises, yet each fails us because our lives can't seem to adapt. So we look to a new diet plan with renewed hope; that, too, places too many demands on us.

However, this book is *not* a diet book. Weight-reduction plans, when recommended by your physician or dietitian, serve an important purpose; and we focus on the nation's obsession with dieting in Chapter 10. While we provide one week's menus to get you started, we do not offer you a new weight-loss diet in this book. What we offer instead is a real life nutrition guide written to accommodate the needs created by your particular life-style. The traditional family meal is important and exists in many homes, but it doesn't represent everyday real life for most Americans today.

What is real life nutrition? It's not three square meals leisurely prepared each day by Donna Reed. We don't have the time to live like that anymore.

Real life nutrition is good nutrition that can be incorporated into our real life situations: family life that often includes both parents working, living alone, and single-parent homes, frequent dining out and travel, exercise squeezed into a day of skipped meals, stress, and a variety of choices offered by the food industry, fast-food establishments, and restaurants.

In this book you will find practical, real life guidelines for good nutrition and fitness that can lead to dramatic improvements in your body composition and endurance capacity. And they can be made at any age. People who look and feel better at forty-two than they did at twenty-two are becoming the norm. Look at the Sally Field of today in her forties and compare her with the Sally Field who played Gidget some twenty years ago. And what about Dolly Parton? Or Cher? These are only three well-known examples. We all have friends who went through similar transformations, often initiated in mid-life, when you begin to come to grips with your own mortality. You begin to think about what you can do to prepare yourself for a long life. And many people today at least say they're doing just that.

Unfortunately, recent surveys indicate that the dramatic nutrition revolution that was going to change the way Americans eat is not happening. A few years ago, a nationwide telephone survey of 1,870 people conducted by *The New York Times* revealed that most Americans, regardless of age, had not responded in a significant fashion to calls for decreasing fat in the diet, reducing sodium, taking in fewer calories, or otherwise eating more healthfully.

More recently, the National Cancer Institute and the Food and Drug Administration interviewed eleven thousand people and found them to have poor diets. Only 49 percent, for example, included vegetables other than potatoes and salad in their daily diets, and more than 40 percent ate at least one serving of luncheon meat or bacon daily.

And a U.S. Department of Agriculture report on the nation's eating habits, which was the focus of the seventy-third annual meeting of the American Dietetic Association in October of 1990, said that current diets contribute to high rates of heart disease, high blood pressure, and diabetes. While the report indicated that Americans' eating habits are improving, it clearly stated that we still eat too much fat, cholesterol, and sodium.

This news is disheartening, because the facts about preparing for a longer life are quite clear. You can learn to manage your stress better and change your work mode to an extent, but the things you can manipulate most easily in your life to stay healthy are what you eat and how much you exercise. And your life-style should dictate your fitness program, rather than vice versa.

"We can no longer afford to ignore the fact that prevention is the single most important factor in maintaining good health," said Dr. Louis Sullivan, Secretary of Health and Human Services, in September of 1990, when he released a report listing 298 national health goals, including losing weight, exercising more, smoking and drinking less. This report was the second to establish ten-year health goals for the nation. Without life-style changes, Dr. Sullivan noted, health-care costs will rise from the $600 billion spent by Americans in 1989 to $1.5 trillion by the year 2000. The report urges Americans to take responsibility for our own life-styles.

In Chapter 1, "Nutrition and Real Life," we begin with a quiz of sorts to get you thinking about your own life-style and how it might affect your health. You'll meet a number of men and women and learn what real life nutrition is for them.

Chapter 2 simplifies all the food facts you need to know, about everything from alcohol and caffeine to calcium and vitamins. It also covers the many hot topics that are a source of conflict among even the most reliable nutrition scientists and offers credible information you can use.

No longer do people get married at age twenty-one and have 2.5 children. In real life, many marry later and have children later, and live in households with both parents working. Another part of real life today is combining two families into one in a second marriage. Some people choose single life or find themselves single due to death or divorce. With the change in family life, eating patterns must adapt as well, and it is this challenge of singles and families on the go that is addressed in Chapter 3.

Shoppers age forty to forty-nine (the core age group of those families on the go) spend more at the supermarket than any other age group, according to the Food Marketing Institute in Washington, D.C. The complex choices facing today's food consumer at the supermarket of the nineties is explored in the next two chapters. In Chapter 4, we look at what concerns America's food shoppers today, and how the supermarket industry has adapted to meet the convenience and the nutritional needs of consumers. You will learn how to use labels and understand the basic dietary principles to guide you toward making the best food choices. Chapter 5 walks you down the aisles of a sophisticated supermarket, from the produce section to the frozen-food counter. Included are comparative charts on milk and cheese products, frozen dinners and desserts, and a list of the fiber content of an array of foods likely to be in your cabinets or refrigerators right now.

The Food Institute, based in Fair Lawn, New Jersey, projects that between 1990 and 1995, people aged thirty-five to fifty-four will spend $13 billion more on food away from home than the same age group spent (as projected) from 1985 to 1990. The reason stems partly from a lack of time to prepare meals at home, and that translates into the fast-food and restaurant industries—the subjects of the next two chapters.

The unlikely marriage of fast food and the fast track is examined in Chapter 6. Here you will find a fast-food industry eager to please a more nutritionally conscious customer. Baby boomers grew up with McDonald's and the concept of fast food, and the cycle is continuing with their families. In this chapter you'll learn how to get a nutritious meal from a McDonald's-like restaurant, and the top five fast-food outlets are rated so you can see how they stack up nutritionally.

Dining out is an American pastime. In Chapter 7, eating out for business or pleasure is the focus. You'll learn how to make nutritious food choices regardless of whether you dine at your neighborhood family spot or at a restaurant specializing in more gourmet fare.

Our real life situations involve travel, national and international. Chapter 8, "The Traveler's Guide to Good Nutrition," discusses the many choices you have to stay on track nutritionally, regardless of where your business or pleasure takes you: regional foods across the United States, airline menu choices, hotel food, spa and cruise fare, and what you can expect from each of these.

Stress is very much a part of real life. We all share the pressure to get the work done while the clock keeps ticking. Chapter 9 explores the nutritional effect of stress in our daily lives: how stress affects the body and what we eat, and conversely, how what we eat affects the way we're able to cope with stress.

Chapter 10 is titled "Diet Mania and the Fuss About Weight Control" for good reason. The problems of obesity and weight control are a serious concern in this country today. While examining America's obsession with food and dieting, this chapter also focuses on the fact that you can be too thin. The compulsive desire for thinness can be as harmful to your health as the compulsion toward overeating.

Chapter 11 covers the effects certain foods and liquids have on us while we engage in various athletic activities. Certainly, the importance of exercise cannot be overstated in any book about maintaining good health and nutrition.

In the final chapter, we enter the twenty-first century. Many products are under development right now that are going to revolutionize the way we're eating and the way our food choices will be made available to us. Chapter 12 offers a glimpse of the future as we base predictions on current trends in nutrition and a little imagination.

The Real Life
Nutrition Book

1

Nutrition and Real Life

Does this sound like you or someone you know?

- A forty-seven-year-old business executive plays basketball instead of having a business lunch, then has a soft drink and a candy bar by mid-afternoon.
- A forty-one-year-old marketing executive has a morning meeting that runs through lunchtime, so she races through an airport trying to make her plane, debating whether she should stop at the concession stand for an ice cream bar or a yogurt.
- A thirty-two-year-old mother is shopping at her local supermarket with her cranky four-year-old and trying to make some sense of the multitude of choices in the frozen-food section.
- A family of four (Mom and Dad are hitting forty; the twins are eight) are arguing about which fast-food restaurant would satisfy everyone; Mom is wondering to herself how she will ever keep her girlish figure with the number of evenings she eats fast food.
- A fifty-seven-year-old investment banker has yet another business dinner with potential clients from out of town; he's thinking about his cholesterol while scanning an expensive French menu

1

that highlights one entree after another sautéed in butter and/or topped with a cream sauce.

In today's busy world, real life for millions of Americans is just like the scenarios described above. The facts are clear. Today, both parents are working, or if Mom doesn't work, she's involved in activities that keep her out of the kitchen. Dining out is increasing: as a unit, families frequent fast-food establishments; singles tend to dine out with friends much more than they eat at home; and wage earners often fill their days dining out for business. To work off some of the stress that has built up from the overscheduled appointments or the back-and-forth car pool for the kids' activities, exercise is generally squeezed into a day of skipped meals. Travel for relaxation is a bigger must, but travel for the job is in full swing.

Whatever your life-style, you do have nutritional choices that can affect how you feel today and how healthy you are down the road. Dining out doesn't have to be an excuse for the extra ten pounds you carry around. Staying at your desk at lunch doesn't have to mean a candy bar or nothing. Frozen dinners don't have to be the alternative to a home-cooked meal just because you can't seem to get home before seven. Certainly your life-style dictates the kind of choices you need to make, but however you live the choices do exist.

What is your life-style, and where does nutrition fit in for you? The following life-style quiz will give you some clues.

Answer yes or no to the following statements:

1. In general, I feel content and satisfied with my life.
2. I enjoy my job and look forward to it each day.
3. Even when I have a great deal to do, I rarely feel rushed and I have no trouble relaxing.
4. I don't smoke cigarettes.
5. I never drink alcohol.
6. Overall, I feel healthy and rarely get sick.
7. I regularly check my cholesterol and blood pressure.
8. I understand the difference between HDL, LDL, and cholesterol.
9. I am at the right weight for my height and build and I never feel a need to diet.

10. I make sure I get regular exercise and I know that my exercise is adequately supported by good nutrition.
11. I am convinced that my diet is nutritionally sound.
12. I regularly eat three balanced meals each day.
13. My evening meal regularly consists of freshly prepared vegetables, whole grains, dairy products, lean fish and chicken and meats, and desserts such as fruits or sorbets.
14. I am knowledgeable about the effects of caffeine, sugar substitutes, and alcohol on one's nutritional state.
15. When food shopping at the supermarket, I always read the labels and understand the nutrient content of the foods I select.
16. I know how to select a nutritionally sound meal at a fast-food restaurant.
17. Regardless of where I dine out, I am able to order a nutritionally balanced meal without adding extra fat and calories to my diet.
18. Even when I travel, I feel confident that my nutrition doesn't suffer.

If you answered "no" to half or more of the above you need to read further, because you probably don't have a clear understanding of nutrition or how nutrition relates to many aspects of your life—or, like most of us, you aren't applying your knowledge of nutrition correctly. You could be doing damage to your health without even knowing it. Poor nutritional habits can be subtle and can impact your behavior, your performance at work and your health, now and in the future. They can even lead to conditions as devastating as atherosclerosis (lesions in the arteries containing fatty deposits) and heart disease. What always may have seemed to you to be a meaningless piece of information—like the difference between a saturated fat and a monounsaturated fat—can make the difference between a healthy life and heart disease.

It's never too late to change lifelong habits. It's never too late to understand nutrition as it relates to your life, and it's never too early to understand nutrition for your children's lives. You may be surprised about what you'll learn in this book. You can prolong your healthy life and get your children off to a healthier start once you make the commitment to become aware of nutritional principles. We promise to make your commitment an easy and even enjoyable one.

In this chapter, you'll learn how to look at and evaluate what you eat in the context of your total diet. You will meet people like yourselves, people who don't lead perfect nutritional lives. In later chapters, you will read about them again, and about others. In their typical lives, their real lives, you'll learn how they can use moderation, balance, and variety in their nutritional habits and common sense about what they eat and how they exercise, and, most of all, how they make the right choices for the kind of people they are and for the kind of lives they lead. You can do that too.

"Nutrition Conscious to a Realistic Point"

Meet Carole Gerber. Carole is a forty-four-year-old freelance writer in Columbus, Ohio, a wife and the mother of two. She is five foot five, weighs 110 pounds, and is generally healthy. She is an ex-smoker, an occasional drinker of wine, a light-to-moderate coffee drinker, and she takes vitamins regularly. She has had her cholesterol checked in the not-too-distant past, and it is normal.

She dines out infrequently, and her typical daily diet looks something like this. She eats bran cereal and juice for breakfast, has pizza twice a week for lunch and either skips the other lunches or has a simple sandwich or salad. For dinner she has a salad, a starch, and grilled chicken or fish. And she is quick to point out that she drinks at least two glasses of milk daily because she is worried about osteoporosis (also known as brittle bones, which will be discussed more in Chapter 2). She snacks with her younger daughter every afternoon, and she admits it is usually some kind of sugary snack.

Carole has never had to diet because she's never been overweight. But because she has had problems with her gall bladder over the past five years, she has tried to limit the amount of fats in her diet. Fast foods are not part of her diet. She says she doesn't like their taste and finds them too salty. Perhaps because she's never had a weight problem, Carole has never been a dedicated exerciser. Just recently she started exercising to a stretch-and-tone videotape three times a week.

Carole is a lot like many people we know. She is bright and aware of most things around her, including her state of health. But she generally eats what she likes out of the variety of foods she believes to be healthy, while adding a few foods from the "less than good for you" category, and has managed to find a balance for her life.

When asked how she sees herself from a nutritional point of view, she said, "I consider myself nutrition conscious to a realistic point. I think it can be overdone. I've read about people on macrobiotic diets and people who've taken up a three-hour daily exercise regime, and I think that's an example of taking things to extremes. I think people should get some enjoyment out of food and not deny themselves everything."

"Nutrition Impaired"—But Not According to the Authors

On the other hand, Judy Markey, forty-seven, a syndicated columnist based at the *Chicago Sun Times,* an author, and a talk-show host on WGN-AM radio, considers herself "nutrition impaired." She's typical of many of you who eat one balanced meal a day—usually dinner—with the rest of the day being catch-as-catch-can, and oftentimes loaded with empty calories.

Working at her computer in her suburban Chicago home, Judy begins her day at 8:30 a.m. with about three cups of coffee lightened by half-and-half. Lunch may be Brie on Triscuits or a half-dozen Pringles with a Coke Classic. For dinner, she'll fix pasta for herself and her teenage son, or they'll order in some Chinese food.

Judy admits she doesn't like to cook and has been known to make herself poached eggs for dinner. "Food is one of the least important areas in my life," she says. Yet when she dines out, she probably has a broader palate than most people. If she's at a Mexican restaurant she has chicken fajitas; if she's in a Japanese restaurant she has sushi; if she's in a Thai restaurant she has beef and chicken with noodles; dining Italian, she'll order carpaccio and a salad. She doesn't eat much deli food like pastrami or corned beef, and she prefers light fare in general because she's small (five feet tall, ninety-eight pounds). But when she orders, she does not think about how the food was prepared or whether it is nutritious. She orders whatever she feels like at the time. And, ironically, her one daily meal tends to be a nutritious one.

Actually, many of Judy's habits are quite nutritious. She's not a regular red-meat eater—she'll have a steak every two or three weeks, either at home or dining out. At home, she prepares her dinner meal from fresh ingredients, produce and meats. And while she calls herself "nutrition-impaired," Judy doesn't have butter in her house now—she uses margarine, though she doesn't have a premeditated reason for the healthy substitution.

Judy says she rarely eats fast foods, but again this isn't for nutritional reasons. "It's just too heavy and sits in my stomach for days," she complains. She is not the least bit embarrassed to tell you she doesn't exercise. "I'm not perfectly toned, obviously, but I can wear a pair of shorts and not embarrass myself. . . . Aerobically, I'm quite a mess," she adds.

She's quite relaxed about most of the things that could affect her health (which she terms "excellent"). She doesn't worry about fats in her diet. She had her cholesterol tested recently for an insurance policy, but she doesn't remember what her level was other than that it was normal. She doesn't take vitamins now, and she never has.

The Corporate CEO: Fitting Priorities into a Tight Schedule

Burt Staniar leads a busy life. At forty-nine, he is chairman and chief executive officer of Westinghouse Broadcasting Company (Group W), a New York–based division of the Westinghouse Electric Company. Group W owns television and radio stations in major cities across the country, along with a production company based in Los Angeles that produces everything from syndicated talk shows to popular cartoon series for children.

Burt is married and has two sons, ages seventeen and nineteen. He lives in Ho-Ho-Kus, New Jersey, and commutes to his Manhattan office by car every day. This interview was conducted, in fact, on his car telephone during his commute to New Jersey after a particularly long day of work.

Burt works in a high-pressured job in a fast-paced business. He participates in a lot of outside activities. He's very involved with his family. He's done a considerable amount of reading about health and nutrition, and he even has a specific philosophy on the subject that he tries to live by. "I've got my regimen figured out," he says. "But I don't execute it well. I execute it partially." Why? "I let the job be the determinant of the time—it's the first priority," he explains. That's to be expected of a corporate CEO. But considering his pace, Burt Staniar bats about a .400.

First, let's look at his typical day and week. During the two or three workdays each week he is in town, Burt is up by 5:30 a.m. and in the office by 7:00. He has a bran muffin and a cup of tea at his desk. For lunch, half the time he'll eat a sandwich at his desk, half the time he'll have a business lunch at a nice New York restaurant. Either way, it's lunch on the run. "I'm either working, or I'm working," he admits. His in-town dinners will be split again, half at home, half out on business.

During his two or three workdays out of town, Burt may eat out three meals a day, and he may be at banquets or industry functions where the meal is preordered. Since he travels a good deal, his in-town weekends are scheduled in order to fit everything in. He spends one-third of the time on business, schedules athletic activities like tennis or racquetball for another third, and spends the rest of the time on family activities. "It's always crowded," Burt says.

But Burt has the energy, enthusiasm, and discipline to maintain a balance that he is happy with. His health philosophy fits into this balance. "I've concluded, from the reading I've done, that there are three things that I can do to, not prolong my life, but make the quality of my life better," Burt explains. "One is fats, two is exercise, three is meditation. Fats, I believe, affect the heart and cancer; so does exercise; and meditation affects the biggest one, stress. Those are my three buttons."

When did he begin this program? "It all started to evolve over the last ten years, and more totally in the past five years. As I hit forty, it was the same time more and more publicity was coming out about [nutrition and fitness], and so the two came together." Hitting forty is not an uncommon time for people, particularly men, to examine their health while finally facing their own mortality.

Burt made some fairly abrupt changes even though his health was excellent and his weight was never a problem. To begin with, he began taking a multivitamin supplement. He stopped drinking coffee completely because it upset his stomach and his nerves. He quit drinking wine with lunch. His family changed how they ate at home. He stopped eating any fast foods.

Let's look more specifically at how Burt lives his three-pronged philosophy. First, he monitors the fats in his diet. "I've learned to eat rolls without butter, and they taste pretty good if they're good rolls. If they're not good rolls, I don't eat them. I still eat ice cream, but I watch how much I do. I love cheese and I still eat it, but I just cut back." He goes off his program on Saturday nights and when out at industry functions where meals are pre-prepared.

His exercise habits are even more difficult to control. "I do not have a regime," he says. "I'd like to, but I haven't been successful maintaining one." Since his job is his number-one priority, it can cut into any exercise time during the work week. "During the week, I'll be lucky to get any serious exercise in more than once or maybe twice." That will take the form of a racquet sport at noon at a New York health club. When he is traveling, he'll try to get in fifteen minutes of random warm-up exercises in his hotel room in the morning. Burt admits his exercise is confined mostly to weekends—and it takes the form of athletics like racquet sports or softball.

To reduce stress, Burt has learned a method of meditation based on a technique described in the book *The Relaxation Response* by Dr. Herbert Benson. He sits in a quiet place, closes his eyes, concentrates on his breathing, and repeats a mantra or a sound, and as he exhales he pushes away the thoughts that come into his mind.

Burt feels he does a mediocre job of carrying out his health philosophy. "I am convinced that if I did a real good job in all three of those areas, there is a reasonable chance I would improve my odds of achieving a better quality of life," he says. "It is insurance worth bothering about, just as the vitamins are insurance."

The Urban Mom Who's Always on the Go

Jane Hartley seems to be typical of the busy urban mother/wife in New York City, a place where people are perpetually in motion. Jane, at forty-one, has two youngsters—a six-year-old daughter and three-year-old son. Her husband is an investment banker. The family lives on Manhattan's Upper East Side and owns a weekend home in the southern Berkshires of Connecticut.

Jane has always worked in demanding jobs. While single and living in Washington, D.C., in the late seventies, she was on the domestic affairs staff in the Carter administration. Since moving to New York in 1980, her career has been in the broadcasting industry. Her most recent full-time job, which she held until her son was born, was as station manager for WWOR, Channel 9 in New York, an independent television station, for which Jane had to commute daily to Secaucus, New Jersey. After working part-time as a marketing consultant for MCA in its New York office, Jane is now a member of the board of directors of Pinelands, Inc., a public company that owns WWOR-TV.

Jane's big-city life-style is typical because of its lack of structure (when there are so many things going on, you can't plan for everything) and its spontaneity (with more commitments, you have to expect to roll with the punches). Dinnertime depends on everyone's schedule. Food shopping is sporadic.

Despite less planning, living in New York has many nutritious advantages. Jane's random shopping consists of walking to a corner market where fresh produce is readily available. "Part of eating fresh foods has to do with living in New York," Jane says. "You have access to fresh produce on every corner. You begin to taste the difference—fresh tastes so much better." And when the time is just too short to prepare a family meal at home, a nearly home-cooked meal is but a phone call away. A take-out meal for home delivery is so simple in New York City, with anything from Italian to Indian food being available.

Whereas nutrition doesn't have to suffer in Jane's life and she has chosen not to let it do so, she and her husband never seem to have the time to fit exercise into their busy schedules—and in this they are quite typical as well. Jane describes herself as "fairly athletic" and says she used to jog. But exercise is the area in her life that has always gone through peaks and valleys. Now she tries to get to an exercise class once every two weeks. She recently bought her husband an exercise bike, but they really haven't used it much. They're "thinking" about joining a Cardio-Fitness Center near her husband's office. "That's what we're striving for. We haven't gotten there yet," she sighs. "Because you can't sluff work off, and I always want to play with the kids when I get home, exercise becomes the first thing to go."

Business Executive and Family Man

Barry Nash struck us as a typical business executive who holds the notion of family near and dear. Along with his dual priorities,

Barry has become increasingly aware of nutrition and fitness as a way of life. He is by no means compulsive at this stage, and in fact there exists an element of contradiction between what he's aware of doing and what he actually does.

At thirty-four years of age, Barry is a partner in a Dallas, Texas consulting firm called Media & Marketing, a firm specializing in marketing television news. Barry's specialty is in training people to be on television. His wife works at his firm, and they have two daughters, ages four and eight.

Barry's job is a demanding one. He travels 60 percent of the time. He sometimes gets home too late to eat dinner with his family. There is always some office work that needs to get done over the weekend. He admits he's pretty compulsive about working and that he often fails to take time to do other things.

Like exercise. For about a year, Barry has made a disciplined effort to exercise nearly every day. But to fit it in, he begins his twenty-to-thirty-minute routine at 6:00 a.m. "If I don't exercise in the morning early, it's tough to get to it," he explains. Barry says he exercises at home rather than at a health club or jogging outside because he feels the need to be near his family. "I guess it's the guilt of the man who travels a lot," he says. "It's real easy to just struggle from waking to sleeping with all the things that press in. But what I'm beginning to understand is the more I exercise, the more stamina I have, the clearer and cleaner I think, and the more I get done."

Barry has come to understand several other things as well. "I'm more and more aware of how quickly the kinds of foods I eat and the amount of food I eat affect my ability to function," he says. Coffee at night is a good example. Barry now limits his coffee intake to one cup a day by cutting out the coffee he had been drinking at night. He says he now sleeps better at night and his stomach doesn't bother him, like it used to, in the morning. He has almost entirely cut out drinking colas. He also noticed that he sleeps a lot better at night if he doesn't have a large or heavy dinner.

He is proud to disclose that he uses no sugar or sugar substitutes in his coffee or tea, but sugar is definitely a staple of his diet. He admits that desserts are his passion and that he probably eats sweets every single day. But he is quick to note that he has made attempts to eat them less. Still, the occasional chocolate milk shake at lunch crops up; the leftover homemade cookies at night are indulged in; and he can't seem to avoid the "overwhelmingly delicious" peanut butter–chocolate chip cookies at a sandwich place near his office where he gets most of his lunches when in town. "I've cut back from three to one of those," he quickly adds, amazed at his own self-control.

The amount of sugar and fat Barry consumes is most evident when you consider that he once stopped eating dessert for four weeks and lost eight pounds without changing anything else in his diet or exercise program. Fortunately, he has an active metabolism, doesn't put on weight quickly, and at five feet eight inches is a proportional 157 pounds.

Barry's family history of heart disease cannot be omitted. His father, who was a diabetic, died of a heart attack when he was only twenty-nine. Three of Barry's grandparents died of heart-related disease as well. This has forced him to be more aware of fats in his diet. But it is here that many contradictions surface.

Barry buys lean meat; he doesn't order bacon and never uses butter. He goes so far as to read the labels of items bought off the shelves for fat content and calculates the percentage of fat. But while he says he seldom eats red meat, he admits to grilling hamburgers twice a week for dinner. If he's on the run during the workday or has a late night at the office, which happens nearly every week, he'll stop at a McDonald's for his lunch or dinner and order a hamburger and french fries. (Fast food in general is not known for its low fat content. It will be discussed in detail in Chapter 6.) When traveling, he often indulges in granola for breakfast—the one breakfast cereal that is surprisingly high in fat, even though it sounds so healthy. His exercise program, while a good one, fails to include a good cardiovascular routine.

But to his credit, Barry has been taking steps in the right direction. The reduction of sweets is one; the inclusion of regular exercise is another. The addition of oat-bran muffins to his morning routine at home is also helpful. And though he typically eats out for three meals a day—and often dines at 8:00 p.m. or later when out of town on business—Barry has resisted many of the temptations facing the frequent business traveler. "I'll find myself in a really nice restaurant with very rich food and large portions," he says. "What I generally try to do is order some kind of fish or chicken, and almost never red meat." Dessert, as you would expect, is hard for him to pass up.

A Health Scare Reformed His Ways

Herb Glimcher grew up in Duluth, Minnesota, eating red meat every day. Along with fats. And sweets.

Actually, from a nutritional standpoint, there are two Herb Glimchers—the pre-Pritikin and the post-Pritikin. But before we get ahead of ourselves, let us introduce you to our last guest in this chapter.

Herb Glimcher, chairman of the company that bears his name, is a national real estate developer specializing in shopping centers, with properties as far east as New England and as far west as the Dakotas. At sixty-two, Herb is married with four grown children, ranging in age from twenty-three to thirty-nine. Nearly ten years ago, prompted by a medical exam, Herb underwent his first heart surgery, triple coronary bypass. Soon thereafter, a friend told him about the Pritikin Program. It was at this point in his life that his eating and fitness habits changed completely.

Prior to his initial surgery, Herb admits, "I ate anything and everything"—he ate red meats daily, sweets, and fried foods. He frequented fast-food restaurants. He snacked on anything. In a nutshell, Herb never watched his diet and didn't concern himself with how foods were prepared. And he did not engage in any consistent form of exercise. The result was that he carried an extra ten pounds on his five-foot-eleven-inch frame.

Now, meet the post-Pritikin Herb Glimcher. He arises at six every weekday, later on weekends; and seven days a week, he spends forty-five minutes or more walking at a fifteen-minute-mile pace on his treadmill. Breakfast will consist of Nutri-Grain cereal, a banana, and skim milk. Whether he is in town or not, lunch will be light—a salad, a turkey sandwich, occasionally no lunch at all. For dinner—again, whether in town or not, whether at home or at a restaurant—he will have a pasta with a light marinara sauce or broiled chicken or fish. His salads are always topped with a wine vinegar or lemon juice instead of salad dressing. He rarely drinks alcohol and never drinks any beverages with caffeine, hot or cold. His cholesterol level stands at 159—the highest it has ever been was 180. On rare occasions, he may have lunch at a fast-food restaurant, but he'll order a grilled-chicken sandwich with lettuce and tomato and no sauces or dressings on the bread. He rarely eats commercial airline food, but if he does it is always the low-cholesterol or vegetarian selection.

What is the Pritikin Program, and how did Herb find himself a convert?

Herb didn't know exactly what the Pritikin Program was when he spent thirteen days at the Pritikin Center in Santa Monica more than eight years ago. He learned to eliminate specific substances and foods from his diet—sweets, fats, oils, red meat, caffeine, and alcohol. He learned how to cook different meals without these items. Lessons in gourmet-type Pritikin meal preparation were offered as well. Herb says he sticks with the basic Pritikin Program and has never gotten tired of it. "I enjoy what I eat. Your taste buds are more sensitive to food once you eat like this than they are when you eat all kinds of garbage." Herb says he is strict about the specific foods he chooses to eat. "I would say I'm about 90 percent Pritikin. I may go off once or twice a year to eat red meat, or I may wind up eating something sweet, but my diet is pretty much Pritikin."

Since his initial visit to Pritikin in Santa Monica, Herb has attended the Pritikin Center located in Florida three times. "If you go back, it's just like taking a refresher course. The more you learn about something, the easier it is to live with it."

You've just met several people who have made different nutritional choices based on where they live, how they work, their family situations, their priorities, and their health status. It is unrealistic to expect everyone's choices to be the same. Each of you must make choices that you can live with from day to day.

Of the people you've met so far, who is right in what he or she does and who is wrong? It's not as simple as that. Balance, variety, and moderation of diet and exercise are "right," but they can be examined only in the context of each individual. The nutritional strengths and weaknesses of the people in this chapter will be discussed at appropriate junctures throughout the book.

For now, we'd like you to think about the reasons for making the right nutritional choices and staying reasonably fit. Some of the people you just met aren't that concerned about maintaining nutritional balance. Some have put exercise low on their priority list.

Some would prefer not to connect *eating* with *nutrition*. Some do, but try not to go to extremes. We all have different levels of concern about our health, proper nutrition, and fitness. Yet we should all be concerned.

Why? There is no doubt that staying fit improves the quality of our lives.

Just look at Noel Johnson. When he turned seventy, he had heart trouble, arthritis, and gout. He drank too much, was fifty pounds overweight and in such bad shape that his son suggested he enter a convalescent home. He lost his weight and began a rigorous exercise program. In 1987, at the age of eighty-seven, he ran his sixth New York Marathon (seven hours, forty-one minutes), then embarked on a tour of Southeast Asia to promote his book, *A Dud at 70, a Stud at 80*.

That kind of remarkable turnaround may not be your typical story, but it does happen. On the other side of the coin, improper nutrition can have serious consequences and can even be life-threatening. Furthermore, a well-chosen diet can lessen the impact of a variety of conditions and diseases, such as heart disease and cancer.

Much is written and preached to the public about proper diet, from quacks and professionals alike. Confusion on many issues exists even for the nutrition experts. But make no mistake about it—diet is one of several important factors promoting health. It is a complicated subject because it requires an understanding of the interrelationship between food and nutrition, and of the variability among individuals of the way food is metabolized and absorbed.

Proper food choices must be available and must adapt to today's trends in life-style. Food manufacturers, restaurants, airlines, hotels, and even workplaces must be responsive to these trends in order to provide the individual with food choices that allow for balance, variety, and moderation in the diet.

While nutrition issues continue to be debated and new food technologies continue to be tested and developed, we now have more complete information about the impact of nutrition on chronic disease. The United States Surgeon General's Report on Nutrition and Health in 1988 reviewed the scientific evidence that relates dietary excesses and imbalances to chronic disease. On the basis of this evidence, it recommended specific dietary changes. Highest priority is to reduce the intake of foods high in fats and to increase the intake of foods high in complex carbohydrates and fiber.

So why should you be concerned about proper nutrition in the first place? Just look at several important relationships between nutrition and disease exposed in the surgeon general's report:

• Getting the right kind and amount of carbohydrates (energy intake) and reducing fat intake helps control diabetes and obesity.
• Controlling cholesterol levels and fat intake helps control cardiovascular diseases, such as atherosclerosis and hyptertension (high blood pressure).
• Proper fiber intake helps treat and prevent constipation and manage chronic diverticular disease (a condition marked by inflammation and irritation along the border of the colon). While inconclusive, evidence suggests that an overall increase in fiber intake might decrease the risk for colorectal cancer, which was estimated to affect 157,500 Americans in 1991.
• Dietary factors that clearly contribute to hypertension include obesity and excessive intake of sodium and alcohol. Some preliminary evidence indicates that a reduction in blood pressure is associated with the dietary intake of potassium, calcium, magnesium, and fiber.
• Adequate intakes of essential nutrients help prevent deficiency diseases such as scurvy, goiter, and anemia.
• Moderation in sugar intake helps prevent dental problems and gum disease.

In the surgeon general's report, one question we all want answered is conspicuous by its absence: Will a proper diet prolong my life? Scientists are furiously studying this question. For lab animals at least, the answer is to significantly cut down calories while keeping nutrients up. In species from water fleas to rats, scientists have found that cutting calories sends life spans soaring and keeps the animals disease-free longer.

A compelling study in favor of nutrition lengthening the life span comes from Dr. Edward J. Masoro, a physiologist at the University of Texas at San Antonio. Masoro's study of aged lab rats is based on the theory that changes in diet somehow retard many of the physiological changes that occur with age. By cutting the caloric—but not the nutritional—intake of the rats to 60 percent of what they would normally eat, Dr. Masoro has extended their average life span by 50 percent, compared with rats on a higher-calorie diet. Masoro's "diet restriction" approach hopes to address just what makes the rats live longer, and what makes normal rats get old, by measuring changes in key hormones, disease, and metabolism.

Studies are now under way to examine the effects of a low-calorie menu on two species of primates, squirrel monkeys and rhesus monkeys, which scientists hope will be more applicable to humans. And an indicator of the level of enthusiasm with the calorie-restriction theory comes from the large financial commitment made in 1990 by the National Institute on Aging. The NIA is spending about $3 million on studies related to the effects of calorie restriction on longevity, compared with the $1 million it committed only three years earlier.

But many scientists realize that genetics plays an important role in the aging process, although studies strongly suggest that physical aging is much less pronounced for those who take care of themselves. A well-known example is that of marathon runner Jim Fixx, a man who inspired thousands of middle-aged Americans to take up the sport. After all, Fixx went from a 214-pound two-pack-a-day smoker into a 160-pound marathoner. With the publication of *The Complete Book of Running* in 1977, and its sequel three years later, the onetime magazine editor tapped into a growing pastime and helped make it a national obsession. He was among the first to argue that running can increase life expectancy and reduce the risk of heart attacks. So there was irony mixed with tragedy when at the age of fifty-two, in August 1984, Jim Fixx died from a heart attack while jogging through a rural village in northern Vermont.

What happened, then, to Jim Fixx? To begin with, he had a family history of heart disease. Fixx's father suffered a heart attack at thirty-five and was dead by forty-three. Furthermore, an autopsy found that Jim had two coronary arteries that were almost totally clogged and a third with a 50 percent blockage. Because the buildup of fatty material in the arteries is usually a slow process, he probably had at least some coronary damage even before he took up running at the age of thirty-five. His history of smoking and being overweight surely contributed to the problem. And the runner was known to be very negligent about seeing doctors—when urged to have a treadmill stress test by his friend Dr. Kenneth Cooper, he refused.

Most likely, jogging did not cause Jim Fixx's heart attack. The connection between sudden death and vigorous exercise is still unclear. In Fixx's case, however, there was pre-existing heart disease, and exercise does put more stress on the heart, which may have led to his attack. Furthermore, Fixx appeared to have had warning signals: he complained of exhaustion a few days before his death, and, more important, he told his family that he felt a tightness in his throat while running, which was probably angina, a telltale sign of coronary trouble.

In general, there's increasing evidence that people who exercise regularly are less likely to suffer from heart disease and more likely to live longer. In the case of Jim Fixx, diet and physical conditioning may have extended his life by ten years.

Several recent studies support this theory. The April 4, 1990, issue of the *Journal of the American Medical Association* reported findings that were among the strongest to show that making a change to a healthy life-style (quitting smoking, eating a low-fat, low-cholesterol diet, and lowering high blood pressure) helps people at high risk for heart disease live longer. The October 6, 1989, issue of the same journal reported findings that were the first to show that hypertension may be preventable among people at risk by making life-style changes such as exercising more, drinking less alcohol, cutting salt intake, and losing weight. High blood pressure is a leading cause of stroke and a risk factor in heart disease.

So while we can't change our genes, we can maximize our potential through proper nutrition and fitness. We can look and feel younger than our years might otherwise indicate. In other words, we can "age" more slowly than our less fit peers.

Look at some of the very visible personalities in their fifties and sixties: Jane Fonda . . . Cicely Tyson . . . Sophia Loren . . . Paul Newman. Despite their fame, these celebrities lead busy lives just like you do. Many of them also have overscheduled workdays and families they try to spend time with. They may travel and dine out frequently. And they are redefining what we used to call "old age."

We hope that in the course of reading this chapter, you have begun to think about your life-style and how it relates to your overall health. Perhaps in the six people you met earlier in the chapter you can see something of yourself. And you now understand that whatever your life-style, you do have nutritional choices, and that those choices can determine the quality of your health and the manner in which you age.

Just like the myths of old age, there are food myths that will shock you. Let's take a look at some of the more controversial food facts and myths in Chapter 2.

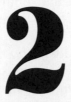

Food Facts and Myths, from Alcohol to Zinc

In the last twenty years or so, we have undergone a revolution of interest and information about our health.

"Nutrition" has become one of society's buzzwords. At cocktail parties, you're as likely to hear about someone's cholesterol count as you are about the ups and downs of Wall Street. Nutritional information is prominently displayed and promoted by today's food manufacturers in their highly competitive efforts to sell their products. Corporations are providing nutritional counseling and exercise facilities for their employees. While not perfect, the curricula of many medical schools now includes at least an elective course in nutrition. Government funding is supporting the investigation of the role of nutrition in the prevention and treatment of major diseases.

And the media have responded as they always do when there is a demonstrated, indisputable cry for information from the masses. National and local television programs cover health as a regular "beat." Every day brings a newspaper report on a new nutritional find that may challenge what we were told just months before. A recent national Gallup survey commissioned by the International

Food Information Council (IFIC) and the American Dietetic Association (ADA) revealed that newspapers and magazines, rather than health professionals, are the most frequently cited sources of nutrition information for most Americans. Unfortunately, the vast amount of information available today has produced an American public that is confused and overwhelmed by seemingly contradictory reports.

Today's mass market for advice on nutrition comes from several personal and societal concerns that are indigenous to our times. First, people are more and more concerned about their health and fitness, and they are taking greater responsibility for their own destiny. They are searching for ways to achieve a better "quality of life." Some hope to prolong their healthful years. Others believe they can add years to their lives.

Second, consumers have become more concerned about the safety of the food and water supply. What Americans eat is jeopardized by many problems that were not recognized twenty years ago. Hazardous chemicals are being identified with alarming regularity in milk, fruit, food packaging, even bottled water. Consumer groups focus public attention on the effects of pesticides, such as alar, sprayed on our fruits and vegetables, or preservatives added to many of our packaged foods, such as sodium nitrite and BHT. Several bacteria, including salmonella and *Listeria,* are under scrutiny. More than half the chickens sold may contain salmonella, and consumers have a one-in-fifty chance of encountering it in an egg. At least twenty-seven pesticides approved for use in the United States are listed by the Environmental Protection Agency as possible carcinogens in humans. The same agricultural chemicals used to rid crops and lawns of pests and provide an abundant food supply present potential dangers to groundwater supplies. Food tampering is another safety issue that can evoke panic. Fear gripped the nation in March of 1989 when two Chilean grapes were found to have been injected with cyanide. Until consumers learn to distinguish between real and perceived risks to health, uncertainty will linger and be perpetuated by misinterpreted information or falsehoods offered by the media.

Finally, many people hold a distrust of the nutritional competence of those delivering health care. While nutritional course requirements vary widely for all health professionals, it is only in recent years that medical schools have been acknowledging the importance of nutrition in their curricula. In most cases, however, these nutrition courses are optional and thus are often passed over.

There is a subtle irony to the nutrition juncture we find ourselves in. On one hand, we have an American public eager for information. On the other hand, we have an American public with varying degrees of knowledge about diet and nutrition and difficulty distinguishing between sense and nonsense.

To make matters worse, our reaction to diet information is often more emotional than intellectual because food appeals to our very basic needs. Food provides nourishment and security. It can calm us and it can stimulate us. That's why we are so gullible when it comes to food. And that is why nutritional quackery abounds.

Nutrition misinformation is certainly not new. Throughout history, outspoken individuals have warned about dietary dangers. Our ancestors were taken in by diet mythology and other forms of health quackery. But today, food faddism may be more sophisticated, and significantly more expensive.

According to the Food and Drug Administration, food faddism is the most widespread form of health quackery in the United States (*Rhode Island Medical Journal*, vol. 69, June 1986). The American Medical Association has estimated that 500 million dollars are spent on nutrition fraud each year, while others have indicated that more than $2 billion is wasted on special foods, supplements, health lectures, and literature of questionable quality (*Heartline*, vol. 16, no. 2, February 1986).

Today's "health food" industry is a multibillion-dollar business which promotes a multitude of products that supposedly can prevent and cure the entire range of human ailments. And it is not alone in its prosperity. The multibillion-dollar diet industry is thriving, too. According to the American Dietetic Association, Americans spend $5 billion a year on diet books, products, and foods. Crash diets are promoted in most women's magazines; best-selling books offer one quick-weight-loss solution after another; weight-loss clinics can be found in every shopping mall; and enough diet gimmicks exist to make your head spin.

Nutrition is not a gimmick. It is not magic. It is a science. Scientific studies are conducted and the facts are examined. But even the facts can be misrepresented by the media and the scientific community. Pulicity concerning some scientific studies of nutrition sometimes includes overenthusiastic statements that stretch research leads into conclusive evidence and turn dietary recommendations into dicta. Our zeal may very well fuel food faddists and damage nutrition as a responsible science.

There very well may be more quacks than real nutrition experts in America today, but this is changing as the public becomes more discerning. The only way you can distinguish the expert from the imposter is to scrutinize credentials. An expert will have a degree in the field of nutrition and diet from an accredited school, and is usually a member of a reputable nutrition organization, such as the American Dietetic Association. With more than sixty thousand members, the ADA is the world's largest association of food and nutrition professionals. Also, most dietitians who belong to the ADA have earned registration status, so they can use the legally protected title, Registered Dietitian, or R.D., after their names. And to protect the public from harm, more than half the states now have licensure laws that govern the practice of nutrition counseling.

While the professionals don't always agree on all the issues, there is agreement on basic nutritional principles, guidelines, and facts. In this chapter, you'll learn about these facts. But first, let's test your knowledge of nutrition science.

The Twenty Biggest Food Myths and Twenty Important Food Facts

MYTH 1: Much of our food has been so processed and refined that it has lost its value for health.
FACT: Most of the changes in food processing—the technological advances, enrichment processes, and fortification programs—have in fact been very beneficial. Taste and textural qualities of food have been improved through HTST (high temperature/short time), UHT (ultra high temperature), pouch processing, refrigeration, and freezing. Through enrichment processes, nutrients not originally present are now added to many commonly eaten foods, such as breads and cereals. Further, there is no scientific evidence supporting the claims that so-called natural or organic products are more healthful.

MYTH 2: Wheat bread and whole wheat bread have the same nutritional value.

FACT: Whole wheat bread is more nutritious than wheat bread because it contains the highest levels of fiber, vitamins, and minerals. In its whole state, wheat offers thirty-seven of the forty-four known nutrients naturally obtained from foods. Wheat bread contains no whole wheat flour and is really white bread with a lot of artificial coloring extracts. Bread labeled "100 percent whole wheat" must be made with whole wheat flour.

MYTH 3: Evidence suggests that even a moderate consumption of alcohol can be nutritionally harmful and lead to disease.

FACT: While heavy drinking has been linked to lung cancer and cancer of the mouth and esophagus (although this could reflect the fact that many heavy drinkers smoke), alcohol consumption of up to two drinks per day has not been associated with disease among healthy male and nonpregnant female adults. There is even some evidence that very moderate daily drinking provides some protection against stroke (which occurs when a clot forms or lodges in an artery in the brain), although this is not conclusive. Researchers speculate that small amounts of alcohol, spread out evenly over time, keep blood from getting sticky and clotting.

MYTH 4: Studies indicate that caffeine consumption causes breast cancer.

FACT: Most studies on the effects of caffeine are inconclusive. There has been some linkage between excessive caffeine consumption and the formation of breast cysts (fibrocysts), but studies have not linked the formation of fibrocysts to breast cancer. Furthermore, the connection between caffeine and breast cysts varies widely among individuals. Moderation, as in all things, is the key.

MYTH 5: Calcium intake is not critical except during the growing years and pregnancy.

FACT: Adequate calcium intake matters during all periods of life. The required daily allowance for this mineral happens to be higher for those between eleven and twenty-four and for pregnant and nursing women (1,200 milligrams), but it is also a requirement for children up to age eleven and adults over age twenty-five (800 milligrams). Women approaching menopause should be certain they are getting calcium, particularly from the foods they eat, to reduce the threat of osteoporosis. An estimated 15 million to 20 million Americans, especially women after menopause, have this crippling affliction in which bone tissue is lost and the bones are susceptible to fractures, particularly in the wrist, spine, and hip.

For the past decade, studies have indicated a strong link between osteoporosis and a lifelong deprivation of calcium in the diet. However, recent evidence indicates that postmenopausal women may be able to slow this bone erosion by increasing their calcium intake to the required daily allowance of 800 milligrams and participating in weight-bearing exercise. Calcium also helps your heart to beat, your muscles to work, your blood to clot, and your nerves to function. Calcium supplements should be taken only to cover what you don't get in your diet because calcium is best absorbed by the body when consumed in food. Foods high in calcium include milk, yogurt, and cheese.

MYTH 6: Because eggs are such a high source of cholesterol, they should be eliminated from the diet.
FACT: One egg yolk contains 213 milligrams of cholesterol, about two-thirds of the 300-milligram daily limit recommended by the American Heart Association. However, eggs are low in fats and a rich source of many nutrients, such as iron, and should not be entirely eliminated from the diet of the average person—which means anyone who does not have a high blood cholesterol level (this is discussed later in the chapter). Moderation is again the key.

MYTH 7: Cholesterol is a substance your body should do without.
FACT: Cholesterol is a substance vitally important to your body. The right amount of cholesterol is essential to provide strength and protection to cells and nerves. Some doctors, however, believe that anyone with blood cholesterol over 200 milligrams should receive attention, although a lot depends on a person's level of other blood components as well (see the discussion later in this chapter).

MYTH 8: If you need to reduce your cholesterol, you need only to reduce your intake of cholesterol-rich foods.
FACT: To reduce your cholesterol, you need to reduce your intake of cholesterol-rich foods *and* saturated fats. Saturated fats have

been shown to contribute to high blood cholesterol. The amount of cholesterol produced by the body and the rate at which it is removed from the bloodstream are controlled in part by saturated fat.

Saturated fat raises the level of low-density lipoproteins (LDLs), the substances in the blood that carry cholesterol and seem to be involved in building deposits in arteries.

MYTH 9: We should remove all fat from our diet in order to prevent heart-related disease.
FACT: Some fat in our diet is healthy and, in fact, necessary, though experts recommend that no more than 30 percent of our calories come from fat. Among its other benefits, fat helps us to absorb vitamins A, D, E, and K and supplies essential fatty acids needed for body processes.

MYTH 10: All fiber is alike.
FACT: There are different types of fiber—soluble and insoluble, which may impact the body differently. Insoluble fiber may play a role in reducing the chance of developing colon cancer, while soluble fiber has been identified in reducing cholesterol levels.

Insoluble fiber, found in wheat bran, whole grains, and vegetables, does seem to reduce intestinal polyps and the likelihood of colon cancer. A study reported in the *Journal of the National Cancer Institute* (vol. 81, no. 17, September 6, 1989) found that a high-fiber diet can shrink the size and number of precancerous polyps of the lower intestine and thus reduce the risk of colon and rectal cancer. A study reported in the April 18, 1990, issue of the same publication suggested that a diet high in vegetables, grains, and fruits may lower a person's risk for colorectal cancer by as much as 40 percent.

Soluble fiber, found in oat bran, beans, barley, and some fruits and vegetables, seems to bring cholesterol levels down. A 1986 Northwestern University study found that oat bran, together with a low-fat diet, lowered blood cholesterol levels by about 3 percent. (A controversial study published in January 1990 in the *New England Journal of Medicine,* however, cast doubt on the unique ability of oat bran to lower cholesterol levels).

Regardless, most dietary authorities, including the National Cancer Institute, recommend 20 to 30 grams of fiber intake a day—most Americans now consume an average of 11 to 12 grams daily.

MYTH 11: Seafood and meats, particularly beef and liver and other animal foods, should be eliminated from the diet.
FACT: Seafood and meats are the major sources of a highly absorbable form of iron known as heme-iron. They are important foods in our diet; their elimination could lead to iron deficiency. Much of the iron we ingest from other foods is not absorbed and is excreted from our body.

MYTH 12: A good multipurpose vitamin to supplement the diet is necessary for good health.
FACT: Anyone who eats a variety of foods in moderation does not require dietary supplements to ensure good health. Unless you are pregnant, modifying your diet to lose weight, or suffering from illness, vitamin and mineral tablets are not the answer to maintaining good nutrition. Vitamins are co-factors that help your body utilize protein, fats, and carbohydrates, the major food components. Adequate amounts of vitamins, as well as all other nutrients, are available in foods. Thus, dietary supplements are not necessary for good health if you concentrate on maintaining a well-balanced diet.

MYTH 13: There is no harm in taking megadoses of vitamins to ensure good health.
FACT: "If some is good, then more must be better" does not apply here. Fat-soluble vitamins (vitamins A, D, E, and K) are stored in the body and over a period of time can be toxic. Even some water-soluble vitamins (such as B6) have been shown to be toxic in large amounts. If you cannot receive enough vitamins and minerals from your food supply, you really need to consult a physician and a registered dietitian.

MYTH 14: Man-made (synthetic) vitamins are not as good as natural vitamins.
FACT: Synthetic vitamins are just as good as natural vitamins, because every vitamin is a specific chemical compound. Vitamin C, for example, is the same whether it comes from rose hips or a chemist's lab. Your body can't tell the difference, but your pocketbook can. Natural vitamins are far more expensive and, from the standpoint of nutrition, needlessly so.

MYTH 15: If I stop adding salt to my foods, I can be assured that my sodium intake is low.

FACT: The amount of sodium already added to prepared foods will surprise you. Convenience items, such as cakes, cereals, breads, and prepackaged dinners, contain high levels of sodium as a preservative, even though they may not taste salty. Removal of the salt shaker from the table is highly advisable, but even that doesn't assure you that your salt intake is low. Be aware of the sodium content in your foods—many soups, cheeses, and prepared meats, for example, contain high levels of sodium. The National Research Council recommends daily intakes of sodium chloride be limited to 6 grams (2.4 grams of sodium) or less.

MYTH 16: Sea salt is more nutritious than regular table salt.

FACT: There is no difference between sea salt and regular table salt other than the price. A low-sodium table salt called Salt Sense, however, provides 30 percent less sodium per teaspoon because it is produced in flake (versus crystal) form. This provides more flavor and less sodium.

MYTH 17: As a substance, sucrose (sugar) is harmful and useless.

FACT: Sugar is a good source of dietary energy, and in small amounts it is harmless. Certainly, a high consumption of sweets is an important factor in the development of dental cavities. And sugar, like any other source of calories, can contribute to obesity if consumed in excess. However, there is no firm evidence that sugar consumption is directly responsible for any disease.

MYTH 18: Honey is more healthful than sugar.

FACT: There is no significant nutritional difference between sugar and honey. They both are composed of sugars, hence are simply concentrated sources of calories. While honey has acquired a special reputation as a nutritional or health food, this reputation is not deserved; it contains only traces of other nutrients. Further, honey has been shown to cause more dental cavities than white sugar. It has also been associated with botulism in infants.

MYTH 19: Zinc is a harmless mineral.

FACT: Too much or too little zinc can depress the immune function. As with many of the trace minerals, the range between too little and too much zinc is narrow. A deficiency of zinc has been associated with the decrease in immune function long accepted as an inevitable part of aging. But too much zinc can also depress the immune function.

Lean meat, eggs, and seafood are the best source of zinc. An average balanced diet of 2,000 calories contains 10 to 15 milligrams of zinc. The recommended daily allowance of zinc is 15 milligrams. Going above this amount is not recommended without medical supervision.

MYTH 20: Products labeled "natural" are better for you than processed foods.
FACT: Many foods labeled "natural" are very deceiving. What sounds healthy may not be so. Many of the foods that claim this virtue, such as granolas, contain ingredients not found in nature. In fact, there is no universal definition of what is meant by "natural." So look beyond the "natural" banner and read the label.

In our discussion of facts and myths, let's revisit the people we met in Chapter 1 and look more closely at their health habits. Many of their beliefs are at least partially accurate, and the ones that are not are quite typical.

She Drinks Two Glasses of Milk Daily to Fight Osteoporosis

Carole Gerber, at forty-four, is concerned about osteoporosis for good reason. This bone-loss disease caused by a lack of calcium in the body affects almost half of all women over forty-five. It is the major cause of spinal fractures in one out of four women over age sixty. Hip fractures due to osteoporosis occur in one out of three women after age sixty-five. By age sixty, almost 40 percent of American women will lose all their teeth due to bone loss in the jaw.

The fact is that bone loss occurs in just about everyone after age thirty-five. The reason for this is that calcium is constantly being added and removed from the bones, where it is stored to carefully regulate the supply of calcium in the bloodstream. Calcium in the blood is critical for the conduction of nerve impulses, heart function, muscle contraction, blood clotting, and the activation of certain enzymes and hormones. Thus, bones are constantly being remodeled by the body; and, assuming that we get enough calcium in our diets, we continue to build bone mass well into our mid-thirties.

After thirty-five, things begin to change. The body's control mechanisms that regulate calcium begin to shift. The result is a gradual thinning of the bone. Moreover, the body becomes less efficient at absorbing calcium as we age, which reduces the amount of calcium supplied to the bloodstream from food.

How can you prevent further bone loss, whatever your age? To begin with, increase your consumption of calcium. The daily recommended intake of calcium is 800 milligrams, with 1,200 milligrams recommended for adolescents through age twenty-four and for pregnant and nursing women. Carole's daily two glasses of milk supply her with 600 milligrams of calcium, so she is on the right track. She can pick up additional calcium from the cheese on her pizzas—one ounce of cheese usually has well over 200 milligrams of calcium. Other alternatives are yogurt (one cup supplies up to 400 milligrams); green leafy vegetables, such as radicchio, leaf lettuce, and endive; and canned sardines or salmon, although the fat and salt content of these foods can be high.

If you don't eat any dairy products, chances are strong that you do need supplementation. Calcium supplements come in the form of calcium carbonate, calcium lactate, or calcium gluconate, all equally effective. Two antacid tablets, such as Tums, contain calcium carbonate and provide about 500 milligrams of calcium.

Another effective preventive measure is to begin a regular exercise program, while this does not preclude the need to consume 800 milligrams of calcium daily. Studies have shown that weight-bearing exercises, especially those where you lift your own body weight, are best. Walking, running, race walking, aerobic dancing, gymnastics, tennis, and weight lifting are all bone builders. Swimming is not good exercise for the bones since it provides weightlessness rather than weight bearing. So even though Carole doesn't have a weight problem, exercise is worth her while if she wants to prevent osteoporosis. And that means she needs to find something more substantial than a stretch-and-tone exercise program.

She Drinks Three Cups of Coffee and a Coke Classic Every Day: The Caffeine Connection

Judy Markey says she would be sluggish and headachy without her caffeine. And for good reason.

In the one thousand years since the coffee plant was first cultivated in Arabia, caffeine has been recognized as a stimulant. It belongs to a group of compounds known as methylxanthines, which trigger the central nervous system to speed up body functions, as evidenced by many who say they can't really wake up without their morning cup of coffee.

Caffeine enters the bloodstream within fifteen to forty-five minutes after it is ingested. Because it also affects the brain, some experts suggest that caffeine helps us think more clearly and perform tasks with greater efficiency. It has been known to improve endurance by facilitating the ability of the muscles to contract, and to make us less susceptible to fatigue.

On the negative side, caffeine stimulates the heart by widening coronary arteries and pulmonary vessels, thus increasing blood flow to the heart. Drinking as few as two and a half cups of coffee can cause extra-fast heartbeats or abnormal heart rhythms (also known as arrhythmia). Caffeine also steps up kidney and bladder action, causing a diuretic effect.

Some people complain that too much coffee upsets their stomachs. Both Barry Nash and Burt Staniar cut out the coffee from their diets for just this reason. Caffeine does increase the secretion of stomach acids and relaxes the muscles along the digestive tract.

In doses higher than 200 milligrams—about three cups of coffee—caffeine can cause trembling, nervousness, chronic muscle tension, and insomnia—symptoms commonly known as "coffee nerves."

Coffee ranks as the single greatest source of methylxanthine, accounting for 75 percent of all caffeine intake, with tea making up about 15 percent. Generous amounts of caffeine are also found in soft drinks (Coke Classic, for one), in chocolate, and in medications for colds, allergies, headaches, and weight control. It is added to certain baked goods, frozen dairy products, and sweets. So even if you don't drink coffee, odds are you're getting plenty of caffeine from other sources.

There are various studies that have connected caffeine to an increase in the incidence of benign lumps in women's breasts (fibrocystic disease) and to heart disease. Other studies have provided conflicting data, however. The most alarming report came several years ago from a study of 1,130 graduates at John Hopkins University Medical School. Researchers found that those who drank coffee had two to three times the risk of heart disease as those who did not drink coffee. But this study did not take into account other risk factors, like diet and a sedentary life-style.

A study reported in the September 1990 issue of the *American Journal of Epidemiology* involved 100,000 people who were part of the Kaiser Permanente health maintenance organization in California. It found a slightly increased risk of heart attacks in people who drank more than four cups of coffee a day. This study, however, did not distinguish between regular and decaffeinated coffee.

A study called the Health Professional's Follow-up Study, of more than 45,000 American men by researchers at Harvard University School of Public Health, was published in the October 11, 1990, issue of the *New England Journal of Medicine*. It produced strong evidence that moderate coffee drinking does not increase the risk of heart attacks or strokes. Even the heavy coffee drinkers, who averaged six or more cups a day, were unaffected, researchers said. Surprisingly, the researchers did find a slight, although only marginally statistically significant, increase in heart disease among moderate drinkers (four or more cups daily) of decaffeinated coffee. This study, it should be noted, involved men who were healthy nonsmokers.

Dr. David Dovmeyer, who has studied the incidence of caffeine-related arrhythmias at Ohio State University, recommends that people who already have heart problems should avoid caffeine completely.

So the answer remains elusive. Moderation, as in all things, continues to be the best solution. And there are alternatives to caffeine if one suffers the jittery side effects. The most obvious low-caffeine choices are decaffeinated coffees and teas and noncaffeinated colas. People who find caffeine a problem, however, should be aware that even decaf coffee contains some caffeine. Further, a chemical known as TCE (trichlorethylene) was once widely used to remove caffeine from the bean. When the National Cancer Institute issued a report that high doses of this chemical produced liver cancer in mice, most companies then switched to alternative decaffeination processes. Today, two methods are used—the water/steam process and the liquid carbon dioxide process. Because some flavor and aroma are lost in the decaffeination process, a stronger bean (robusta bean) is used, which may have an effect on cholesterol absorption and utilization. New studies on this subject are inconclusive.

Some heavy coffee drinkers who decide to give it up entirely may experience "withdrawal" symptoms, as Judy Markey described, such as headache, drowsiness, and nervousness, usually about twelve to sixteen hours after their last dose of caffeine. To avoid these symptoms, it is often advised to reduce caffeine intake gradually. Cut back by a cup or two a day.

A Multivitamin Supplement Is His Insurance

Burt Staniar takes a multivitamin supplement as insurance for his three-pronged health philosophy of reducing fats in his diet, increasing his exercise, and reducing his stress through meditation.

At least a third of the adults in the United States take some form of vitamin or mineral supplement regularly, according to the Council for Responsible Nutrition, a trade association. So Burt is one of an estimated 60 million Americans who take vitamins. Carole Gerber, who also takes vitamins, said she specifically takes 2,000 milligrams of vitamin C (the daily requirement is only 60 milligrams) and 400 milligrams of vitamin E (the daily requirement is only 8 milligrams for women, 10 milligrams for men). If we are the best-fed people on earth, why are so many of us popping vitamin pills?

The answer is that despite our wealth in terms of foods to choose from, most of us are still not certain whether or not we are getting a proper supply of vitamins. So we take a pill to be sure. The market for vitamin and mineral pills amounted to $2.7 billion in 1988.

An important fact must be stated here: vitamins are not the end-all. They do not work alone. They work in concert with the proteins, fats, and carbohydrates coming from the foods you eat. In other words, skipping meals but taking a daily vitamin supplement will not keep you healthy.

The best place to get vitamins is from the food we eat. It is crucial that a person's diet provide adequate amounts of the fabled "thirteen essential vitamins." Why? Vitamins act as helpers in our bodies. They regulate metabolism, convert fats and carbohydrates into energy, and assist in forming bone and tissues.

The Federal Food and Drug Administration has established United States Recommended Dietary Allowances (U.S. RDAs) for vitamins, referred to on most food labels; but it is important to remember that these figures are guidelines for a mythical "average" person. They are a good tool for beginning to measure how much you need, but they are not the final word. For instance, if you are sick or recovering from a disease, surgery, or an injury, your need for certain vitamins may increase.

Also, you may be clinically well but have life-style habits or characteristics that interfere with how well your body utilizes vitamins. Cigarette smoking, heavy drinking, and simply getting older are relevant factors. From calculations based on several studies, the vitamin C requirement of smokers has been estimated to be as much as twice that of nonsmokers.

Diseases stemming from specific vitamin and mineral deficiencies, such as rickets and scurvy, have practically disappeared in this country. But that's not to say inadequacies in vitamins and minerals don't exist. Recent government surveys point out that some portions of the population appear to have low intakes of vitamin C, calcium, iron, and fluoride. Furthermore, some women in their reproductive years were found to have less than the required daily allowance for vitamin E, calcium, magnesium, vitamin B6, iron, zinc, and folic acid.

The vitamin or mineral inadequacies that result from failing to eat a balanced diet regularly don't produce full-blown illness, yet they compromise your general health. These inadequacies are caused by many other factors as well, including the drugs you take, whether you drink or smoke, whether you're dieting or are under emotional stress.

People over age sixty-five should not assume that common, troublesome maladies are the unavoidable legacy of aging. Problems such as loss of appetite, insomnia, headaches, or even lack of enthusiasm can be caused by nutrient shortages and not necessarily by age itself.

At any given time, some 25 percent of the United States population is on some kind of weight-reduction diet. Every one of the ten most popular diets is well below the average daily requirement in at least one essential vitamin.

Most of us sooner or later will hit a period in our lives when our diet intakes are low in vitamins. If it becomes evident that you are low in one or more vitamins and you are unwilling or unable to resolve it through dietary changes, we recommend a general vitamin supplement that provides 100 percent of the recommended nutrients for all vitamins and minerals.

Burt Staniar seems to eat a well-balanced diet and probably doesn't need a supplement. However, there's no harm in taking a general all-purpose supplement each day for "insurance." But there doesn't seem to be a good reason for Carole Gerber's megadoses of vitamin C or E, which can only be toxic over a period of time.

He Craves Sweets and Rarely Passes on Desserts

Dessert is a passion for Barry Nash, and he manages to sneak sweets into his day in a variety of ways—a chocolate milk shake with lunch, some homemade chocolate-chip cookies at night that happen to be left over from the weekend, the mouth-watering desserts following his frequent business dinners on the road.

It is absolutely okay to like sweets. Most of us do. What is not okay is the quantity of the sweets consumed, especially if they are replacing more nutritious foods in your diet. The average person consumes 600 calories from sweets a day, not including fruits and other natural sources of sugar.

Eating too much sugar does not necessarily predispose a person to be overweight. In fact, studies show that overweight people eat less sugar than thin people.

Sugar is "generally recognized as safe" by the Food and Drug Administration, so food companies can use any amount of it they choose. Sugar is added to just about everything from soup to nuts because, along with providing a good taste, it helps foods retain moisture (as in breads and cakes), prevents spoilage (in jellies and jams), and improves texture and appearance (as in the browning of muffins). So even without his desserts and cookies, Barry Nash is getting a lot of sugar.

The only certain health risk associated with sugar consumption is tooth decay. But there are a couple of gray areas that could have an effect on Barry, given his particular history. First, Barry's father was diabetic. While sugar cannot be said to cause diabetes, people who are genetically susceptible to this disease should curtail a high intake of sugar. Second, Barry has a strong family history of heart disease. While heart problems can't be pinned on eating too much sugar, people who tend to accumulate large amounts of triglycerides (artery-damaging fats) in their blood may be prudent to limit their sugar intake.

Barry needs to make different choices, given his craving and his life-style. While sorbets and fresh fruit are often not placed on dinner menus, many restaurants do have them available upon request. At home, he could stock up on frozen fruit bars, replace his cookie jar with a fruit bowl, and keep ice milk or frozen yogurt on hand when he's in the mood for milk shakes or ice cream.

Sugar-free sweeteners are worth mentioning here. Aspartame, marketed as NutraSweet and Equal, is currently the most talked-about artificial sweetener. One year after its approval for soft-drink use by the U.S. Food and Drug Administration, aspartame sales increased from $74 million to $336 million. NutraSweet is now used in more than seventy-five products, ranging from soft drinks and cereals to vitamins and laxatives. It is even in orange drinks and may soon be found in yogurt and ice cream. The product has been readily accepted by consumers because it has 180 times the sweetening power of sugar with only one-tenth the calories.

As the sales of aspartame have increased, so have the protests by researchers, who say the basis for FDA approval may not be entirely valid. The scientific community has been concerned by reports that a small percentage of users have suffered severe adverse reactions to aspartame, some involving the brain, including dizziness, depression, behavior changes, headaches, and seizures. Although there is no direct evidence, a few scientists believe that aspartame may cause subtle imbalances in brain chemicals that influence mood and alertness.

We keep returning to the concept of moderation in the diet. That goes for sugar and sweeteners alike. There's nothing wrong with *some* sugar in your diet. Remember, one teaspoon of sugar is only 16 calories. The one exception would be people with diabetes, who have difficulty processing sugar and must control how much they consume. If you're trying to cut out sugar, there's nothing wrong with *some* artificial sweetener in your diet.

Two Men at Risk of Heart Disease: Two Approaches to Fats

We thought it would be instructive to closely examine the lifestyles of two individuals who, when it comes to heart disease, have more to worry about than the average person. Herb Glimcher and

Barry Nash share what experts would consider some level of risk of coronary heart disease. Their dietary approaches, however, are quite different.

Herb Glimcher has already suffered from some heart disease. In 1982, he had arterial blockages and underwent a triple coronary bypass operation. He subsequently underwent a total lifestyle change that he has been committed to ever since.

Barry Nash, at thirty-four, is just more than half Herb's sixty-two years. And while he has no indication of any heart disease, his family history points in that direction. As you may recall, Barry's father died of a heart attack at age twenty-nine, and three out of four of Barry's grandparents died of heart-related disease. Genetically, Barry is definitely at risk.

Herb's approach is a rigid one. There are not many people who are as disciplined and committed as Herb Glimcher when it comes to their health and fitness. Regardless of whether Herb eats at home or dines out, travels for business or pleasure, he holds to his basic interpretation of the Pritikin dietary program. He drinks no caffeine and very little alcohol; he stays away from red meat and desserts; he eats his pasta with an oil-free marinara sauce and has his chicken or fish usually broiled, plain. For salad dressing, he chooses lemon juice or just vinegar.

His weight is just right for his height and build. He exercises seven days a week on a treadmill. He works hard to keep his cholesterol low and is quick to point out that the highest it has been is 180. His knowledge of nutrition only extends, however, to the type of foods he eats since he only allows himself specific foods.

Maybe one needs to be single-focused about diet and nutrition to be successful on a program as restrictive as the Pritikin diet. It seems hard to comply with a diet that is so low in fat, but Herb has managed quite well. And for someone with heart problems, extreme measures may be prudent. Herb may have made the best choice for himself.

On the other hand, Barry Nash is not compulsive about his diet. And perhaps he may be too flexible about what he eats. Barry does drink coffee and tea, but he's cut coffee consumption down to one cup daily, and tea is occasional. He allows himself a glass of wine at dinner averaging every other dinner. He prides himself on staying away from red meat, but he does have a hamburger at least twice a week. He would like to limit his desserts and sweets, but he craves sweets. While he says he is really conscious of fats in his diet, some of his food choices—desserts, muffins, granola, hamburgers, fast food—do contain fair amounts of fats.

Like Herb, Barry is at his desirable weight for his height. And he regularly exercises, maybe five or six days of the week. He says his cholesterol is "not an alarming number" but doesn't recall what it is. Barry regards himself as nutrition conscious, but not compulsive about it.

Barry's awareness about nutrition seems to be one that is slowly evolving. Since he is still relatively young, the potential risk of heart disease may seem remote to him. Research does indicate, however, that the earlier one can make the necessary dietary changes, the better. Heart disease develops over time. Altering its course takes time as well.

The statistics are grim. One out of every two Americans will die of heart attack, stroke, or other cardiovascular disease. More than 1.25 million people (two-thirds of them men) suffer heart attacks annually, and 500,000 die as a result (Surgeon General's Report on Nutrition and Health, 1988).

Which brings us to the issue of cholesterol.

The Facts (or Fats) and Myths of Cholesterol

There are two arguments on cholesterol: one says the cholesterol risk is overrated for many; the other suggests that the benefits of lowering cholesterol levels are obvious. Most experts do agree that Americans need to reduce their consumption of fat, cholesterol, and calories, and that the reduction of the risk of heart attack is just one of the benefits of such a diet.

However, two recent books—*Heart Failure* by Thomas J. Moore (Random House, 1989) and *Balanced Nutrition* by Dr. Frederick J. Stare, Dr. Robert E. Olson, and Dr. Elizabeth M. Whelan (Bob Adams Inc., 1989)—argue that while cholesterol is a risk factor for heart disease, it is only one of several, including heredity, smoking, and obesity. And the authors are concerned that most of the evidence showing that the risk of heart attack can be reduced by lowering cholesterol comes from studies done on middle-aged men. They contend that many of the scientific studies were inadequately designed or misinterpreted and that the public has thus been oversold on the need to lower their cholesterol. Both of these books have been criticized for omitting important clinical trials and data that do not support their claims.

The facts about cholesterol, gathered by the National Heart Association and the National Heart, Lung and Blood Institute from dozens of large-scale scientific studies and laboratory experiments done over the last thirty years, do tell us:

- In middle-aged men, high blood cholesterol levels are causally related to atherosclerosis and to an increased risk of coronary heart disease.
- The progressive clogging of the arteries in heart disease can be reversed by cholesterol-lowering drugs or, in some cases, just by life-style changes such as regular exercise, low-fat diet, and stress management.
- Dietary intervention may improve at least one of the known coronary-heart-disease risk factors, namely obesity, and over a lifetime may improve several risk factors to the extent that life expectancy is increased.
- Populations that customarily follow high-fat diets have higher cholesterol levels and higher heart-disease death rates than populations that follow low-fat diets.
- The effects of lowering cholesterol in women, the elderly, and the young have not been explicitly studied. The advice to them to lower cholesterol is by analogy from middle-aged men, who have the highest risk of premature heart attacks.
- The long-term health effects of cholesterol-lowering drugs are unknown.
- Whether there are health problems stemming from cholesterol reduction is unknown.

So you see, the subject of cholesterol is not a simple good-versus-evil issue. Someone recently asked if everything one needed to know about cholesterol could be stated in just one sentence. The response is not what you might expect—i.e., "Cholesterol causes heart attacks" or "Cut down on your eggs and bacon in the morning." Instead, by summarizing the facts about cholesterol, a one-sentence answer could only be: "Cholesterol is a substance vitally important to your body—if it's in the right place, at the right time, and in the right amount."

Of course, such a reply only prompts more questions, because the real answer is to learn how your body uses cholesterol and how to keep the right amounts circulating in your bloodstream. Just as with many other topics in nutrition, you need to know the whole story to understand all the intricate parts of that story.

Since cholesterol is the most controversial topic in nutrition, we developed answers to the ten most-asked questions on the subject, going all the way back to the very basics:

The Ten Most-Asked Questions About Cholesterol

1. WHAT IS CHOLESTEROL? Cholesterol is a waxy yellow substance found only in animals and manufactured by your body as well. It is one type of fat: triglycerides and phospholipids are the others (more on them in a bit).

Your liver can manufacture cholesterol from these other fats as well as from carbohydrates. Even if you could cut every single milligram of cholesterol from your diet, your liver would still be able to produce enough to satisfy all your body's needs—it typically sends out 1,000 milligrams of cholesterol a day through the bloodstream to be used by the cells.

Some substances needed for digesting food are made from cholesterol and are produced by the liver. Cholesterol is also used to make vitamin D and hormones. Cholesterol is an essential component of the coating that provides strength and protection to cells and nerves. This is why cholesterol itself is not a bad thing. It is a necessary substance, vital to the everyday functions and smooth operation of your body.

2. WHAT IS THE DIFFERENCE BETWEEN "DIETARY" CHO-LESTEROL AND "SERUM" CHOLESTEROL? The distinction is important. Dietary cholesterol is found only in the foods we get from animal sources, such as meats, dairy products, eggs, and fish. Egg yolks, shellfish, and liver contain the greatest amounts. Fruits, vegetables, grains, cereals, and nuts do not contain any. (See the chart "Cholesterol Values in Common Foods," page 40.)

Serum cholesterol is what you need to be most concerned about, because it's the amount circulating in your blood, carried along by various protein-based molecules. Your serum cholesterol level is a key indication of whether or not you're at risk for heart disease. It can be affected by what your body makes and what you eat.

Cholesterol Values in Common Foods

Food	Amount	Cholesterol (milligrams)
Whole milk	1 cup	33
2% fat milk	1 cup	18
Skim milk	1 cup	5
Yogurt, plain, low-fat	8 oz	14
Natural cheddar cheese	1 oz	60
Mozzarella cheese, part skim milk	2 oz	32
Lean ground beef patty, cooked	4 oz	106
Pork loin, lean, roasted	4 oz	100
Liver, beef, cooked with fat added	4 oz	496
Chicken, roasted	4 oz	96
Cod fillets, broiled	4 oz	70
Shrimp, steamed, shelled	4 oz	234
Egg, medium-sized	1	213

3. HOW MUCH SERUM CHOLESTEROL IS TOO MUCH? As far back as 1986, the National Heart, Lung and Blood Institute stated that total blood cholesterol should be below 200 milligrams; that at 200 to 239 milligrams, a person is at moderate risk for coronary artery disease; and that at more than 240 milligrams, at high risk. By October of 1987, the National Cholesterol Education Program was launched "to reduce the prevalence of elevated blood cholesterol in the United States and thereby contribute to reducing coronary heart disease morbidity and mortality." This national cholesterol screening program called on the authority of physicians to prescribe a medically supervised regimen of treatment based on the National Heart, Lung and Blood Institute's cholesterol guidelines. But, as is to be expected with such a historic medical intervention effort, it became embroiled in controversy, with some experts saying that the cholesterol numbers were too low and that many people were needlessly being sent to their physicians for treatment.

The June 14, 1990, issue of the *New England Journal of Medicine* reported that lowering cholesterol may be more important for people with existing heart disease than for healthy people who want to prevent the disease. The study led some experts to suggest a revision of cholesterol guidelines so that people with previous heart trouble should keep their counts below 170 or 160 milligrams. Nonetheless, studies have shown that for every 1 percent reduction in serum cholesterol, there is a 2 to 4 percent reduction in the risk of heart attack.

4. WHAT HAPPENS WHEN SERUM CHOLESTEROL LEVELS ARE HIGH? When too much cholesterol circulates in your blood, its protein-fueled carriers leave deposits (or plaque) on the lining of the artery walls. If your blood levels are allowed to remain high over a period of years, these deposits can accumulate to the point where the flow of blood is impeded, a disorder termed atherosclerosis. Eventually the deposits can get so thick that they can trap a blood clot, or the artery closes completely. If the blockage occurs in a major coronary artery, the result will be a heart attack. (A "stroke," or cardiovascular accident, the brain's equivalent of a heart attack, results when plaque blocks the carotid arteries in the head and neck, so low cholesterol is equally important in preventing stroke.) In some people, high serum cholesterol levels are offset by other factors, some known and some unknown, that protects them from developing heart disease.

5. WHAT IS THE RECOMMENDED INTAKE OF DIETARY CHOLESTEROL? The American Heart Association recommends that we limit cholesterol intake to 250 to 300 milligrams per day (see the chart on page 40). However, the AHA, the National Institutes of Health, the National Academy of Sciences, and other prestigious health organizations and medical experts believe it is not enough to cut out foods that are rich in cholesterol, like eggs and organ meats. They point to another, more important, culprit—saturated fat.

6. WHAT IS SATURATED FAT, AND HOW DOES IT AFFECT YOUR SERUM CHOLESTEROL LEVEL? Saturated fat is found mostly in animal products like lard, meat fat, butter, and other whole-milk products. Solid at room temperature, saturated fats give us that velvety texture so pleasant in ice cream, cheeses, and rich sauces. Poultry and fish also contain it, though usually less than red meats.

Three vegetable oils—palm oil, palm kernel oil, and coconut

oil—are among the most highly saturated and artery-damaging fats and are often used in processed foods such as cake mixes, nondairy creamers, and vegetable shortenings. One tablespoon of palm kernel oil or coconut oil contains more saturated fat than butter or lard, yet it is free of cholesterol.

Extensive and consistent research studies show that saturated fat raises blood cholesterol more than anything else in the diet. The U.S. Surgeon General's 1988 Report on Nutrition and Health recommended we lower our overall fat intake as well as our saturated fat intake. The National Institutes of Health, the American Heart Association, the National Research Council, the American Cancer Society, and the American Diabetes Association, among others, recommend that total fat intake should be no higher than 30 percent of our daily calories, with only 10 percent coming from saturated fat.

What is important to emphasize here is that the amount of saturated fat in a particular food is just as ominous as, and perhaps more so than, the amount of cholesterol. Saturated fat in our diet literally produces cholesterol in our bloodstream. *So the ideal foods to eat would be those containing very small amounts of both cholesterol and saturated fats.* Examples of such foods include white fish such as sole, cod, and halibut; water-packed tuna; and poultry without the skin. Foods originally thought forbidden due to high cholesterol content, such as shellfish, can also be quite acceptable. The reason for this is that while shellfish have high amounts of cholesterol— some as much as twice that of poultry and red meats—its saturated fat content is extremely low, making it as healthy a food choice as poultry without the skin.

More and more, experts are looking at four elements and their relationships to each other to assess someone's risk of heart disease. They are the amounts of cholesterol, high-density lipoproteins (HDLs), low-density lipoproteins (LDLs), and triglycerides.

7. WHERE DO THE HDLS, LDLS, AND TRIGLYCERIDES FIT INTO THE CHOLESTEROL STORY? High-density lipoprotein is commonly referred to as the good fat. It's actually a group of proteins that helps carry excess cholesterol in the bloodstream back to the liver for disposal. Research has shown that someone with high cholesterol values, who ordinarily might be in danger of heart disease, is endowed with special protection if the levels of

HDL in his blood are high. Increasingly, experts, such as Dr. William P. Castelli, medical director of the long-term heart-disease study conducted by the federal government in Framingham, Massachusetts, are recommending that a far better gauge of heart-disease risk is the ratio between total cholesterol and HDL. To calculate the ratio, the total cholesterol value obtained in a blood test—let's say 200 milligrams—is divided by the HDL value—we'll use 40 for simplicity. The higher the ratio—in this case it would be 5.0—the greater the risk of heart disease. The average risk of heart disease in Americans is 4.5. Those with a ratio less than 4.5 probably do not require any treatment.

LDL, on the other hand, appears to promote the buildup of atherosclerotic plaque. When there is more cholesterol circulating than your cells can use, the LDL carriers deposit the excess on the artery walls. High levels of LDL can point to potential heart disease.

Finally, triglycerides are another form of fat in the blood totally different from cholesterol that have been implicated in the formation of atherosclerotic plaque on artery walls, the cause of angina and heart attacks. As with LDL, high triglycerides can suggest potential problems even though cholesterol and HDL values are normal.

Dr. Kenneth Cooper, author of *Controlling Cholesterol* (Bantam Books, 1988), compiled a comprehensive chart assessing all blood lipids based on sex and age and assigned low, moderate, high, and very high risk categories. (It is reproduced on the next two pages.) Experts do disagree about precise lipid levels and the risk of developing heart disease, however, since there is great variability from one person to another.

Furthermore, one recent study, reported in the March 23, 1990, *Journal of the American Medical Association,* found that reducing the overall amount of fat in the diet is more important than changing the kinds of fats consumed when it comes to protection against atherosclerotic heart disease. Life-style factors, such as diet, exercise, and smoking, play a role in the development of heart disease, in addition to hereditary factors.

8. HOW DO I LOWER MY LDLS AND TRIGYLCERIDES AND RAISE MY HDLS? The majority of research indicates that cholesterol levels and LDLs can be lowered by eating less saturated fat and more monounsaturated fats and polyunsaturated fats (unsaturated fats). The scientific understanding of the effects of fats and

Assessing Your Blood Lipids

Experts disagree about precise lipid levels and the risk of developing heart disease. There is also great variability from one person to another, and such things as smoking and hereditary factors play a role in addition to diet and exercise. This chart was compiled by Dr. Kenneth H. Cooper based on his research and that of other experts.

Lipids	Age	EXCELLENT PROTECTION 25TH PERCENTILE		MODERATE RISK 50TH PERCENTILE	
		Male	Female	Male	Female
Total	20–39	162–179	157–176	180–202	177–197
Cholesterol	40–59	186–209	186–209	210–233	210–235
mg/dl	60+	189–213	205–227	214–240	228–252
LDL	20–39	100–117	90–108	118–137	109–127
Cholesterol	40–59	119–140	110–118	141–162	132–140
mg/dl	60+	122–143	126–149	144–165	150–175
HDL	20–39	> 51	> 63	37–51	45–63
Cholesterol	40–59	> 52	> 69	37–52	49–69
mg/dl	60+	> 60	> 74	40–60	50–74
Triglycerides	20–39	71–93	58–77	94–133	78–106
mg/dl	40–59	89–121	73–98	122–170	99–140
	60+	83–110	82–110	111–154	111–146
Total	20–39	3.6–2.3	2.8–1.9	5.1–3.7	3.6–2.9
Cholesterol/	40–59	4.2–2.6	3.0–2.0	6.0–4.3	4.0–3.1
HDL ratio	60+	4.0–2.5	3.2–2.0	6.0–4.1	4.8–3.3

Lipids	Age	HIGH RISK 75TH PERCENTILE		VERY HIGH RISK 90TH PERCENTILE	
		Male	Female*	Male	Female
Total	20–39	203–225	198–220	> 226	> 221
Cholesterol	40–59	234–257	236–259	> 258	> 260
mg/dl	60+	241–262	253–276	> 263	> 277
LDL	20–39	138–159	128–149	> 159	> 149
Cholesterol	40–59	163–183	156–181	> 183	> 181
mg/dl	60+	166–190	176–198	> 190	> 198
HDL	20–39	< 37	< 45	—	—
Cholesterol	40–59	< 37	< 49	—	—
mg/dl	60+	< 40	< 50	—	—
Triglycerides	20–39	134–195†	107–146†	> 195	> 146
mg/dl	40–59	171–231†	141–190†	> 231	> 190
	60+	155–206†	147–206†	> 207	> 207
Total	20–39	6.1–5.2	4.2–3.7	> 6.1	> 4.2
Cholesterol/	40–59	7.4–6.1	4.9–4.1	> 7.4	> 4.9
HDL ratio	60+	6.9–6.1	5.5–4.9	> 6.9	> 5.5

*Due to the lack of data, one may question whether HDL cholesterol levels in women in this range truly mean high risk. However, at this time, this is the best estimate of risk.
†Triglycerides at this level do not warrant drug therapy. Consult your physician for dietary, weight loss, or exercise therapy.

Source: *Controlling Cholesterol* by Kenneth H. Cooper, M.D., M.P.H.

oils is still evolving, however, so that newly published studies continually challenge old recommendations.

Polyunsaturated fats are liquid at room temperature and are found primarily in cooking oils of vegetable origin. At the top of the list, in descending order of preference, are safflower, sunflower, corn, sesame, and soybean oil, for they are lowest in saturated fats and highest in polyunsaturated fats. Cottonseed oil and generic vegetable oil—generally a blend of oils, such as soybean and cottonseed—are at the bottom of the list because they are more saturated. While polyunsaturates reduce the amount of cholesterol and the level of LDL lipoprotein in the blood, they also reduce the "good" HDL as well. No more than 10 percent of total daily calories should be polyunsaturated fats.

Monounsaturated fats, on the other hand, reduce only the damaging LDL carrier and have no effect on the protective HDL. Found in high amounts in olive, rapeseed (also called canola), and peanut oils, monounsaturates remain liquid at room temperature but become viscous or hard when refrigerated. Most research has been done on olive oil, less on rapeseed, while the research findings on peanut oil are conflicting. Monounsaturated fats should be limited to 10 to 15 percent of total daily calories.

Your body needs both monounsaturated and polyunsaturated fats.

Cardiologists have found that two of the best ways to reduce triglycerides are to get down to the ideal body weight for your age and sex and to engage in regular aerobic exercise. The relationship between triglycerides and diet is still unclear.

Exercise also seems to increase HDL levels, but researchers do not yet understand why.

9. WHERE DOES FIBER FIT IN THE CHOLESTEROL PICTURE?
Certain components of dietary fiber have been shown to reduce blood cholesterol levels, but studies have been inconclusive. There is some indication that one type of fiber, lignin, lowers blood cholesterol. Further, pectins and gums, two sticky fibers, seem to help lower blood cholesterol and fat in the same way that lignins do— they bind the bile salts and thus help them pass out of the body.

Lignin can be found in bran and whole-grain cereals, peas, tomatoes, cabbages, pears, peaches, strawberries, and peanuts. Pectin can be found in apples, bananas, beets, carrots, grapes, okra, oranges, and potatoes. Gums are found in dried beans, oat bran, oatmeal, and sesame seeds. (You can find a chart listing the fiber content of common foods in Chapter 5.)

Many researchers believe, however, that adding fiber to reduce cholesterol goes hand in hand with cutting back on fat.

10. WHAT ARE OMEGA-3 FATTY ACIDS, AND DO THEY LOWER BLOOD CHOLESTEROL? In 1985, researchers reported that Greenland Eskimos have a low incidence of heart disease. Since Eskimos eat large amounts of oily fish and blubber, scientists hypothesized that a unique type of fatty acid—omega 3—found in oily fish and blubber protects the Eskimos from heart disease. And because fish is generally low in saturated fat and cholesterol, the report supported the growing evidence that lowering saturated fat in your diet can reduce your risk of heart disease.

A number of studies using supplements of omega-3 fatty acids have indicated a lowering of blood levels of cholesterol and triglycerides, particularly if they are initially high. However, researchers are uncertain whether isolated fish oil is solely responsible for the cardiovascular benefits of eating fish.

Keep in mind the inconclusiveness of the studies, but the best sources of omega-3 fatty acids can be found in mackerel, herring, lake trout, sturgeon, albacore tuna, and pink salmon.

Earlier in this chapter, we discussed why food myths come about. We also said that we are easily fooled when it comes to food and that nutritional misinformation can get expensive for the gullible consumer. Fiber's suggested role in lowering cholesterol and the inconclusive evidence on omega-3 fatty acids are two cases in point.

Shortly after the new interest in omega-3 fatty acids, a variety of fish-oil supplements were introduced. Many of these supplements have been promoted as an easy way to increase the amount of those fatty acids you consume and, therefore, to reduce your risk of heart disease. But long-term clinical studies of these supplements have not yet been completed. It is too early to judge the potential merits and possible dangers of fish-oil supplements. Yet many Americans have joined the bandwagon to buy these supplements because they believe the hype.

The announcement about soluble fibers, particularly when a

specific fiber—oat bran—was touted, prompted even less restraint from food companies, advertisers, and American consumers. Soon oat-bran muffins became *the* health food. By 1989, sale of oat-bran cereals rose to $247 million, up 240 percent from the previous year. Actually, anything containing oat bran was touted, and if a product (like potato chips) didn't have oat bran, it was added, and *then* the product was touted.

But oat bran by itself cannot offset the effects of a high-fat, high-cholesterol diet. The great majority of research over the past twenty-five years shows that oat bran simply gives an extra boost to a low-fat, low-cholesterol diet.

Fully 30 percent of the $3.6 billion in annual U.S. food advertising now includes some type of health message (see *Business Week*, October 9, 1989). Food companies are claiming health benefits everywhere. They are finding previously hidden virtues in old products. Cheerios are now advertised as an excellent source of oat bran. Miracle Whip is now labeled "cholesterol free," although it has always been cholesterol free.

Messages often are incomplete, which can further mislead the naive consumer. Yes, Crisco is taking out the palm oil, but it's still made from hydrogenated (highly saturated) oils. Cookies and crackers made from vegetable oil don't have cholesterol, but many still contain partially hydrogenated oils, again adding saturated fats. (Finally last year, the Food and Drug Administration, under Commissioner David Kessler, began ordering companies to remove misleading health claims from food labels.)

And so it goes. Food myths and mistruths may always be alive and well in some form. One reason is that today's facts may become tomorrow's myths as new information continues to challenge present scientific beliefs. But the best dietary advice is the most straightforward and the easiest for you to remember: moderation, variety, and balance.

Let's deal with this age-old maxim in Chapter 3 as we tackle the nutritional challenge inherent in eating at home.

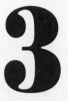

3

A Nutritional Challenge to Eat at Home

Where is the traditional family meal heading? Sitting down to a meal with the family used to be a daily ritual that fed the soul as well as the body and provided a rhythm for the day. A family meal, for many, provided relief from stress.

To be sure, the family meal has always validated the importance of the family. It provided a forum for communication, a time when the kids could get the undivided attention of their parents, and vice versa. Mealtime offered everyone some sense of continuity and security. But the family meal hour is changing for at least some segments of the population.

The traditional American family of a homemaker-wife, a breadwinner-husband, and 2.4 kids represents only 15 percent of all families today. One-fourth of all households are one-person households. Currently, nearly 60 percent of married women are employed outside the home. An interesting outgrowth of this life-style trend is that 52 percent of teenage girls spend two hours per week shopping for family groceries. Nearly half of all grocery shoppers are men, and most of them are shopping for the family. The good news is that everyone is pitching in.

The bad news is that eating habits in this country have gone berserk, and some feel conventional meals are the biggest casualty. We often don't know where the next meal will come from, when or with whom. Breakfast may be a doughnut or a biscuit from a fast-food restaurant. Lunch is consumed off the dashboard or out of the office candy machine. Dinner is often whatever can be grabbed from a store shelf at 6:00 p.m. "Grazing"—what snacking has been called for the last few years—has gone out of control. Today, sitting down to a meal no longer ranks with sleeping and bathing as a necessary daily routine. There has been a shift in attitudes in some segments about the role and importance of food. Yet to many, it is still a family priority to break bread together—a priority that has become more challenging due to time constraints caused by Mom's lack of time to prepare dinner, the children's early-evening activities, either parent's late night at the office, or all of the above.

Regardless of what "family" is to you, a traditional family gathering at mealtimes, particularly at dinner, is here to stay. Certainly, new technologies in the future will allow the way we prepare food, as well as our specific choices of foods, to change (more of that in Chapter 12); but rest assured that the family dinner hour is not marked for extinction. We hope that this book will turn many of you who eat on the run into careful cooks by making you more health-conscious while working within your time constraints.

In the last chapter, we discussed many important nutritional facts. In this chapter, let's build on those facts as we give you the tools to win the challenge of eating nutritiously in your own home.

Balance, Moderation, and Variety

At home, you do have a head start. Home is where you have the most control over eating what you want when you want it, the size of your portion, and the kinds of foods and ingredients you use. In the last chapter, we discussed the Surgeon General's Report on Nutrition and Health released in 1988. After reviewing all the scientific evidence available, this landmark report gave us proof that dietary excesses and imbalances do lead to chronic diseases. In fact, these diseases account for more than two-thirds of all deaths in the United States.

In plain language, that means you need to look at all the foods you eat each day and do your best to maintain a balanced diet, to eat all things in moderation, and choose a variety of foods. Without this total diet approach, you are jeopardizing your health. That is a fact. Proper nutrition, after all, is a matter of common sense. But, as we have seen earlier, our reaction to food is often quite emotional. So when it comes to nutrition, we can't assume common sense applies. Let's give you some tips now on how to achieve balance, moderation, and variety in your diet.

Most of us fight a continual battle between self-control and self-indulgence. Balance lies somewhere in the middle. It shouldn't be feast or famine, all or none. Balance for some may be having low-fat cottage cheese and fruit, salads, and broiled chicken or fish during the week, and splurging a bit on appetizers, sauces, and desserts offered at weekend social gatherings. That's okay. Balance for others may be exercising vigorously, then rationalizing the french fries, ice cream, and fudge brownies. This has been called the work out/pig out syndrome. That's *not* okay.

Another aspect of balance in the diet has to do with the types of foods you eat each day. A proper balance of protein, carbohydrates, and fat in your diet provides you with the right amount of vitamins, minerals, and other nutrients that you need to stay healthy. If you never eat any dairy products, chances are you're not getting enough calcium. If you never eat any meat, fish, poultry, or vegetables, you probably aren't getting enough iron. If you have juice and a muffin for breakfast, a salad for lunch, and no dinner, you're short on nutrients and total calories for the day. The concept here is getting what you need—not too much and not too little.

You can achieve a balance in your diet by trading off one food item for another. In other words, if you can't resist the candy machine at work at 3:00 p.m., pass on dessert after dinner that night so you don't have too many calories or too much sugar and fat that day. Don't have a three-egg cheese omelet for breakfast and an eight-ounce cheeseburger for dinner—it's just too much fat and cholesterol in one day. But you don't have to feel guilty every time you reach for a candy bar or enjoy your favorite cheeseburger. You can have your cake—just limit the amount you eat, and eat it on a day when you trade off other items that might be high in sugar, fat, and calories. It's that easy.

Now let's take a look at how you can achieve moderation in your diet. Most important, you need to know what normal portions are. Here are some guidelines. A portion of milk is one cup, and the same goes for a portion of yogurt. Hard cheeses, on the other hand, are measured by one-ounce portions. The individually wrapped cheese slices are generally ¾ ounce per slice (or 1⅓ slices per 1-ounce serving.) One portion of most vegetables is considered ½ cup, while fruit portions are more variable. Half a banana, one small apple, half a grapefruit, and half a cup of orange juice are each considered one portion. One slice of bread is considered one portion, as is ¾ to 1 cup of ready-to-eat cereal. One serving of fat, in general, is 1 teaspoon whether it is butter, margarine, or oil.

A single portion of meat, poultry, or fish is usually three or four ounces, which is about the size of the palm of your hand. In fact, experts recommend no more than six ounces a day of animal protein; yet at restaurants you are often given at least twice that amount in one meal. In 1989, meat consumption averaged more than eight ounces of meat a day, according to an Agriculture Department report.

At home, you can control portion size. To get familiar with the portions mentioned, try to weigh and measure portion quantities until you are able to actually visualize what a portion looks like. Eating in moderation—eating normal-sized portions—allows you to eat more kinds of foods.

And eating a variety of foods is extremely critical to your health. You need about forty different nutrients to stay healthy. While most foods contain more than one nutrient, no single food item supplies all the essential nutrients in the amounts that you need. So the greater the variety of your diet, the less likely you are to develop either a deficiency or an excess of any single nutrient. Furthermore, we still are not aware of all the properties in the foods we eat and all the nutritional requirements. To maintain the proper variety, choose foods every day from each of the four major food groups: grains, milk and milk products, fruits and vegetables, meat, fish, and poultry, and meat alternatives, such as beans, tofu, and other vegetable proteins. Particular weight should be given to grains, and fruits and vegetables, to maintain the proper balance in your diet. (See Chapter 4 for suggested servings of each food group.)

"There's Never Enough Time!"

While balance, moderation, and variety are the basis of healthy eating, most families today have busy schedules. Mothers who work outside the home and single parents are particularly short on time and energy to prepare meals. Working women in a 1989 survey by *Better Homes and Gardens* and the Food Marketing Institute spent less time preparing dinner (about forty-nine minutes) than women who didn't work (about sixty minutes). Feeding a large family can also be exhausting. But it doesn't have to be.

Here are some tips to help you plan nutritious meals in a busy household:

- **Plan ahead.** Discuss meal planning with the whole family and come up with menus for a whole week at a time. Divide up the jobs, from shopping to putting groceries away to cooking and cleaning up.
- **Stock the basics.** Sometimes we race for a fast-food chain or pull out a frozen dinner because we don't have the ingredients in the house to make a quick and tasty meal. Keep your cupboards stocked with staple foods, such as pastas, cereals, rice, tomato paste, lemon juice, canned beans, tuna, salmon, peanut butter, seasonings and condiments, and oils low in saturated fat.

  Keep whole wheat breads, peas, corn, and fruits in your freezer, along with boneless, skinless chicken breasts and fish fillets. Vegetables such as cabbage, cauliflower, turnips, and carrots and reduced-fat cheeses and eggs will keep for three to four weeks in the refrigerator. Have skim milk, low-fat yogurt and cottage cheese, and a variety of fruits and vegetables on hand; they will keep for at least a week in the refrigerator.
- **Cook extra on the weekends.** Double whatever you make on Saturday and Sunday (or any day of the week you happen to have more time to cook) and eat it again later in the week. Or roast a turkey on the weekend, use it for cold sandwiches on Monday, and put it in a soup or casserole on Tuesday. Freeze individual servings and, with the help of your microwave, have a quick nutritious meal on a night you're really pressed for time.
- **Do some meal preparation, if possible, before bedtime for the next day or before you leave for work.** Chop up some vegetables

for a stir-fry or for a salad or take out the nonperishable ingredients you'll be using for the next meal. Store all perishables (including meats and diary items) in the refrigerator before you leave for work.

- **Get someone to help you with meal preparation and/or grocery shopping.** A member of the family or even a baby-sitter might help out. Many exciting and nutritious recipes just require that extra time for basic cutting-up of vegetables or meats. If everything is ready when you get home, many recipes can be prepared in minutes!
- **Eating solo:** If you're living alone, finding the motivation to cook and learning how to shop for one can be additional nutritional challenges. The above tips do apply to you, however. And since you may have a bit more time on your hands, you might consider boosting your cooking skills a notch or two. Try to prepare many of your weeknight meals on weekends. Casseroles, soups, and stews are all foods that can be prepared ahead and frozen or refrigerated for later.

Cooking Methods: Fast, Healthy, and Fun

Even the best intentions of healthy-minded cooks can go awry. It is most important to choose cooking methods that do not add fat to otherwise low-fat foods. Fortunately, the most healthful cooking methods are often the fastest. Let's look at some specific cooking methods through the eyes of a professional chef who was trained in nutritional cooking. For that purpose, we spoke with chef Robert Briggs.

Chef Briggs teaches nutritional cooking at the Culinary Institute of America in Hyde Park, New York. The CIA, long known as one of the pre-eminent institutions for the culinary arts, established an innovative nutrition program in the mid-1980s. Later, in 1989, the school unveiled the $2.75 million General Foods Nutrition Center, which houses a classroom, a library/learning-resources center, and a production kitchen with many unique design concepts. The center also is the home of St. Andrew's Cafe, one of the institute's four student-staffed public restaurants, which serve "good food that's good for you."

After spending six years in the kitchen of the Greenbriar Hotel in West Virginia, Chef Briggs saw the need for nutritional cooking firsthand. "Every night, we had a list of special orders—no oil, no butter, no salt," he remembers. "I could see then that this was going to be the new trend in American cooking, and I wanted to be a part of that."

The approach at St. Andrew's Cafe is a moderate one, since it is a restaurant open to the public, but it is much stricter than the average restaurant in every way. First, each meal contains approximately 800 calories, with just under 20 percent of the calories coming from protein, under 30 percent coming from fat, and 50 percent from carbohydrates (no more than 10 percent of those come from simple sugars). Sodium is kept under 900 milligrams and cholesterol no higher than 150 milligrams per meal.

"The bottom line is control and moderation," Chef Briggs explains. Their entree portion size is only three and a half ounces, but the entree is not the main event: it is accompanied by a vegetable and a starch, and all are presented on the plate together.

Great effort is taken to keep the St. Andrew's kitchen just like any other restaurant kitchen. To accomplish this, the staff uses regular restaurant equipment and works with real ingredients like butter and cream rather than substituting margarine and low-fat milk, but these are calculated into the recipes so that the correct balance of nutrients is maintained. "Our students can go into any restaurant with existing food items and equipment and be able to incorporate nutritional techniques," Briggs says. At home, you can be more flexible—you don't have sophisticated computers to calculate nutrients, and you can have food items on hand that allow you to substitute one item for another. But more on that in a bit.

Before sharing his quick and healthful cooking methods, Chef Briggs makes a plea to the cook at home that will lead to quicker, tastier, and healthier cooking: "The most basic and healthy cooking you can do is to make a chicken stock and a fish stock." Chef Briggs suggests making the stock in quantity because it can be frozen indefinitely. He insists that fresh stock takes little effort, only requires cooking time, and that it adds so much flavor, minus the sodium, to foods.

Consult your favorite cookbook for basic chicken and fish stock recipes. You can freeze the stock in airtight quart-size containers. Briggs suggests freezing the stock in ice-cube trays, then breaking them up into a Ziploc freezer bag so you can grab whatever amount you need at the time you need it.

Chef Briggs objects to the use of canned chicken broth or clam juice instead of homemade stock, unless you just can't keep some homemade stock on hand. He tells his students that these canned products greatly increase the sodium content of the food and don't taste as good.

While quick to point out that no one method can or should be used for every food, Chef Briggs offers five fast and nutritious cooking techniques: dry sautéing, poaching, broiling/grilling, stir-frying, and microwaving.

"*Dry sautéing* is one of the most interesting methods because we'll sauté with no fat. We take a sauté pan, rub it with a little bit of oil, heat the pan up until it's smoking, and season it. Then wipe out the excess oil so there's only an ultra-thin coating of fat in the pan. Heat the pan back up to the smoking point and add the meat. First, the meat will stick; it grabs right away. But as it sits there, it caramelizes; some fat renders out of the product and it becomes nicely browned. Turn it over, brown the other side, and it's done.

"Dry sautéing works pretty well with fattier meats like beef, pork, veal, chicken, and lamb. It will also work well with fatty fish like salmon. It won't work with lean items like sole, turkey, or vegetables. With those leaner items, we can afford to add a bit of fat and still stay within our guidelines, but this would not be a dry sauté.

"Lean toward the monounsaturated oils, like extra virgin olive oil, which also have a lot of flavor. In using so little fat, our goal is to get as much flavor as possible from the oil we use. Cooking sprays made with olive oil are acceptable, but the cooking pan should still be wiped.

"We use normal aluminum sauté pans found in all restaurants because they hold up better," says Chef Briggs. The Culinary Institute has found that the nonstick pans tend not to caramelize as easily as the aluminum pans. Nothing can stick to those nonstick pans, and in order to get a nice browning, the meat needs to stick for a few seconds.

Poaching is a quick, low-fat cooking method. It also enhances seasoning, since with a shallow poach you can reserve the liquid in the poacher, reduce it, and add it to your sauce to help preserve that flavor without adding a lot of salt.

Chef Briggs suggests this method of poaching a 3½-ounce portion of salmon: Put the fish in a pan and bring a mixture of half white wine, half fish stock, and some chopped shallots one third the way up the fish. Warm it on your range, but don't bring it to boiling; then cover the pan with parchment (or foil) and put it in the oven to poach at 350 degrees for 3 or 4 minutes. Remove the fish onto a warming platter, then reduce the poaching liquid (it will take about 10 minutes to thicken), and pour it over the salmon. For some color, you can top the salmon with some chives and/or strips of carrot and you have an appetizing main course. Chef Briggs says that chicken breasts and lean fish, such as sole and flounder, do well with poaching.

Broiling and grilling really do the same thing to food in terms of reducing the fat content—broiling heats from the top, grilling heats from the bottom. Cooking time is also quite similar—a 3½-ounce portion of chicken breast cooks in just a few minutes. Chef Briggs uses a charcoal or mesquite grill in the St. Andrew's kitchen since it enhances the flavor (and with less cleanup afterward).

To keep food moist while cooking and to add flavor, Chef Briggs recommends marinades for meat, fish, and poultry. He suggests marinating a chicken breast in some apple cider with some shallots and garlic. Or squeeze some lime juice onto a piece of fish and add some cilantro and pepper. Chef Briggs cautions against using oil-based marinades that leave food floating around in fat. And he stresses the importance of grilling or broiling close to the heat source and of getting your food right out when it's done—don't overcook.

"Remember, grill, broil, or dry sauté the fatty fish; poach the lean fish," Chef Briggs instructs.

"*Stir-frying* is a cooking method I'd like to put a caution flag next to," Chef Briggs explains. "Most people equate stir-fried food with healthy food, but often the fat content in stir-fried items is high. Americanized Chinese or Japanese food uses so much oil that the food is actually greasy." So stir-frying can be a good method as long as you don't use too much fat. Measure the amount of fat you use, and use as little as possible.

Chef Briggs's stir-fry method looks like this: Cook the meat in a pan without any oil (dry sear). As you add the vegetables, add a few drops of chicken stock. When the liquid hits the hot pan, it steams the vegetables. You can stir-fry in a sauté pan or in a wok;

just limit the fat you use by adding a small amount of stock to steam the vegetables. Stay away from MSG, and if using soy sauce, dilute it with water to reduce the sodium content, or use light soy sauce, which cuts the sodium in half.

Microwaving is a good low-fat cooking method, and it is very quick. The problem with the microwave is that it is a relatively new cooking method. While it has been around for forty years, it first caught on over the past ten to twenty years. "People tend to think you can cook anything in it, but that's not the case," says Chef Briggs. "You don't grill every item, you don't poach every item, and you don't microwave every item, either. It is fine to use the microwave for what it is good for." It's good for some vegetables and some starches and to reheat soups; but, according to Chef Briggs, microwaves can dehydrate and dry out meats, fish, and chicken without giving the foods time to absorb any herbs or seasonings.

We would like to note here that recent attention has been given to the potential cancer risk caused by cooking any meats or fish at high temperatures for a long time (by grilling, frying, or broiling). Some of this risk, which is not conclusive, can be reduced by precooking those meats (poach, boil, or microwave) for a few minutes, pouring off the juice derived from the meat, then finishing by grilling or broiling. Remember, as in all things, moderation is the key.

Cooking with Your Favorite Recipes: Low-Fat Cooking Techniques and the Art of Substitution

We've discussed the total diet approach necessary for healthful eating, given you tips on beating the time issue, and introduced you to fast and nutritious cooking methods to try out in your kitchen. Let's go one important step further. You need to be skilled in low-fat cooking techniques and the principle of substitution. You need to know how to modify recipes to reduce cholesterol, fat, salt, and sugar. Once you understand this principle, it will become second nature to you. And it will enable you to have confidence that the meal you're preparing is a healthy one.

The whole idea is that when you eliminate a food or cut back on it, you use something similar in taste or texture to take its place, but always something with less fat, salt, and sugar. There are certain standard substitutions that people who have more than a passing interest in fat are familiar with: substitute low-fat or nonfat dairy products for whole milk products; use margarine instead of butter; replace egg yolks with egg whites. But we need to get a little more specific here.

Let's start with eggs. A single medium-sized egg yolk contains 1 teaspoon of fat and 213 milligrams of cholesterol. We saw in the last chapter that the American Heart Association recommends our daily intake of cholesterol be no more than 250 to 300 milligrams. One egg yolk nearly gets us to our daily quota! Fortunately, egg whites don't have any cholesterol; so you can substitute one and a half or two egg whites in place of each whole egg specified in some recipes. If you want a three-egg omelet, for example, you can use two egg whites and one whole egg, cutting the cholesterol by two-thirds. Or you can use egg substitutes: there are several of these products available in your local supermarket, in either the frozen-food or the refrigerated section. (We offer you a supermarket tour in Chapter 5.) They consist almost entirely of egg whites, with a little fat added to emulsify them. Baking recipes often require egg yolks, but they do specify when an egg substitute can be used. Heartland now offers a low-cholesterol egg, available in some grocery stores today.

Butter is high in both cholesterol and saturated fat and is another easy place to make substitutions. The best is to switch to a soft margarine, in tubs or soft sticks. The softer the margarine, the less saturated fat it is made from. The difference between butter and soft margarine is significant. One tablespoon of butter has 33 milligrams of cholesterol and 7.5 grams of saturated fat. One tablespoon of several regular and reduced-calorie soft margarines contains no cholesterol and less than a gram of saturated fat. When lard or shortening is specifically called for in a recipe, substitute vegetable oils low in saturated fat (such as canola) or regular soft tub margarines.

Since many of us have never lost our love for sandwiches, it is important that you learn more about three items that go into many sandwiches—peanut butter, mayonnaise, and Miracle Whip. While peanut butter contains no cholesterol, it is about half fat, as are all nuts. The fat in peanut butter, however, is less saturated than animal fat; still, you should use moderation because of the high fat content. Mayonnaise and Miracle Whip are each a little more than two-thirds fat. Fortunately, there are substitutions available that often have as much as one-half less fat, and some with no fat or cholesterol. Miracle Whip Light and Hellmann's Light are low-fat, no-cholesterol products. Kraft has recently come out with fat-free and cholesterol-free Miracle Whip and mayonnaise.

We've seen that some cuts of meats are major contributors of fat, saturated fat, and cholesterol in the diet (see Chapter 5 for more detail). If you're watching your cholesterol, the best recommendations here are: buy the select grade of lean cuts of beef (which has less fat than choice or prime), and trim as much visible fat as possible; stay away from all organ meats, because they are extremely high in cholesterol; remove all skin and visible fat on poultry; and select ground sirloin (10 percent or less fat) instead of regular ground beef (30 percent fat) if you're a hamburger fan.

Cheese tends to be a very high-fat product. Cheddar cheese, the cheese of choice for most people, is even higher in fat than many kinds of meat. There are alternatives to the cheeses made from butterfat. Many cheeses are being made with skim milk and vegetable oils, especially soybean oil. They still contain considerable fat, but much less saturated fat and very little cholesterol.

Ice cream is another product that needs to be selected carefully, and perhaps saved for special occasions. Almost all ice creams contain high levels of fat and cholesterol. Low-fat substitutions may include ice milks; sorbets; low-fat frozen yogurt; sherbet; nonfat frozen dairy desserts, such as those offered by Borden, Edy's, and Sealtest; and Simple Pleasures, which uses Simplesse, a natural fat substitute made from egg white and milk protein. Tofutti and Tofutti Lite are nondairy desserts which contain some fat (soybean oil).

To make substitutions a regular part of your cooking habits, you need to have the lower-fat products available in your kitchen— nonfat or low-fat milk, nonfat yogurt, low-fat cottage cheese, olive and safflower oil, margarine, and the like. Have artificial sweeteners on hand. Use nonstick pans and vegetable-oil sprays in cooking whenever possible. Learn what those red-flag food items are and be prepared to use an alternative. And keep all your recipes—the idea is to change those recipies to fit your healthier eating habits.

That is exactly what Tracy Ritter, chef at the Golden Door Spa in California, does. During the twelve years she spent as a chef learning her craft before coming to the Golden Door Spa, Ms. Ritter never cooked with the amount of cream, butter, or fats that most chefs use. Her culinary training was at the French Culinary Institute in New York, and her early years as a chef were spent mostly in diverse restaurants in New York. Now in her fourth year at the Golden Door Spa, Ms. Ritter looks daily for even more ways to infuse her cooking with the depths of flavor previously provided by butter and cream. Most of her discoveries are easily translatable to home cooking. "The main issue for the person at home is understanding where the fats are coming from," she says. "Generally, whether at a restaurant or at home, you're getting your higher amounts of fats from your sauces and your vinaigrettes, as opposed to your actual cooking process." Ms. Ritter is well versed on all the standard substitutions described earlier. She creatively incorporates many others, and, as she says, "the possibilities are endless."

Here are some interesting ways to have your sauces and your salad dressings without the fats:

- When roasting a chicken or turkey, remove the skin. Don't baste with butter or pan juices: use a mixture of white wine, water, and chicken stock, or a light glaze of olive oil. Cover with an aluminum foil tent. You may not have a crispy outer skin, but you will have a good flavor.
- To add flavor when broiling a piece of salmon or flounder, cover the foil you place the fish on with vegetable oil spray. Put the fish on the foil, then sprinkle with white wine and lemon juice and top with some fresh herbs.
- Poached fish works very well in the microwave, according to Ms. Ritter. Place a piece of fish in a glass dish, sprinkle it with a little white wine, some pepper, fresh herbs, and some mustard or horseradish, and top with some thin slices of tomato. Seal it tight with a glass cover or cover with wax paper and cook for 2 minutes. When the fish poaches, it forms its own liquid, and that becomes its sauce.
- Use mustard as a thickening agent when reducing a sauce. Ms. Ritter offers this sample sauce recipe that can be used over meat, chicken, or fish and serves six people: Cook together, slowly, ½ cup white wine, 4 chopped shallots, and an herb, like tarragon or thyme; reduce it down to 1 tablespoon; add 1 cup of chicken stock to that, bring it to a boil, and reduce it by half. Into that, whisk 3 tablespoons of a grain mustard, which will thicken and form the sauce.
- Or instead of mustard, use fruit as a thickening agent. To pre-

pare Ms. Ritter's pineapple-ginger sauce, start with ½ cup white wine and some shallots or onion and reduce the liquid down to 1 tablespoon. Add 1 cup of chicken stock, bring it to a boil, and reduce it again by half. At the very end, whisk in 3 tablespoons of pureed fruit and a 1-inch cube of ginger, chopped. (You can make vegetable purees as well by following the same procedure but adding some finely chopped vegetables at the end and letting them cook down a bit.)

- Additional thickening agents are oatmeal, rice purees, cornstarch, and arrowroot, but you cannot boil the latter because it gets too pasty. Ms. Ritter says that thickening agents are the number-one key to sauces.

- In some recipes, you can make a cream sauce by replacing heavy cream with nonfat buttermilk, which adds a tang. The difference is significant—1 cup of buttermilk made from nonfat milk contributes 88 calories and almost no fat, while 1 cup of heavy cream is 832 calories and 36 percent fat. Any cream sauce can begin with 1 cup of buttermilk, thickened by 1 tablespoon of cornstarch. Then flavor the sauce with 3–4 tablespoons of tomato sauce or mustard or pesto. If you want a lighter sauce, use ½ of your flavoring ingredient.

- Use a teaspoon to a tablespoon of olive oil to finish off sauces based on vegetable purees made without fat. This provides a smoother consistency and adds a sheen for a nice finish, along with added flavor.

- Marinate meat, poultry, and fish in a savory mixture for a few hours to replace flavor lost when fat is removed. Ms. Ritter offers two marinades as examples.

Orange-ginger-sesame marinade: 1 cup of fresh or frozen orange juice; 1-inch cube of fresh ginger, chopped; ½ teaspoon of dark sesame oil; half a chopped onion; a pinch of black pepper; and ¼ teaspoon of red pepper flakes. This keeps well in the refrigerator, and if you make extra, you can cook the extra marinade over the stove, reduce it, and form a glaze for chicken.

Stir-fry marinade: Blend together 1 cup of low-sodium soy sauce; ½ teaspoon of sesame oil; 1 ounce of rice wine vinegar or apple cider vinegar; 1 chopped shallot; 1 chopped garlic clove; 1 chopped scallion; 1 tablespoon of lemon juice; and a 1-inch piece of ginger, chopped. This keeps well in the refrigerator and works well for vegetables, chicken, or fish.

- Traditionally, salad dressing is 3 parts oil and 1 part vinegar. Cut it back to 1 part oil, 1 part vinegar, 1 part water or juice, and 1 part mustard and fresh herbs, such as dill, basil, tarragon, and cilantro. If the herbs are not available, just use more mustard. You add flavor by using flavored vinegars and flavored mustards, like tarragon mustard or green peppercorn mustard. The mustard will also act as the emulsifier and will produce a creamy-type dressing without the eggs.
- Use high-flavored condiments (like horseradish) or full-bodied cheeses (like blue cheese) in salad dressings. A small amount of cheese can go a long way, like in this quick salad dressing recipe of Ms. Ritter's: 1 cup of buttermilk, thickened with a bit of cornstarch, to which is added a bit of mustard, a small amount of lemon or capers, a dash of Worcestershire sauce, and 1 ounce of blue cheese.
- Vegetable juices can be used as bases in salad dressings. To make a mock French dressing, blend 6 ounces of V-8 juice and two heaping tablespoons of cottage cheese, then flavor with thyme or tarragon.

When Snacking Is the Only Answer: The Art of "Grazing"

If you love to nibble and nosh all day long, hate the idea of sitting down to three meals a day, or are just on the run from dawn to dusk, you may be what the media masters call a "grazer." The Snack Food Association says Americans snack to the tune of $8 billion every year. Nibbling whatever's at hand, whenever it's convenient, can throw the four food groups, the recommended daily nutrients, and balanced nutrition out the window. It doesn't have to.

In fact, grazing may be better for the heart than gorging, if that's what you find yourself doing when you sit down to a meal.

The *New England Journal of Medicine* (October 5, 1989) reported that snacking all day rather than eating three big meals may lower blood cholesterol. Researchers led by Dr. David J. A. Jenkins, a professor of medicine and nutritional sciences at the University of Toronto, reported that cholesterol levels may be lowered by an average of 9 percent by increasing the number of meals eaten, provided there is no change in the type or amount of food consumed. The report suggests that the reduction in the cholesterol level may be caused by the nibbling diet's effect on insulin secretion. A sudden rise in blood sugar after each meal normally prompts the secretion of insulin, and this hormone stimulates the liver to produce cholesterol. Nibbling was found to result in the release of smaller amounts of insulin. High blood levels of cholesterol and insulin are both believed to play a role in the development of heart disease.

If there's one problem with grazing, though, it's that many people go at it haphazardly, grabbing whatever is within arm's reach—a cookie here, a doughnut there, some potato chips or fast food on the run. Needless to say, random grazing can be nutritionally unwise as well as fattening. It doesn't have to be. In fact, if you plan what you snack on, and when, you can not only maintain your weight and nutrition, but even lose weight if that's your goal.

An effective grazing schedule looks something like this. Divide the traditional three meals into smaller parts. The mid-morning hunger pangs can be eliminated by breaking breakfast into two parts: have the cereal with fruit first and save the bran muffin for later. Likewise, eat a salad for lunch and save the crackers for a mid-afternoon nosh—or divide your sandwich in half and have part of it at lunch and the rest at mid-afternoon. If you work late into the afternoon or early evening, it would be a good idea to keep an extra apple, half a sandwich, or carrot sticks on hand to avoid overindulging in the evening.

Here are a couple of tips to get you into a healthy grazing pattern:

- Eat a variety of foods from the four food groups.
- Eat more starch and fiber, which can be found in fruits, grains, and vegetables.
- Avoid excess fat and cholesterol. To get adequate protein without all the fat and cholesterol, eat more dried beans, fish, and poultry, fewer eggs and less red meat.
- Avoid excess salt and sugar—both are found in abundance in many popular snack foods. Read the label to know what's in the foods you choose, and select fresh foods when possible.
- Eat when you're hungry and stop when you're satisfied.

20 Good-for-You Snacks, 150 Calories or Less

Celery (3 stalks), 10
Broccoli, raw (3 stalks), 25
Carrot, raw, 30
Peach, raw, 40
Graham cracker (one whole), 50
Orange juice (½ cup), 55
Cantaloupe (half), 60
Bread, whole wheat (1 slice), 65
Apple, 80
Egg (1 boiled), 80
Cottage cheese, 1 percent fat (½ cup), 80
Peanuts (2 tbsp), 105
Cheese, cheddar (1 oz), 115
Muffin, 120
Milk, low-fat (1 cup), 125
Tuna, in water (½ cup), 130
Turkey, white meat (3 oz), 135
Potato, baked (plain), 140
Yogurt, Weight Watchers (8 oz), 150
Chicken breast, broiled (½ breast), 150

In this chapter, we've tried to give you the tools to effectively manage the challenge of eating nutritiously at home. Balance, moderation, and variety in your diet can be achieved by trading off one food for another, knowing what one portion of a food looks like, and eating from each of the four major food groups every day. (We get even more specific in the next chapter.) You've learned about food preparation, cooking methods that prove to be fast and nutritious, and how low-fat cooking techniques can translate your favorite recipe into a nutritious meal. In Appendix A, we recommend cookbooks to help you meet your challenge. And if all the above fails, you now have the skills of effective noshing.

In the next chapter, we'll get you ready to stock your shelves and turn you into a more intelligent food shopper. You'll be introduced to the supermarkets of the nineties; you'll learn how to read a food label; and you'll understand the basic dietary guidelines enabling you to make healthy choices wherever you buy your groceries.

4

A Guide for Today's Supermarket Shopper

You've finally gotten yourself organized to plan quick and nutritious meals for yourself and your family at home. List in hand, you head for your nearest supermarket for your weekly excursion to stock your shelves.

What you're likely to find, however, is a plethora of food choices that leaves you in a daze. There are some appealing shortcuts—frozen meals requiring only a microwave oven, prepared foods you just warm and serve, even a take-out section with a drive-through window—and you're starting to get sidetracked from your shopping list. To make matters worse, almost everything has a label on it with words that are confusing to you. You're not even sure what to look for or what dietary guidelines to follow. . . .

Sound familiar?

Food shoppers, still pushing for the family dinner hour, have demanded more convenience from their stores. Supermarkets have addressed those demands by developing new stores and improving old ones.

As a result, the corner grocery store has faded to a memory. Sure, there are specialty stores where you can buy meats or gourmet items, and some nieghborhood groceries are still around. But changing life-styles and intense competition among supermarkets have brought U.S. grocery stores into a new era. More and bigger is the name of the game today.

The growth in size is coupled with the more than twenty-four thousand different food items available in the average supermarket. Stores are catering to every consumer whim to survive in a business yielding $640.2 billion in national supermarket and grocery sales each year, according to *Progressive Grocer*'s 1990 figures. So while the intimacy of grocery shopping is mostly a thing of the past, the consumer reaps other benefits, such as variety and top-quality food products.

If you consider yourself a typical grocery shopper, then your food choices will be based on taste, price, convenience, and nutrition. Taste is individual, and people's pocketbooks vary as well, but the quests for convenience and nutrition are becoming universal priorities.

Searching for Convenience

The busy life-styles of the nineties have produced consumers who want high-quality meals that don't require time-consuming cooking. We gave you the tools to meet that challenge in the last chapter. But on the days when preparing a nutritious meal is impossible, you do have an alternative. Food companies today are producing ready-made items, frozen, refrigerated, or for your pantry shelf, that are low in sodium, cholesterol, and fat. Increasingly, your local supermarket offers you an abundance of take-out foods that eliminate a lot of the fuss of preparation while maintaining freshness. Some of these foods are prepared with the health-conscious shopper in mind.

A 1987 study for the Food Marketing Institute (FMI) and the Campbell Soup Company found that 81 percent of American households bought take-out food in a four-week period. While that study, "Shopping à la Carte," is several years old, the FMI believes that this take-out trend continues today and will continue in the future.

On the average, the study found, buyers purchased take-out food one and a half times each week. Take-out foods included prepared hamburgers (purchased by 73 percent of the respondents), pizza (72 percent), prepared chicken (49 percent), deli meats/cold cuts (34 percent), sandwiches (28 percent), baked/fried fish (22 percent), and prepared salads (20 percent). About half of the buyers (49 percent) said they had bought ethnic take-out food, particularly Chinese (33 percent) and Mexican (18 percent).

When buyers were asked to name places that come to mind for take-out food, 85 percent mentioned fast-food restaurants, 65 percent mentioned pizza parlors, and only 18 percent mentioned supermarkets. Yet 30 percent of the buyers in this 1987 survey reported that they purchased take-out food at supermarkets during the preceding three months.

Since this study, however, ready-made "take-out" meals are just one of the changes that have been made in today's supermarket. Today's supermarket may offer home shopping and delivery service for groceries, food catering, video rentals, and photo finishing. Many provide delicatessen items, gourmet and specialty foods, fresh pizza and ice-cream-shop ice cream. You can call in and order ahead from a take-out section that offers an appetizing ethnic array of hot, nutritious foods. These foods vary from the "hot to go" items (prepared in the supermarket's kitchen and taken from the store in a heat-proof bag), to partially cooked foods (marinated or seasoned and ready to be warmed up at home), to foods you can "heat and eat" (refrigerated precooked meals that need only to be popped into the microwave or oven). While the ingredients used in these items are typically not identified on a label, customer inquiries can be made to the supermarket chef. Many stores now employ a chef. Some supermarkets have even developed prepared foods for the nutritionally conscious shopper: often, nutritional information in the form of brochures or pamphlets accompanies a prepared item.

Some supermarkets are trying to make traditional fast food available for their customers. Kroger, among the nation's largest supermarket chains, based in Cincinnati, has begun selling 1- and 3-pound packages of the same meat that goes into Wendy's Old Fashioned square hamburgers. This joint marketing effort between Kroger and Wendy's International, the fast-food company headquartered in Columbus, Ohio, trades on the name recognition of Wendy's burgers. Other fast-food-type products have appeared in selected supermarkets, including frozen White Castle burgers and Cincinnati's Skyline Chili.

Besides fast food, supermarkets are increasingly carrying gourmet-type foods, and some supermarkets are attracting gourmet shoppers exclusively. Gourmet-to-Go sections have been available in many of Giant Food Inc.'s stores in Maryland, Virginia, and Washington, D.C. Seattle-based Larry's Markets has employed master chefs to prepare ready-to-go entrees. Buffalo's Wegmans has offered pizza with fifty varieties of toppings, from Thai with cilantro to Mexican with cumin, hot pepper cheese, olives, and coriander. Other gourmet operations include Tom Thumb's "Simon David" in Dallas, Byerly's in Minneapolis, and New York's D'Agostino chain, which hired a graduate chef from the Culinary Institute of America to oversee its new prepared-food operation.

The availability of ready-made, take-out fast-food and gourmet items addresses the shopper's need for convenience. But let's next take a look at what supermarkets and food companies have done to appeal to the shopper's nutritional concerns.

Nutritional Concerns of Today's Food Shopper

Every year, the FMI conducts a "Trends" survey to track shoppers' attitudes toward food products and supermarkets. In 1989, the most significant change took place in the response of shoppers to the importance of having nutrition and health information available to them as they make their shopping decisions. Jumping a full 10 percentage points from the previous year, 84 percent of the shoppers polled in 1989 said this was an area of importance to them. This result was the same in the 1990 survey, and was 86 percent in 1991. Only one in ten shoppers was confident enough to say that his or her diet was "as healthy as it could be" (9 percent in 1989, 12 percent in 1990, 10 percent in 1991). In 1989, two-thirds of the shoppers (66 percent) expressed a high degree of interest in having their supermarket provide them with nutrition-related information and, as a result, many of the innovative programs we discuss in this chapter were developed at this time.

Supermarket chains have developed innovative ways to provide nutrition information for their customers. The programs range from general nutrition information pamphlets and recipes to food-safety materials to color-coded shelf tags which identify foods suitable for calorie-controlled, fat-modified, or sodium-restricted diets. Here are some particularly innovative examples that have been developed.

Cholesterol and blood pressure screenings as well as Lifescan, a computerized health-hazard appraisal that helps customers learn more about their health risks, have been offered at the Copps Corporation (Stevens Point, Wisconsin) stores. Copps customers also received free monthly health and nutrition pamphlets with topics like "Osteo . . . What?," "Serving Seniors," "Foods for Kids," and "Dental Diet." All information has been reviewed by a group of thirteen health professionals.

D'Agostino Supermarkets (based in New Rochelle, New York) has created the *Good Food Newsletter* with artwork from children in a Manhattan school district. Distributed to ten thousand families in Manhattan, the newsletter encouraged children to eat "power breakfasts" that provide good nutrition. This community project also promoted the breakfast program in the schools and was translated into Spanish and Chinese.

Giant Food of Washington, D.C., has developed one of the most comprehensive programs to educate consumers. Its "Eat for Health" guides, developed with the National Cancer Institute, are useful for finding foods low in fat, calories, cholesterol, and sodium, and high in fiber. Shelf tags, recipe cards, and stickers displayed in the meat department are also part of this unique program. Giant Food also provides a 27-page consumer guide, *Fat, Cholesterol and Your Heart,* which encourages diets low in fat and cholesterol to reduce the risk of heart disease. It focuses on monitoring blood cholesterol and includes "heart healthy" recipes and shopping tips. The guide coordinates with Giant's in-store shelf labeling, which identifies the content of fat, cholesterol, and fiber in various foods. In-store brochures and booklets at Giant stores feature a variety of topics, such as sodium, calcium, fats, and cholesterol; seniors; pregnancy; nutritious lunches; meats, cheese, seafood, and poultry. As they check out, Giant customers can pick up a bright yellow-and-blue bulletin that discusses how to safely handle some favorite summer foods. The bulletin offers handling tips for fresh and frozen meats and dairy products in case of loss of refrigeration due to an electrical storm, as well as advice on food preparation and refrigeration. Finally, Giant has offered Tel Med, a call-in service of more than 250 recorded messages on health, nutrition, and medical concerns.

Hyde Park Cooperative (based in South Elgin, Illinois) has registered dietitians available to answer consumer questions on food and nutrition. A weekly recipe sheet features nutritional analyses of the recipes. A monthly newsletter offers a wide variety of consumer, food, and nutrition information. Special diet shopping lists have been developed for sodium-restricted, fat-modified, calorie- and gluten-controlled diets.

Price Chopper Supermarkets (Schenectady, New York) has offered the "Call on Our Cooking Specialist" (COOKS) Hotline, which answers inquiries on nutrition, food preparation, recipes, and food safety from 9 a.m. to 9 p.m. seven days a week. The hotline was co-sponsored with a food product manufacturer, McCormick Spices. Price Chopper also operates a hotline manned by local dietitians and conducts bimonthly aisle-by-aisle tours to show shoppers how to trim fat, limit cholesterol and sodium, and add fiber to their diets. This free program was developed with the local affiliate of the American Heart Association.

SNAP is Safeway's Nutrition Awareness Program (Safeway is based in Oakland, California). One component uses bright yellow shelf tags for consumers to easily spot foods low in calories, sodium, fat, and cholesterol, and rich in fiber; and an in-store guide lists brand-specific foods along with their nutrient values. Another SNAP component is a bimonthly nutrition magazine that is available in both English and Spanish.

Wegmans Food and Pharmacy (based in Rochester, New York) developed labels to indicate the percentage of leanness on its ground beef. Each meat department was equipped with leaflets to implement the program.

These are only a few of the unique nutrition information programs now available through supermarkets across the country. Many stores nationwide even offer videotapes in produce sections that show shoppers how to select, store, and prepare various produce. In Appendix B, you'll find a full directory of supermarket nutrition and health programs as of 1989 compiled by the Consumer Affairs Department of the Food Marketing Institute.

Food manufacturers have also joined the nutrition bandwagon. Along with the labeling of their food products (which will be discussed in detail in the following section), food companies have also begun to produce foods low in sugar, fat, cholesterol, and sodium. These items can be found on a shelf aisle, in the freezer section, or next to the meats in the refrigeration area of your local supermarket.

For ultimate convenience, two products—Top Shelf by Hormel and Impromptu Lite by Kraft—offer complete lines of main-course entrees that stay fresh indefinitely on your pantry shelf without the use of preservatives. Each entree is sealed in an airtight dish and then heat-sterilized to retain the taste and safety of the food.

Impromptu Lite products cook for 2 to 3 minutes in the microwave and 10 minutes in a conventional oven. Entrees are all under 300 calories and are generally low in fat (but a bit high in sodium— one entree went as high as 1,170 milligrams), and chicken selections tend to predominate. Entrees include Glazed Chicken in Sauce with Vegetable Rice, Vegetable Lasagne, Turkey Tetrazzini, Chicken à la King with Rice, Sweet and Sour Chicken with Rice, Chicken Cacciatore with Fettuccine, and Chicken Breast and Vegetables in Wine Sauce with Noodles.

Top Shelf entrees can be ready within 2 minutes in the microwave and under 10 minutes on the range top. These too are high in sodium (more than half of the selections have more than 1,000 milligrams) but low in fat; calories ranged from 210 to 360 per dinner. Top Shelf offers a greater variety of selections: Glazed Breast of Chicken with Vegetables and Skin-on Potatoes in Wine Sauce, Cheese Tortellini in Marinara Sauce, Tender Beef Roast with Potatoes and Vegetables in Burgundy Wine Sauce, Spaghettini with Meat Sauce, Vegetable Lasagna with Zucchini, Salisbury Steak with Potatoes in Gravy, and Italian-style Lasagna with Spicy Italian Sausage and Five Cheeses (this dinner was highest in calories, fat, and sodium).

In the freezer section, there are more product lines to choose among. Shoppers who watch their calories have several products available, the most popular being Weight Watchers (now offered in microwavable dishes) and Stouffer's Lean Cuisine (with meals under 300 calories). Alongside these products are Armour Classic Lites and the Budget Gourmet Light entrees and dinners, both providing meals under 300 calories.

More recently developed product lines are less focused on calorie counting, although they generally stay around 300 calories, and promote "healthier" eating by cutting down on fat, cholesterol, and sodium. These product lines include Stouffer's Right Course, Healthy Choice by Con Agra Frozen Foods, and Campbell's Le Menu Light Style.

Le Menu Light Style claims to be "nutritionally designed for healthy eating" with controlled calories, sodium, cholesterol, and fat. All Le Menu Light Style meals take about 10 minutes in a microwave and 40 minutes in a conventional oven. Calorie counts range from the Sliced Turkey at 210 to the 3-Cheese Stuffed Shells topped with tomato and mushroom sauce and seasoned broccoli florets and the Salisbury Steak, both at 280.

Healthy Choice provides the most extensive nutritional information on its package. It promotes its dinners as "low fat, low cholesterol, low sodium meals" that can be part of a diet that "meets the recommendations of the National Cholesterol Education Program [see our discussion in Chapter 2] for people with high blood cholesterol who must limit their intake of saturated fat and cholesterol." Each Healthy Choice dinner package lists the National Cholesterol Education Program's recommended daily percentage averages for total fat (less than 30 percent), saturated fat (less than 10 percent), polyunsaturated fat (up to 10 percent), and cholesterol (less than 300 milligrams) and shows how the meal inside compares with these guidelines.

All Healthy Choice dinners take from 6 to 8 minutes in a microwave, 30 to 35 minutes in a conventional oven. Meals are particularly appetizing and innovative, like the Mesquite Chicken Dinner, with white rice au gratin, corn with carrots, and apples in cinnamon raisin sauce (310 calories); the Shrimp Marinara Dinner, with green zucchini and red peppers in butter sauce, and apples in cinnamon raisin sauce (220 calories); or the Oriental Pepper Steak Dinner, with broccoli and water chestnut medley in butter sauce, and apples in plum sauce (290 calories).

Finally, Right Course offers "entrees to healthier living." It bases its nutrient guidelines on the American Heart Association's recommendations. Percentage of calories from fat are included; calorie counts range from 220 (home-style Pot Roast) to 320 (Chicken Tenderloins in Peanut Sauce); and sodium levels do not exceed

600 milligrams. Meals are appetizing and inventive, like the Fiesta Beef with Corn Pasta (270 calories) or the Beef Dijon with Pasta and Vegetables (290 calories).

While products in the supermarket's refrigerator section must be used fairly quickly, usually within two days of purchase, these product lines promote freshness above all. In fact, Nestlé came out with a line called FreshNes: it offers a wide variety of meals, from Chicken Salad Oriental and Cajun Seasoned Pasta and Chicken Salad to Beef Fajitas, Pork Dijon, and Rigatoni. Calorie counts vary (most are under 300 calories), and sodium content is on the high side. But FreshNes meals can be microwaved in less than 5 minutes, so they're especially attractive for picking up on your way home and heating up for that night's dinner.

Tyson offers marinated chicken breast fillets with flavors that include lemon pepper, butter garlic, barbecue, Italian style, and teriyaki. Each 3.75-ounce serving is about 130 calories, and marinades are low in sodium. You can throw them on the grill or in the oven when you get home. Again, here's a product that leaves you feeling like you're not completely sacrificing freshness.

All of these products, from Top Shelf to the frozen Healthy Choice to FreshNes in the meat section, are attempting to provide nutritionally balanced and convenient meals for shoppers.

Labeling: Your Key to Nutrition

The constant dilemma facing the food shopper is how to make the healthiest choices, particularly with the quantity of choices available in today's supermarket. As we discussed earlier, many supermarket chains have responded by expanding their activities to provide nutrition-information programs in the store, and several food manufacturers have even come up with meals low in fat, sodium, and cholesterol.

Many food manufacturers also have reacted to consumer demand by providing nutritional labeling information on their products. Food labels can sometimes be found on meats and in the produce section of your average supermarket.

How do most food shoppers react to nutrition labeling? In the 1989 and 1990 FMI "Trends" surveys, more than a third of the shoppers said they read labels for ingredients and nutrition just about every time they shop. The 1990 survey broke down this question further. Fifty-three percent said they read for ingredients the first time they shop for a product, and 49 percent read labels for nutrition information the first time only. (This question was not repeated in the 1991 survey.) Shoppers who have never read labels state most often that they don't have time. Of those who do read labels, just more than half (1989 survey) find the information adequate.

Some of the people you met earlier in the book are typical of those surveyed in the FMI report. Carole Gerber says she doesn't take time to read a label; "I just buy the brand I like," she admits. Herb Glimcher, who is on the rigorous Pritikin Program, buys specific foods. "I don't read labels because I don't buy packaged foods," he says.

On the other hand, Jane Hartley reads the labels on baby juices and baby foods to make sure they contain little or no sugar, and she checks the ingredients of packaged pasta sauces or other "fresh" packaged items. Barry Nash goes even further, checking fat and calorie content and, on occasion, sodium content. As you might expect, Burt Staniar's executive life leaves him little time for grocery shopping, let alone label reading. If he had the opportunity to do so, he says, he might be inclined to read the label, but not "fanatically."

Predictably, label reading by most people is based on personal concerns. But we all need to be more diligent, because a food product label, very simply, is the most basic tool we have to make the best nutritional decisions in the supermarket.

Unfortunately, in the fifteen years since nutrition labels began appearing on food products in the United States, many people remain confused about what's inside a box or a can. Judy Markey's response is typical. "It's too complicated," she says. "I decided not to worry about it. I know the basics." In the FMI "Trends" survey, those who felt similar to Judy Markey thought labels could be improved by making the information clearer and providing more information on calories, salt content, and saturated fats.

The Food and Drug Administration, which oversees the majority of food products sold in supermarkets (except for meat and poultry), now requires only basic information on all food labels, such as the identity of the food, the net amount, and the manufacturer's name and address. In 1990, however, Congress passed the

Nutrition Labeling and Education Act, which gives the FDA until May 1993 to standardize food labeling for more than 14,000 foods.

While almost all products require a listing of ingredients, nutrition information is only required under special circumstances today. While there may be changes in the near future, nutrition labeling is mandatory only (1) when a nutrient, such as a vitamin or mineral, is added to a food product (enrichment/fortification); (2) when the label or advertising claims some nutritional value, such as "rich in vitamin C"; or (3) when special dietary use is specified, such as for infants or for purposes of weight reduction. As a result, roughly half of the foods purchased by Americans carry nutrition labeling. On those labeled foods, you will find two types of information—nutrition information and ingredients.

Nutrition information provides the total calories, grams of protein, total carbohydrates, total fat, and the milligrams of sodium per serving. Potassium is sometimes included, as are various vitamins and minerals. The United States Recommended Daily Allowances (U.S. RDAs) of these vitamins and minerals are listed as percentages to help buyers compare the nutritional content of foods. A food must contain at least 10 percent of the recommended allowance to be considered a good source of a nutrient.

Also provided are the serving size and the number of servings per container. A word of caution—note the serving size carefully. Products often use different serving sizes, so a high-salt, high-fat, high-sugar, or high-calorie product may be masked by providing an extremely low serving size. For example, calories of a granola-type cereal may not seem too high until you realize that one serving is only ¼ cup and has more than 100 calories. Most cereal portions are 1 cup and have only 100 calories, so this granola cereal is about four times as high in calories!

Ingredients are itemized in descending order by weight, but that can be misleading if you don't know what many of the ingredients are. For example, by listing the various types of sweeteners in a breakfast cereal separately, you may not realize the fact that sugar is the main ingredient.

As you read the list of ingredients on nutrition labels, look for acceptable and unacceptable ingredients. Sometimes the amount of an unacceptable ingredient is low enough (it is listed near the end rather than the beginning) so that the product overall is acceptable.

But even while more than half of all foods currently carry nutrition information and a listing of ingredients, many consumers feel nutrition labels are inadequate. According to FMI's 1989 "Trends" survey, 42 percent of the respondents who said they read nutrition labels most of the time told the researchers that not enough information is provided. To that we would add (and most nutrition experts do concur) that the information is often misleading, inconsistent, and not up to date with current scientific data. It is time to reorganize and coordinate the entire system of food labeling so that we can make food choices based on clear and useful information. One case in point: scientists have recommended that Americans eat less saturated fat and sugar and more fiber and complex carbohydrates, but current labels list only total calories, grams of protein, carbohydrates, and fat, milligrams of sodium, and other specified minerals and vitamins. Labels in the future will include total dietary fiber, cholesterol, saturated and unsaturated fat, complex carbohydrates and simple carbohydrates (sugars).

Consumers often are confused by reading the amounts of fat per serving. Health authorities are telling people to limit the amount of fat in their diets to 30 percent or less of their total calories, but people don't know what this means. It would be more helpful to provide the number of calories coming from the fat content, since people are more aware of approximately how many calories they consume each day. If an afternoon snack has 300 calories from fat, for example, and you typically consume 1,500 calories a day, that one snack is providing 20 percent of your total calories from fat, leaving you little room for fat calories at mealtimes.

Also not helpful is the present practice of providing only the total fat content on the label. As you read in Chapter 2, saturated fats have been scientifically proven to raise the cholesterol level in the blood and thus contribute to heart disease. Under our current labeling system, you'll often see "and/or" labeling of fats and oils, like "coconut and/or soybean oil," which could be either highly saturated coconut oil or polyunsaturated soybean oil. The full disclosure of fat content and composition (total fat, saturated fat, and unsaturated fat) in the nutrition label is needed to allow consumers to make wise and informed decisions related to their fat intake. That too will be available in the future.

Be aware of the foods or ingredients that are very high in saturated fats. Some common examples are butter, cheese, chocolate, coconut, coconut oil, egg yolks, lard, whole milk, palm oil, and vegetable shortening. Poultry and beef are high in saturated fats, while fish is a source of polyunsaturated fats. Other sources of polyunsaturated fats are almonds, corn oil, canola oil, margarine, mayonnaise, pecans, safflower oil, soybean oil, and sunflower oil. Monounsaturated fats are found in avocados, cashews, olives and olive oil, peanuts and peanut oil, and peanut butter.

You can't always judge a food by its label, especially if you rely only on the bold print. Proper food choices are difficult when terms such as "high," "reduced," "low," "no," "lite," "lean," "natural," and "organic" are not based on standard definitions. "Light" or "lite" can mean lighter in color or flavor, or it can mean reduced in salt or calories. "Dietetic" means that at least one ingredient has been changed or restricted, but that may mean fewer calories, less sugar, less salt, or less fat. A food can contain any level of fiber and still call itself "high fiber."

"Natural" has no legal definition except on a meat label, where it means there are no artificial ingredients and no added coloring. Otherwise, it means that the food is found in nature and is not artificially synthesized by humans. Caffeine is a natural chemical compound, and granola is naturally high in fat, sugar, and calories. So "natural" is not synonymous with "good for you."

You need to read the label closely. While the word "fat" may not appear on the label, the following ingredients are all forms of fat: glycerides, glycerol, esters, shortening, hydrogenated oils. And as we mentioned earlier, often different sweeteners are listed separately in breakfast cereals and other food products, but they all add up to "sugar." All the following words mean sugar: glucose, fructose, sucrose, lactose, maltose, sorbitol, mannitol, dextrose, honey, syrups, molasses, sweeteners.

"Salt" is another word often in disguise. A label might say "no salt added" or "unsalted," which means only that no salt is added in processing. The food could have naturally occurring sodium, and there could be sodium present from sources other than salt, such as soy sauce or sodium compounds such as monosodium glutamate (MSG), sodium benzoate, or disodium phosphate. Brine, baking powder, and baking soda also raise the sodium content of foods. Packaged cake and flour mixtures, for example, are not thought of as salty products, yet they contain preservatives with a sodium base.

Beyond inadequate food labels, consumers can be most misled by food companies' bold health claims that appear on their food packages. Since the fall of 1987, when the FDA lifted its ban on such claims until detailed rules could be set (which are now pending), claims quickly began appearing on food packages, from assertions that high-fiber breakfast cereals and even doughnuts with oat bran could reduce cholesterol, thus helping to prevent heart attack, to the "no cholesterol" labels on products high in saturated fat, like cookies and potato chips. A "no cholesterol" claim should not be allowed unless the food is low in total fat and saturated fat. Also, if a food does not naturally contain cholesterol (for example, fruits, vegetables, peanut butter, vegetable oils), "no cholesterol" claims should not be allowed.

Misleading health claims on labels and in advertising often lead to the food myths we discussed in Chapter 2, and add to the general consumer distrust of the credible scientific research about diet and health. Inadequate and useless nutrition labeling only adds to the public's confusion.

The new FDA labeling regulations aim to clarify and standardize the labels on virtually every food product sold in the United States, including uniform definitions for controversial terms such as "low fat" and "fresh." At the same time, the U.S. Department of Agriculture announced that it will overhaul its own labeling rules for meat and poultry, products that are not governed by the FDA and not covered by the congressional Nutrition Labeling and Education Act. Ideally, the Agriculture Department will harmonize its regulations with the newly emerging rules from the FDA. Mandatory, uniform labeling is essential if consumers are to eat more healthfully.

Know Your Dietary Guidelines and Make Healthy Choices

All the labeling in the world, however, won't help you if you don't understand the key nutritional principles underlying a healthy diet. So read on!

Foods are made up of three major nutrients—carbohydrates, protein, and fat—plus small amounts of minerals and vitamins. These are the only sources of calories. Carbohydrates and protein have 4 calories per gram. Fat has 9 calories per gram—more than twice as concentrated. Most Americans consume too many fat calories, which explains why obesity is a national concern. The caloric density of fat can be simply illustrated: a cup of flour (carbohydrate) has just over 400 calories, while a cup of oil (fat) has almost 2,000 calories.

Remember, from Chapter 2, that the American Heart Association says fat should constitute 30 percent or less of your total daily calories, with under 10 percent of it coming from saturated fats. Saturated fats are found primarily in foods of animal origin and certain oils (palm, coconut, hydrogenated vegetable), and they cause cholesterol levels to climb. Ideally, protein choices should constitute 12 to 15 percent of your calories. Two 3-ounce servings of protein are all the average adult needs on a daily basis, according to the American Heart Association. The majority of daily calories (55 percent) should come from complex carbohydrates, which are low in fat and calories, cholesterol free, and rich in vitamins, minerals, and fiber.

Let's look at this a bit more closely. Say a hypothetical Jane Doe is five feet four inches tall and weighs 118 pounds. On the average, she takes in 1,500 calories daily to maintain her weight. (Caloric needs are based on your age, sex, weight, body composition, activity level, and metabolism. The more you weigh, the more calories you need; the more you exercise, the more calories you burn.) If fat should not exceed 30 percent of total calories, Ms. Doe shouldn't consume more than 450 calories from fat. Since every gram of fat has 9 calories, she should eat about 50 grams of fat each day. This leaves 225 calories (15 percent of 1,500 calories) for protein and 825 calories (55 percent of 1,500) as carbohydrates. These categories needn't be so exact but are approximate daily values.

Ideal Daily Intake of Nutrients for Jane Doe

	CALORIES	GRAMS
Fat	450	50
Protein	225	56
Carbohydrates	825	206

What happens to Ms. Doe's daily intake when she has a cheese-burger and a cup of skim milk for lunch? The cheeseburger has four ounces of ground meat and one ounce of cheese. The meat has about 310 calories, 28 grams of protein, and 22 grams of fat. The cheese has 100 calories, 7 grams of protein, and 8 grams of fat. The bun provides 136 calories, 30 grams of carbohydrates, and 4 grams of protein. One cup of skim milk has 89 calories, 12 grams of carbohydrates, 8 grams of protein, 1 gram of fat. (If you have an urge to know the nutrient value of the foods you eat, you might check *Bowes and Church's Food Values of Portions Commonly Used*, fifteenth edition, by Pennington and Church [Harper and Row, 1980]. There are also pocketbook-size books with this type of information available at most bookstores.)

Total calories from this lunch add up to about 635. Jane Doe will have consumed 31 grams of fat, 47 grams of protein, and 42 grams of carbohydrates. Let's work this into calories, remembering that fat has 9 calories per gram, and protein and carbohydrates each have 4 calories per gram. Her lunch provided 279 fat calories, 188 protein calories, and 168 carbohydrate calories.

**Cheeseburger, with 4 ounces of meat,
1 ounce cheddar cheese, and a bun, and
a cup of skim milk:**

	CALORIES	GRAMS
Fat	279	31
Protein	188	47
Carbohydrates	168	42

As you recall, to maintain her weight, Ms. Doe consumes about 1,500 calories a day. Let's look at how her lunch fits into her daily allotment of the key nutrients. First, it contributed nearly 42 percent of the daily calories. Fat calories came to 19 percent of total daily calories. Understanding that, for the total day, fat should be kept down to 30 percent of one's total calories, we see that this one meal contributed to more than half of Ms. Doe's daily allowance. Making careful selection of low fat food choices is essential for the remainder of the day. Protein calories added up to just over 12 percent of total daily calories—protein intake from this one meal approaches the 15 percent daily guidelines. Finally, carbohydrates were a mere 11 percent of the lunch.

	% DAILY CALORIES	DAILY GUIDELINES
Total lunch calories	42%	100% (= 1,500 in this example)
Fat calories	19%	30% or less
Protein calories	12%	12–15%
Carbohydrate calories	11%	55%

This lunch is not atypical—in fact, some people would have a milk shake and french fries with their cheeseburger, and probably some mayonnaise or ketchup on the burger, adding quite a bit to the fat and calories categories. Our sample lunch was a conservative one, and yet, for Jane Doe, one high in calories, high in fat, and low in carbohydrates. The changes we need to make are clearly illustrated in this example: increase your complex carbohydrates (fruits, vegetables, grains, beans) and decrease the fats and protein from your diet.

But, more important, what specifically should you eat to stay healthy? There's so much conflicting advice about what foods we should or shouldn't eat. Many prestigious organizations which support specific diseases, such as heart disease, cancer, or diabetes, suggest guidelines for Americans to follow. The 1990 Dietary Guidelines for Americans issued by the U.S. Department of Agriculture and the U.S. Department of Health and Human Services (*Nutrition and Your Health: Dietary Guidelines for Americans,* 3rd edition) are the most current, comprehensive and useful of these. Let's look at their seven recommendations for a healthier diet:

1. EAT A VARIETY OF FOODS. Dietitians have long espoused this principle as the basis of a healthy diet. This is because each of us requires forty different nutrients for good health and no one food has all the nutrients. For example, milk, Mother Nature's "almost perfect food," has plenty of calcium but little iron. Required nutrients include vitamins, minerals, amino acids (derived from protein), fatty acids (derived from fat), and calories (derived from protein, fat, and carbohydrates). Vegetables and fruits provide vitamins A and C, folic acid, minerals, and fiber. Breads and cereals supply B vitamins, iron, and protein. Whole grains give us fiber. Meat, fish, and poultry offer B vitamins, iron, and zinc.

Experts agree that most of us can get what we need from food without having to rely on supplements of any type. Exceptions may be pregnant women, breast-feeding mothers, and some women of childbearing years who may need iron supplements or other supplements to meet increased nutritional requirements. Those who eat little food for whatever reason and older people who take medications that may interact with nutrients may also be candidates for various types of supplements.

To get all the nutrients you need each day, choose different foods from each food group. Use the following as a daily guide for selecting foods (serving size for each group is detailed later in this chapter):

FOOD GROUP	SUGGESTED SERVINGS
Vegetables	3–5 servings
Fruits	2–4 servings
Breads, cereals, rice, and pasta	6–11 servings
Milk, yogurt, and cheese	2–3 servings
Meats, poultry, fish, dry beans and peas, eggs, and nuts	2–3 servings

2. MAINTAIN A HEALTHY WEIGHT. Americans are becoming more aware of the importance of this guideline, since people who are too fat or too thin have a greater risk of developing health problems. Because of the importance of desirable weight, we have devoted Chapter 10 to this topic.

Determine whether you are at the appropriate weight for your build by using the weight chart provided in Chapter 10. If your weight is not appropriate, reasonable goals should be set. A gradual loss (or gain) of one or two pounds per week until you've reached your goal is realistic. Your goal should be long-term success, which includes balancing food intake and physical activity.

Maintaining your weight is indeed a balancing act. Healthy people should maintain their physical activity at a moderately active level, improve their overall physical fitness, and moderate their food intake to maintain an appropriate body weight. Overweight people should increase their physical activity and reduce their caloric intake. Use the chart in Chapter 11 to estimate how many calories you burn in various activities. To decrease your calorie intake, select foods low in fat and sugar and eat more fruits, vegetables, and breads and cereals.

3. CHOOSE A DIET LOW IN FAT, SATURATED FAT, AND CHOLESTEROL. There is much scientific evidence concerning the detrimental effects of dietary fat, saturated fat, and cholesterol on your health. (Chapter 2 discusses this in detail.) While authorities may disagree with the validity of some of these studies, few dietitians or other health care professionals would disagree with this guideline. Choosing a diet low in fat and cholesterol helps you maintain a desirable weight and level of blood cholesterol (below 200 milligrams).

The first step to help you comply with this guideline is to have your blood cholesterol measured. Next, limit total fat intake to 30 percent or less of your total calories; limit saturated fatty acid intake to under 10 percent of total calories and the intake of cholesterol to less than 300 milligrams daily. The intake of fat and cholesterol can be reduced by substituting fish, poultry without skin, lean meats, and low- or nonfat dairy products for fatty meats and whole-milk dairy products; by choosing more vegetables, fruits, cereals, and legumes; and by limiting oils, fats, egg yolks, and fried and other fatty foods.

Here are more specific suggestions for a diet low in fat, saturated fat, and cholesterol:

Fats and Oils:
- Use fats and oils sparingly in cooking.
- Use small amounts of salad dressings and spreads, such as butter, margarine, and mayonnaise. One tablespoon of most of these spreads provides 10 to 11 grams of fat.
- Choose liquid vegetable oils most often, because they are lower in saturated fat.
- Check labels on foods to see how much fat and saturated fat are in a serving.

Meat, Poultry, Fish, Dry Beans, and Eggs:
- Have two or three servings, with a daily total of about 6 ounces. Three ounces of cooked lean beef or chicken without skin—the size of a deck of cards—provides about 6 grams of fat.
- Trim the fat from meat; take the skin off poultry.
- Have cooked dry beans and peas instead of meat occasionally.
- Moderate the use of egg yolks and organ meats.

Milk and Milk Products:
- Have two or three servings daily. (Count as a serving 1 cup of milk or yogurt or about 1½ ounces of cheese.)
- Choose skim or low-fat milk and fat-free or low-fat yogurt and cheese most of the time. One cup of skim milk has only a trace of fat; one cup of 2-percent-fat milk has 5 grams of fat, and one cup of whole milk has 8 grams of fat.

4. CHOOSE A DIET WITH PLENTY OF VEGETABLES, FRUITS, AND GRAIN PRODUCTS. Eating fruits, vegetables, and grains and cereals is the way to help you achieve a varied low-fat diet. This guideline recommends that each day we eat three servings of vegetables, two servings of fruits, and six servings of grain products (breads, cereals, pasta, and rice). Along with reducing fat and adding variety to your diet, these foods also help you increase your fiber intake. Dietary fiber is part of plant foods and is abundant in whole grain breads and cereals. Once again, it is important to emphasize variety, since these foods contain different types of essential fibers.

For a diet with plenty of vegetables, fruits, and grain products, have daily:

Three or more servings of various vegetables. (Count as a serving 1 cup of raw leafy greens, ½ cup of other kinds of vegetables.)

- Have dark-green leafy and deep-yellow vegetables often.
- Eat dry beans and peas often. (Count ½ cup of cooked dry beans or peas as a serving of vegetables or as 1 ounce of the meat group.)
- Also eat starchy vegetables, such as potatoes and corn.

Two or more servings of various fruits. (Count as a serving 1 medium apple, orange, or banana; ½ cup of small or diced fruit; ¾ cup of juice.)

• Have citrus fruits or juices, melons, or berries regularly.
• Choose fruits as desserts and fruit juices as beverages.

Six or more servings of grain products—breads, cereals, pasta, and rice. (Count as a serving 1 slice of bread; ½ bun, bagel, or English muffin; 1 ounce of dry ready-to-eat cereal; ½ cup of cooked cereal, rice, or pasta.)

• Eat products from a variety of grains, such as wheat, rice, oats, and corn.
• Have several servings of whole-grain breads and cereals daily.

Vegetables, fruits, and grain products are generally low in calories if fats and sugars are used sparingly in their preparation and at the table.

5. USE SUGARS ONLY IN MODERATION. Sugars, such as table sugar, honey, and syrup, as well as foods containing large amounts of sugar, should be used sparingly. This is especially true if you have low caloric requirements. Sugar has the most negative effect on the teeth, contributing to tooth decay. Even starchy foods (carbohydrates), when ingested, are broken down to simple sugar. Watch your between-meal snacking, and be certain to brush and floss your teeth regularly.

6. USE SALT AND SODIUM ONLY IN MODERATION. High blood pressure is common in the United States. It is estimated that one out of every three adults has high blood pressure. While most people are aware of the relationship between high blood pressure and salt intake, many automatically reach for the salt shaker even before tasting their food. Factors such as obesity and excessive drinking of alcoholic beverages also contribute to this health risk; but too much table salt and high-sodium foods are the major culprits.

Table salt contains sodium and chloride, both essential in the diet. But most of us consume too much, especially since sodium is also found in most foods (as a preservative) and beverages. Sodium is found in everything from pickled foods to packaged mixes to salad dressings and sauces, and in many other convenience items.

To comply with this guideline, have your blood pressure checked. Normal blood pressure for adults is less than 140 millimeters Hg systolic and less than 85 millimeters Hg diastolic. If you find that you need to lower your blood pressure, here are some tips for reducing your salt and sodium intake:

- Use salt sparingly, if at all, in cooking and at the table.
- When planning meals, consider that:
  - fresh and plain frozen vegetables prepared without salt are lower in sodium than canned ones.
  - cereals, pasta, and rice cooked without salt are lower in sodium than ready-to-eat cereals.
  - milk and yogurt are lower in sodium than most cheeses.
  - fresh meat, poultry, and fish are lower in sodium than most canned and processed kinds.
  - most frozen dinners and combination dishes, packaged mixes, canned soups, and salad dressings contain a considerable amount of sodium. So do condiments such as soy and other sauces, pickles, olives, ketchup, and mustard.
- Use salted snacks, such as chips, crackers, pretzels, and nuts, sparingly.
- Check labels for the amount of sodium in foods. Choose those lower in sodium most of the time.

7. IF YOU DRINK ALCOHOLIC BEVERAGES, DO SO IN MODERATION. Alcoholic beverages contain calories but very little of anything else. If you choose to drink, moderation is the watchword. This means that women should have no more than one drink a day, and men no more than two. While some studies have suggested that moderate drinking may be linked to lower risk for heart attacks and strokes, the consequences of too much alcohol are life threatening. Pregnant women, children and adolescents, alcoholics and those predisposed to alcoholism, individuals who plan to drive (or engage in other activities requiring skill or attention), and those taking medication should be particularly careful of their intake of alcholic beverages.

Many factors contribute to good health. Food alone cannot make you healthy. Factors such as heredity, environment, health care, exercise, and smoking all play important roles. But a diet based on the above guidelines can keep you healthy, and may improve the quality of your life.

Today's supermarket offers you an abundance of choices, along with information, through in-store brochures, shelf tags, food product labels, and more, to help you make the right selection. Now you should be ready to make practical use of this information as we visit a typical supermarket, aisle by aisle, in the next chapter.

5

Touring the Supermarket,
Aisle by Aisle

The first essential step to understanding the fundamentals of good nutrition is translating your nutrition knowledge into food choices in the supermarket, aisle by aisle. Here are some suggestions that will help you before you go shopping.

First, make a list. Determine in advance what items (or at least, what categories of food) you need—and then stick to your list. Avoid impulse buying; it leads to mistakes that are costly in both nutrition and money.

Second, begin your shopping in the produce section. Stock up on fresh fruits and vegetables, and you'll be less likely to fill your basket with prepared foods that are sources of saturated fats, sodium, and other unhealthy ingredients.

Finally, try not to shop for food when you're hungry. That's when your willpower is lowest.

So pick up your shopping cart and we'll go along with you, aisle by aisle, to give you suggestions for food choices that will lead to longer, healthier lives for you and your family.

Aisle 1: Produce

You literally can't go wrong in this aisle. The displays of fresh, colorful fruits and vegetables which are such a treat to the eye are also gold mines of nutritional values. Fruits and vegetables are low in calories (usually no more than 50 calories per serving), contain negligible fat and sodium, are excellent sources of vitamins (particularly A, C, and B-complex), minerals (such as potassium, magnesium, and iron), and fiber. Many supermarkets give nutritional information on fresh fruits and vegetables, either on the packaged items themselves or on the bins. So go for variety in this aisle. It's easy to do: the average produce section may have 250 or more different items—a significant increase over the past twenty years.

Here are some things to keep in mind:

- Many fruits and vegetables contain substances that may help the body protect itself against certain forms of cancer. These include deep-colored fruits and vegetables (deep green, orange, red, or yellow), which are high in beta carotene and vitamin A, and cruciferous vegetables (the cabbage family), including brussels sprouts, broccoli, cauliflower, kohlrabi, radishes, mustard greens, and collard greens. As this book goes to press, the National Cancer Institute is researching these and other foods to the tune of $20 million.
- Be adventurous! Notice fruits and vegetables that are new to you and give them a try. Many produce departments provide recipes and preparation tips to help.
- Select a variety of crisp greens and other items for salads. The old standby iceberg lettuce is always a good choice for salads. Spinach leaves, butter lettuce, leaf lettuce, romaine, endive, alfalfa sprouts, watercress, and cabbage also add interesting flavor and nutrients to your salad base. Broccoli and cauliflower florets, fresh pea pods, green onions, and cherry tomatoes make convenient additions. If you're cooking for one and you don't need salad ingredients in quantity, you might want to prepare a salad at the store's salad bar. It can save you time and money.
- Citrus fruits, as well as red peppers, spinach, and collard greens, contain lots of vitamin C, an essential nutrient.
- Carrots, in addition to being high in beta carotene, are also a

good source of fiber. Dip them in a low-calorie dressing or balsamic vinegar for a delicious and healthy snack.

- Potatoes are surprisingly low in calories—about 100 in a medium-sized potato. It's the butter and sauces you use on them that add fat and calories. Add some mustard to a baked potato instead of butter and sour cream. Or grill the potatoes and vegetables in a little olive oil and sprinkle on some dill.

- Ginger root gives zest to a dish and helps replace the need for salt. Try adding a small amount to your stews and soups instead of salt.

- Dried fruits are also located in the produce section, and they are generally a good source of potassium. In addition to the usual selections of raisins, prunes, dates, dried apples, and peaches, you may find dried papaya, pineapple, and bananas. Again, read the labels. Some of these have added sulfites to prevent browning, and added sugar, which makes the food almost a candy. And some even have coconut and/or palm oil added. Avoid these.

POSSIBLE CULPRITS

- Though avocados are rich in vitamin A, they are also high in calories and fat (30 grams), while the fat is primarily the more beneficial monounsaturated. If you can afford the calories—about 306 in the average-size avocado—use them in moderation.

- Avoid coconut, or use it sparingly. It has no cholesterol, but it's high in saturated fat.

- Fresh nuts and seeds are often found in the produce section. But as you guessed, be careful here. While they are a good source of protein, vitamins, minerals, and fiber, they're also loaded with fat and calories (130–200 calories per ounce). You'll be less likely to eat too many if you buy them in the shell. And when you select nuts, choose those which are lowest in saturated fats, like walnuts, pecans, almonds, pistachios, peanuts, and hickory nuts.

Aisle 2: Meat, Poultry, Fish

Your selections in this aisle are good sources of vitamins, minerals, and protein. Red meat is a good source of iron; fish is high in omega-3 fatty acids, substances shown to reduce serum cholesterol and decrease the risk of developing blood clots.

While variety is still important here, the balance should weigh more on the fish and poultry side. The American Heart Association tells us to eat no more than 6 ounces of animal protein per day, and to have at least two fish meals per week. Ideally, it's best to have no more than two 3-ounce servings of animal protein per day.

You may say that 3 ounces sounds like a child's portion, particularly in light of the 8- to 16-ounce portions of steak that are offered by most restaurants; but 2 to 3 (cooked) ounces is a healthy and moderate serving when it comes to red meat. Try to fill up on salads, vegetables, and potatoes (prepared without heavy sauces and dressings, of course).

A common misconception is that people need large amounts of meat to get enough protein. Not so. You get protein from dairy and vegetable products as well, and most Americans consume at least twice as much protein as their bodies really need.

In the meat section of this aisle, choose lean cuts of beef (select is the grade with the lowest fat content), lamb, veal, and pork, with the least amount of visible fat. The meat industry has responded to nutritional concerns by making animals leaner through new breeding and feeding techniques and also by closer trimming of fat (down to ¼ inch and closer). Among the leanest cuts of beef are eye of round, round tip, and top round; also top loin, tenderloin, and sirloin (all of which contain less than 8 grams of fat, 76 milligrams of cholesterol, and 180 calories per 3-ounce serving).

You are likely to find a small new section of the meat case devoted to beef with brand names like Coleman, Golden Trim, Larsen, and Maverick. This beef, which the industry refers to as "branded" or "designer" beef, usually costs more than supermarket cuts, sometimes contains less fat, and often comes from cattle raised without hormones or antibiotics. But despite the brand names and the special packaging—and the higher prices—this new niche in the beef market is not significantly different in terms of fat content or cholesterol from well-trimmed supermarket beef of the same grade.

Veal and lamb are also lean; lean cuts include well-trimmed loin and leg. You might consider pork a poor choice when you're trying to cut down on fat and cholesterol. Not so. In addition to being a good source of thiamine (vitamin B1), 3 ounces of cooked pork tenderloin has only 4 grams of fat, 79 milligrams of cholesterol, and 141 calories. Look for nutritional information on packages or bins.

Canadian bacon and lean ham are also low-fat meats, but they contain lots of added salt. Some companies offer reduced-salt cured products with one-third less salt than the regular product. That's an improvement, but it still may be too much salt for you. If salt is a concern, use high-salt meats sparingly, if at all.

What about the popular ground meats? Of the usual variety in the meat section, ground round is the best choice. The label states it's 85 percent lean. That's 15 percent fat (by weight). A 3-ounce cooked portion provides 225 calories, 24 grams of protein, 13.5 grams of fat, and 84 milligrams of cholesterol. That's not bad at all. So for those of you who are trying to cut down on fat, you can have your ground round and eat it too!

Proceeding down the aisle, we come to the processed meats. New reduced-fat versions of familiar products like turkey or chicken appear almost weekly. Read carefully! Look at the serving size listed on the label, the grams of fat, the calories, the milligrams of sodium. In many regular deli-type meats and hot dogs, it's common for 80 percent of the calories to come from fat. And they're high in salt.

See the "Lunch Meat" chart at the end of this chapter (page 118) for selected processed-meat comparisons. If the label claims "reduced fat," it is—but is it low enough? Some do have less than 30 percent fat calories. Others use a smaller serving size to make the product appear lower in fat than it really is, so be sure you're comparing the same portion sizes. An easy way to determine if you're in the 30-percent-or-less fat range is: for every 30 calories, the fat content should be 1 gram or less.

As an alternative to the processed luncheon meat, try preparing your own. Marinate lean cuts of fresh meat and poultry with a variety of herbs, spices, and marinades. Roast or bake, let cool, then slice thinly. You'll love the results!

In the poultry section, choose freely. Skinless and boneless chicken breast is a tasty choice that is low in fat and quick to prepare. White meat has less fat than dark meat. Try substituting ground chicken or turkey for ground beef, lamb, or veal.

In the fish section, you can more or less let your taste be your guide. Fresh fish is an excellent lean, protein-rich food. The fish that are highest in the beneficial omega-3 fatty acids mentioned above are salmon, bonito, mackerel, pompano, shad, whitefish, albacore, and bluefin tuna.

Shellfish are extremely low in fat. They have a reputation for being high in cholesterol, but faulty laboratory analysis techniques for cholesterol previously elevated their true cholesterol content. In general, shrimp, crayfish, and squid are the highest in cholesterol, but there's no need to avoid them entirely. Clams, lobster, scallops, mussels, and oysters are extremely low in fat and fairly low in cholesterol.

Surimi is a fish product made from pollack, flavored and shaped to resemble either crabmeat, shrimp, lobster, or scallops. It's very low in fat, calories, and cholesterol—and inexpensive too. The only drawback is that it's loaded with sodium—715 milligrams in 3 ounces. See the "Fish and Shellfish" chart (page 121) for details on calories, fat, and cholesterol content of selected fish and shellfish.

Also in the meat department, probably next to the fresh products, you will find many ready-cooked meats, chicken and turkey parts, and prepared fish dishes, some vacuum packed, some ready for the microwave. Just check the labels for the presence of unwanted ingredients and the amount of added salt.

POSSIBLE CULPRITS
- Most lunch meats are high in fat and sodium, so stick with turkey and chicken.
- Remember that both regular hot dogs (all beef as well as beef-and-pork) and chicken franks are very high in fat.
- Red meat, including pork, can be a high source of fat. Select lean cuts, trim visible fat, and cook simply (roast or broil), then drain fats. All ground beef items are high-fat products—even the extra-lean ground beef gets more than 53 percent of its calories from fat! Rinse and drain—or try ground turkey.
- The skin of fresh poultry is the culprit with regard to fat. Remove the skin before cooking and you cut the fat by more than half.
- Organ meats—liver, heart, sweetbreads, kidney, and brains—are low in fat but high in cholesterol and are to be avoided if you are watching your cholesterol.
- Duck and goose are both high in fat.
- Many processed or prepared meats, poultry, and fish are very high in salt, including: corned beef, dried beef, and chipped beef; chicken and turkey rolls; canned, dried, or smoked ancho-

vies, clams, crab, herring, kippers, oysters, salmon, sardines, shrimp, and tuna. You can rinse to reduce sodium.
• Ready-to-cook products such as breaded fish sticks and stuffed chicken breasts may have hidden fat. Beware of the high fat content in meat loaf with gravy, barbecued ribs, or fried chicken.

Aisle 3: Dairy Products

Here's an aisle filled with calcium! In fact, it would be difficult to meet your body's calcium needs without consuming ample amounts of dairy products. It is also an aisle in which fat lies in ambush, cunningly disguised, pervasive, insidious. Your skill in making the proper selections is especially important.

In the milk section, low-fat milk or nonfat milk are the best choices. Nonfat milk has virtually zero fat; 1 percent milk has 3 grams of fat per serving; 2 percent, 5 grams; and whole milk has 8 grams. Buttermilk is low in fat but high in salt. (See the "Milk" chart, page 123.) Nearby, the cottage cheese is also offered in four alternatives, from the traditional 4 percent fat to a low of less than one-half of 1 percent fat.

Likewise, plain yogurt is offered in three alternatives: whole milk, low fat, and nonfat, ranging from a high of 11 grams fat and 190 calories per cup to a low of zero fat and 110 calories. Weight Watchers and Yoplait are delicious nonfat brands. Your best choice is a nonfat, nonflavored yogurt; then add your own fruit, flavoring, and sweetener to suit your taste.

Here's a tip. Use plain nonfat yogurt in place of sour cream. In cooked recipes, simply add 1 to 3 teaspoons of cornstarch for every cup of nonfat yogurt to help thicken the sauce. Lactaid brand milk (generally 1 percent fat by weight) is available if you cannot digest lactose (milk sugar). You may find low-lactose cheeses and frozen desserts as well.

Butter is high in saturated fat and cholesterol. New buttery spreads are made with dairy products and vegetable oils. They have less saturated fat and cholesterol but are still loaded with lots of calories.

In the spice section of the store you will find some exceptional butter substitutes without fat or cholesterol. They can either be sprinkled onto moist foods or be made into a liquid butter sauce.

Brand names include Butter Buds, Butter Bud Sprinkles, Molly McButter, Molly McButter with Sour Cream, Molly McButter with Cheese, and McCormick's Best O'Butter.

Margarines vary in the amounts of unsaturated and saturated fat they contain. It's best to choose a margarine that has at least twice as much polyunsaturated fat as it has saturated fat. The label usually does not list the monounsaturated fat, which is assumed to be the remainder.

Liquid vegetable oil (safflower, sunflower, soybean, or corn) should be listed as the first ingredient on margarine labels. But all margarines contain some hydrogenated vegetable oil; that's what makes them solid at room temperature, and so it's an acceptable second or third ingredient. When hydrogen is added to a liquid oil, the oil becomes more saturated and more solid. Liquid margarines contain less saturated fat than tub margarines, and tub margarines contain less than stick.

Follow the same rules to select a "diet," "light," or "reduced fat" margarine, but note that the first ingredient in diet margarine is water, so the calorie content will not be as high as in regular margarines. And remember, the source of fat does not affect its calorie count. In fact, whether it's margarine or butter, 1 tablespoon equals 100 calories. So if the extra calories don't bother you and you don't have a cholesterol problem, an occasional pat of butter is an option. Just remember, you're always better off staying away from saturated fats.

Let's move to the egg section. If cholesterol is a problem for you, limit your intake of eggs—egg yolks, that is. Since all of the cholesterol is in the yolk, the easiest and most economical way to do this is to use just the egg whites in place of all or part of the whole eggs. However, an occasional egg yolk is okay for most people.

Other choices include prepared egg substitutes, which are basically egg whites with added ingredients such as skim milk powder, oil, coloring, seasonings, and agents to control product consistency. There are a variety of low-sodium egg substitutes, including Dried Egg Whites by Ballas, Chono Imitation Whole Egg Powder by General Mills, and Second Nature by Avoset. Medium-sodium egg substitutes are Egg Beaters by Fleischmann and Morningstar Farms Scramblers.

You need to be most cautious in the cheese section. It takes 9 to 10 pounds of whole milk to make 1 pound of most cheeses, so they are very high in saturated fats, which raise blood cholesterol. (Usually 70 percent of their calories come from fat!) Recently, however, lower-butterfat cheeses became available. Read the labels, keeping in mind that a "nonfat" label means the product is under 1 percent fat by weight and a "low fat" label means 2 percent fat by weight. (See the "Cheese" chart beginning on page 124 for comparisons.)

Processed cheeses like Borden's Lite-Line, Kraft Light n' Lively, and Weight Watchers have less that 2 grams of fat and 50 calories in an ounce (1⅓ slices). The bad news is that like other processed cheese, they are also high in sodium.

Kraft, Weight Watchers, and several other companies make "light" naturally aged cheeses with two-thirds the fat and calories of the regular products. Labels generally show the nutrient comparison of the light and the regular products, including the percentage of fat calories.

Mozzarella cheese made with part skim milk is a good choice. Farmer cheese is another.

Parmesan cheese is a case where a little goes a long way. Although as much as 59 percent of its calories come from fat, 1 tablespoon has only 1.5 grams of fat and 23 calories. Use a little of the stronger-flavored cheese as seasoning, or to add flavor when milder low-fat cheeses are used.

So know your cheese, make the right selection based on your total diet, and use it moderately.

POSSIBLE CULPRITS
- Whole milk. Remember: 1 cup of whole milk has as much fat as 2 pats of butter!
- Most natural and aged cheeses, including American, havarti, blue, Brie, Swiss, cheddar, and provolone. These contain 8 to 9 grams of fat per ounce and get 65 to 80 percent of their calories from fat. (See the "Cheese" chart for some healthy alternatives.)
- Parmesan cheese. It's a little lower in fat than the above, but very high in sodium, with 450 to 500 milligrams per ounce (two tablespoons). It's hard to avoid Parmesan cheese when you're sitting down to pasta; just be aware of its sodium content and use it sparingly.
- Pasteurized process cheeses such as Velveeta are high in both fat and sodium.
- Don't be fooled by labels on cheeses which say "lite," "low choles-

terol," or "low fat"; most of these still get half their calories from fat and are high in sodium. Pay special attention to cheese products labeled "light." These products may be light in sodium only and still contain regular amounts of fat and cholesterol.

- In eggs, the yolks are the culprits. Egg whites have no cholesterol and only 16 calories per egg, while the yolks have 213 milligrams cholesterol and 60 calories. Try using egg substitutes in a frittata and you won't be able to taste the difference. Substitute two egg whites for one egg when cooking.

- Margarines may have a high percentage of saturated fat. Tub margarines in general contain less than stick margarines. Read the labels and pick those that list a liquid oil first among the ingredients.

- Cream cheese is high in fat—90 percent of its calories come from fat! Even the new "light" cream cheeses, such as Neufchâtel, still derive 75 to 78 percent of their calories from fat. Here's a tip— try pureeing cottage or farmer cheese and add some chives as an alternative.

- Most imitation coffee creamers are generally high in saturated fat; imitation creamers typically are made with coconut or palm oil and should be avoided. For powdered creamer, use powdered skim milk, Weight Watchers Dairy Creamer, or regular evaporated skim milk.

- Fruit-flavored yogurts are high in sugar. Try plain or vanilla yogurt and add your own fruits.

- Chocolate milks have a lot of sugar, too. Use a small teaspoon of Hershey chocolate syrup or other flavoring extracts instead.

- Sour cream has about one-fifth the calories of butter or margarine. But even the so-called "imitation" kind still contains fat—so use it sparingly.

Aisle 4: Breads, Cereals, Pasta, Rice, and Other Grains

For today's fast-track people, dietitians and nutritionists emphasize carbohydrates, and, of course, we are bombarded with exhortations to consume enough fiber. So linger in this aisle!

According to the National Cancer Institute, the average American takes in only 11 to 12 grams of fiber daily. Yet we need 20 to 30 grams of fiber per day, from a wide variety of sources. (See the chart "Dietary Fiber per Serving of Commonly Eaten Foods," page 130.) If you are on a diet of 1,200 to 1,500 calories per day, 20 grams of fiber is sufficient. If you eat more than that, then you should increase the amount of fiber proportionately.

Just to give you an idea of what foods you could eat to reach your fiber quota, we'll give you a sample game plan. Start off your morning with a serving of raisin bran topped with a banana for 8 grams of fiber. If you have an apple and an orange during the day for snacks, you're adding 5½ more grams. For dinner, along with whatever meat dish you choose, eat one potato with the skin, ½ cup of corn, and another vegetable. You've met your requirement.

Here are some more tips: Eat the skins of fruits and vegetables. A potato with the skin has almost twice as much fiber as one without. Eat plenty of fruits with edible seeds, like kiwis, figs, blueberries, and raspberries. Include more of the stems when preparing vegetables like broccoli and asparagus. Peel grapefruits and eat sections with their membranes.

Although you are unlikely to consume too much fiber—especially if you obtain it from a variety of sources—be cautious in beginning a high-fiber diet too quickly. There can be too much of a good thing for those who take things to extremes—50 to 75 grams a day of fiber can cause intestinal problems and can cause loss of minerals and vitamins because of poor absorption. Fiber intake should be increased gradually over four to six weeks to lessen the possibility of cramping and bloating.

On the bread shelves, the most encouraging product developments to meet consumer concerns are whole wheat breads and breads featuring stone-ground whole wheat flour, cracked wheat, wheat berries, sprouted wheat, and oatmeal. Again, check the label and buy breads that list whole grain flour as the first ingredient. The ideal bread for nutrition and flavor is one that is made with whole grain flour, has less than two grams of fat per 1-ounce serving, and uses added ingredients that are low in saturated fat. It provides the carbohydrates and fiber we seek and also is a good source of some of the B vitamins and iron.

Let's look at label terms. "Enriched flour" means that the thiamine, riboflavin, and niacin that are removed during the refining process are selectively added back. It helps, but it's not the best deal around, because fiber and some nutrients still are lost. Enriched wheat flour, unbleached flour, and unbleached wheat flour are all products that have been refined.

The words we want to see on our loaf of bread are: "100 percent whole wheat flour," "stone-ground whole wheat flour," "whole wheat flour," "wheat berries," "sprouted wheat," "oatmeal," "rye," "millet," or any other whole grains.

Variety is still desirable. If you really like white bread, have it occasionally—especially if it contains no fat. Zero-fat breads include French bread, Italian bread, Vienna bread, kaiser rolls, pita bread, water bagels, and corn tortillas (not fried).

Many loaves are sliced thinner to attain fewer calories "per serving." Others have used various fibers to add bulk without adding calories.

Breads that are made with a combination of white-enriched flour and whole grains with appropriate amounts and types of added fat are acceptable. They also provide a nice compromise or transition for the person who really doesn't enjoy the texture and flavor of 100 percent whole grain breads. No one says you must change your preferences today. Just keep moving in a positive direction!

Frozen whole grain breads are a pleasant surprise you'll find in the frozen-food aisles. Pritikin ready-to-eat whole grain breads are kept frozen to preserve freshness. There are several brands of frozen bread dough that contain at least part whole wheat flour and only partially hydrogenated soybean oil.

Among cereals, the biggest product development is bran-type breakfast foods. Cereal manufacturers have gone to great lengths to highlight nutritional information on their boxes. In general, choose whole grain cereals. But read more than the promotional banners on the front! (For example, the Post Grape-nuts box proclaims on a banner, "Natural Wheat Cereal." Sounds healthy? As it turns out, the cereal is made from toasted white flour.)

In general, choose whole grain cereals without added fat. Most cereals, except the granola variety, are low in fat, but they may contain salt or sugar in varying amounts. Try the new müesli-type cereals which combine several grains, fruit, and nuts; unlike granolas, they have no added fats. But always check the labels to determine if these are the ingredients you want.

Many new cereals cater to the nutrition-conscious consumer as evidenced by such terms as "fiber-rich," "100 percent RDA," and "no sugar added." Puffed Rice, Puffed Wheat, and Shredded Wheat are low in salt.

Wheat germ, while containing more salt, is an excellent source of fiber, vitamins, and minerals. Cooked cereals (now complete with microwave instructions) are low in fat and salt. Instant (add hot water) oatmeal is just as nutritious as the old-fashioned kind. Oat-bran cereal is particularly rich in water-soluble fiber, which has been shown to help lower blood cholesterol and blood sugar. Among children's cereals, Nabisco Frosted Wheat Squares (which are lightly sweetened bite-size biscuits) have about half the sugar of some other types and have no added fat.

Pasta is a favorite of the nutrition-minded consumer, and it comes in a wide variety of shapes and colors. Try the whole wheat pastas and noodles. Pastas generally do not contain eggs; noodles do, but there are "no yolks" products to choose from.

Rice, including brown rice, has regained popularity as a great source of carbohydrates. Even the long-cooking brown rice is no trouble at all to cook in the microwave. It requires little of the cook's attention, and it's perfect every time without boiling over or sticking. Brown rice and white rice are nutritionally the same. Contrary to popular belief, brown rice contains no additional nutrients.

That southern favorite corn grits (or polenta, as the Italians call it) is a tasty, nutritious starch dish with meals. And don't forget about an old-fashioned favorite, hominy.

Beans and legumes provide a nice blend of water-soluble and insoluble fibers. Different types of fibers have different health benefits. (See the "Fiber Sources and Benefits" chart, page 131.) Many of the new health-conscious cookbooks feature innovative, delicious recipes. One of our favorites is a thick chili, rich in beans, served over pasta or rice and topped with low-fat cheese, green onions, and chopped fresh tomatoes.

If you're short on time, you may prefer to use canned products instead of cooking dried beans and legumes. But you sacrifice low salt for speed. You can reduce the salt content considerably by rinsing the canned products under running water.

Some boxed entrees that meet our goal of 30 or less fat calories include cheese pizzas by Appian Way, Chef Boyardee, and Contadina. Feel free to dress them up with extra vegetables and lean meat such as turkey. You can even make a mock sausage using ground turkey or chicken breast by flavoring it with sage, pepper, or any other seasonings.

POSSIBLE CULPRITS

- Sweet rolls, Danish pastries, biscuits, crescent rolls, fruit breads, muffins, and croissants contain high amounts of saturated fats and calories.
- Granola-type cereals often contain three times as many calories as plain cereals, and some have four grams of fat per ¼ cup serving (or 16 grams per cup—about the same as four pats of butter!). Furthermore, the fat may be in the form of coconut or palm oil, or shortenings, which are high in saturated fat. General Mills makes several varieties of granolas without coconut pieces or tropical oils (coconut, palm, or palm kernel oils) in any form; corn oil is the added fat. Breadshop offers several varieties of granola sweetened with fruits and juice concentrates instead of sugar, uses canola oil for the added fats, and contains low amounts of sodium. These are better choices than other similar cereals. An option is to make your own lower-fat version of granola using the most desirable ingredients.
- Some bran cereals and some mix-and-eat cooked cereals are high in added salt.
- So are seasoned noodle or rice mixes. Toss plain pasta, noodles, or rice with low-fat margarine or olive oil and herbs, and add panache with some mushrooms, zucchini, and/or carrots.
- Some high-fiber cereals contain more bran than is probably healthy to eat in a bowl of cereal. Don't go overboard in getting your fiber from one source or at one sitting. Remember: moderation and variety.

Aisle 5: The Freezer Section

Frozen items are ideally geared for those in a hurry or not in the mood to pick up a pot or pan. The good news is that portion control is often built-in. The bad news is that many frozen foods are laden with sodium, flavor enhancers, and sauces high in fat and calories. (See the "Healthier Choices for Shelf-Stable, Refrigerated, and Frozen Dinners/Entrees" chart, beginning on page 132.)

Manufacturers have for several years provided many dinners under 350 calories. But not all low-calorie dinners are also low in fat; many still have more than 50 percent of their calories coming from fat. We discussed the new frozen products now on the market that are low in sodium, fat, cholesterol, and calories in the last chapter. Consumer demand will continue to trigger improvement in this area.

If the frozen dinner you choose is high in salt, make your other choices of food that day low in salt to compensate—in other words, that would not be the day to have a bowl of soup, a ham sandwich, and a glass of tomato juice at lunch. For balance, try perhaps a low-salt cereal and fruit at breakfast and a fresh sliced turkey sandwich with lettuce, tomato, and onion, some fruit, and milk at lunch. The trade-offs discussed in Chapter 3 do work; it just takes a little planning—but planning allows for flexibility and good results.

A wide variety of frozen vegetables is now available. Choose the most convenient packages for your needs. They range from packs of single-serving frozen vegetables to boxes with three and four portions, and of course the loose-pack plastic bags. Some have butter and sauces; some are plain. Choose the plain and add your own seasonings.

New combinations of vegetables and vegetables with rice or pasta appear frequently. Products containing dark green and deep yellow vegetables are the best nutritional values. Again, it's best to choose those without added butter and sauces to keep your total and saturated fat low. But for variety, better choices with sauces include Budget Gourmet Side Dishes and Stokely's Singles, which have less than 5 grams of fat and less than 400 milligrams of sodium.

Most of us enjoy french fried potatoes. There are a couple of lower-fat options. One is to prepare fresh potatoes or buy plain frozen potato sticks, coat them very lightly with a little oil, then bake in the oven until crispy and lightly browned. Placing oil in a small spray bottle helps distribute a thin layer of fat on foods; some people like spraying their food with either plain or butter-flavored nonstick cooking spray. Preparing Ore-Ida Lites Crinkly Cuts in the oven is another option, since they use less fat than most and contain 80 calories and two grams of fat (23 percent fat calories) in a three-ounce portion.

You'll find frozen fruits often next to ready-to-bake pie shells;

ready-to-heat, ready-to-thaw, or ready-to-bake pies; cakes, cookies, doughnuts, waffles, pancakes; and frozen whipped toppings. The healthy choices are fresh fruits without added sugar. These include whole unsweetened strawberries, blackberries, raspberries, blueberries, peaches, and fruit mixtures including melons. Enjoy! The flavor and texture seem best when served slightly frozen. If you haven't frozen your own blueberries for year-round use, buy them frozen in handy plastic bags. Pour out just the amount you need for a delicious addition to cold or hot cereal, homemade whole grain muffins, whole grain pancakes, or mixed fruit cups.

Most prepared pies or pie shells contain lard and/or coconut, palm, or palm kernel oils. If you really want a pie, it's best to make your own crust, using oil or an acceptable margarine. Lower in fat than a regular crust is a crumb crust, using any dry cereal or graham crackers. Better yet, for a fat-free shell, make a meringue.

Frozen part-dairy and nondairy whipped toppings are high in saturated fats, so try to use them sparingly. Again, while there's no cholesterol in nondairy toppings, they contain—even worse—highly saturated coconut, palm, or palm kernel oils. If you want a whipped topping, consider a boxed whipped topping mix made with skim milk (such as Estee's sugar-free, fat-free whipped topping—usually found with other "dietetic" foods). Tip: a little vanilla extract improves the flavor of all the nonfat whipped toppings. Following the trend for reduced-fat products, there are now several "light" whipped toppings with less than 1 gram of fat per tablespoon. The fat is still saturated, but more important, the amount of it is greatly reduced.

Other fat-free toppings include whipped marshmallow creme (high in sugar), sweetened nonfat yogurt (flavored with vanilla, other extracts, spices, sugar, or sugar substitute), and low-fat vanilla pudding. So, you see, there are healthier options!

POSSIBLE CULPRITS
- Frozen dinners with cheeses and creamy sauces. Look around—there are other tasty and nutritious choices.
- Frozen meat and cheese pizzas. There are a few fairly low-fat cheese pizzas—see the "Healthier Choices for Shelf-Stable, Refrigerated, and Frozen Dinners/Entrees" chart, page 132.
- Dinners that include fried items such as deep-fried potatoes or

high-fat meats such as fried chicken, Salisbury steak, and sausages.

- Mexican dinners and entrees. Lard or shortening (high in saturated fat) is a common ingredient added to the meat or bean mixtures. With added cheese and sauces, these meals generally are high in total and saturated fat.
- Most frozen vegetables with butter, cheese, and sauces. Season your own with healthy choices such as herbs, spices, onions, garlic, a little unsaturated margarine, low-calorie butter substitutes, olive oil, or a low-fat sauce.
- Deep-fried foods such as potatoes, french fries and similar potato products, onion rings, zucchini, cheeses, okra, and mushrooms.
- Baked stuffed potatoes, fried rice, and macaroni and cheese.
- Frozen part-dairy and nondairy whipped toppings.
- Frozen pies, pie shells, cakes, cookies, doughnuts, waffles, pancakes, and even healthy-sounding muffins presently contain lots of saturated fats. Kellogg's Nutri-Grain and Roman Meal offer frozen waffles that contain whole grain flours, but both contain partially hydrogenated oils. One waffle of Kellogg's Nutri-Grain contains 130 calories and 5 grams of fat (34.6% fat), while one Roman Meal waffle has 120 calories and 6 grams of fat (45% fat). While less than perfect choices, they are better than some.

Aisle 6: Ice Cream and Other Frozen Desserts

If you can afford the extra calories and fat (after meeting your basic nutritional needs with selections from fruits and vegetables; grains and cereals; poultry, meat, and other protein foods; and dairy products), an occasional serving of ice cream is certainly acceptable. But there are a variety of tempting low-fat frozen desserts available today. Most ice creams, ice milks, and other frozen desserts are, of course, concentrated sources of sugar. (See the "Frozen Desserts" chart, beginning on page 140.)

A nice mix of dairy and nondairy products is available. Some of the low-fat, milk-based choices include Weight Watchers frozen dairy desserts, various brands of ice milks (some with as few as 100 calories and 2 grams of fat per ½ cup), sherbets, Dannon low-fat frozen yogurt and bars, regular and sugar-free Fudgsicles, and Sealtest low-fat frozen yogurt.

Ice creams made with fat substitutes (Simplesse, for example) are good possibilities if you love to eat ice cream but must watch your fat intake. Sugar content (and calories) is still high.

Low-fat nondairy choices include fruit and juice bars, gelatin pops, regular and low-calorie Popsicles, fruit ice, Rice Dream (made from brown rice), and certainly soy-based frozen desserts. Tofutti Lite is low in fat (90 calories and 0.2 gram of fat—2 percent fat calories—in ½ cup), but regular Tofutti is high in fat (220 calories and 12 grams of fat—49 percent fat calories, so it is not a healthy choice).

POSSIBLE CULPRITS
- Gourmet ice creams are highest in fat (around 55 percent fat calories).
- Regular ice creams (around 50 percent fat calories).
- Dove Bars and Häagen-Dazs Bars contain more than 500 calories per bar.
- Regular Tofutti—the label says "no cholesterol," but that certainly does not mean low fat (see above).
- Ice cream sandwiches, chocolate-coated ice milk bars, and Jell-O Brand pudding pops contain saturated palm and/or coconut oil. Pudding pops, however, have only 23 percent of calories from fat and each bar is low in calories (80).
- Ice milks with added ingredients high in saturated fat (such as chocolate pieces, coconut, and buttery sauces).
- Always check the labels of so-called diet or dietetic ice cream. The terms mean little. There may be no table sugar in the product, but it still contains calories, and it may be higher in fat and calories than the regular product. Look for low-fat products.

Aisle 7: Canned Foods

From a nutritional standpoint, fresh fruits and vegetables are best, frozen are next-best, and canned rank third in preference. Convenience, shopping frequency, and storage space may determine which works best for you. Use the following tips for making good selections.

- Regular canned vegetables are high in sodium. You can reduce the salt content dramatically by rinsing them in cold water, but you also lose other nutrients. Most stores now carry those without added salt—but they don't have much taste, either.
- Canned fruits are convenient to have on the shelf. They keep well and offer an alternative between fruit-growing seasons when the quality of fresh fruits may not be optimal. Choose canned fruits that are packed in juice (best choice), water, or extra-light syrup.
- Canned soups are now available that are low in fat when prepared with water or skim milk. This includes most broth-based soups. To reduce fat further, chill your can of soup in an upright position in the refrigerator. Open the top end and lift off any fat that you see; then prepare.
- Canned soups frequently contain 800 to 1,200 milligrams of sodium per 1-cup serving. For added flavor without added salt or calories, dilute regular soups with unsalted chicken or beef bouillon. The unsalted canned bouillons have a better flavor than salt-free bouillon cubes, which contain the bitter potassium chloride used to replace the salt. Campbell's makes a "Special Request" line of soups which have one-third less salt than its regular products. Campbell, Estee, Dia-Mel, and Pritikin all make soups that have no added salt. If an unsalted soup tastes just too flat to eat, consider adding just a few sprinkles of salt to take the edge off. After you've cut down on salt considerably, you'll be surprised how well you can taste just a trace of salt. Another way to cut down on salt is to add a small amount of sugar to unsalted foods, as long as you don't need to avoid sugar. This makes the absence of salt less noticeable.
- Choose canned fish and shellfish packed in water rather than oil. As a rule, this will save you more than one-third of the calories and preserve some of the valuable omega-3 fatty acids that might be transferred to the oil. Rinse canned fish to reduce salt. Chicken of the Sea makes water-packed tuna with 50 percent less salt. Featherweight makes water-packed salmon and tuna with no added salt.
- Canned entrees are often high in salt, but there are several choices that are low in fat. Most of the La Choy entrees are good low-fat choices. Many of the Chef Boyardee pasta with meat or cheese entrees have less than 30 percent fat calories. The pasta is

always made from refined flour, however, and the salt content is substantial. These are far from "perfect" choices, but ease of storage and preparation makes them nice additions to the "emergency" shelf in your cupboard. They can add variety with a reasonable fat content, even though we would not suggest them as regular selections.

• A new twist to the canned-food selection is the introduction of shelf-stable, single-serving, microwaveable entrees. The Dial Corporation introduced Light Balance for the nutrition-conscious brown bagger who wants a hot lunch that's quick, low in fat, and moderate in sodium. There are also Top Shelf Entrees from Hormel, with tempting selections like Chicken Cacciatore and Cheese Tortellini in Marinara Sauce. See more about them in the "Healthier Choices for Shelf-Stable, Refrigerated, and Frozen Dinners/Entrees" chart, page 135.

• Canned milks are also in this aisle. Choose skim evaporated milk. Use it anytime in place of cream or milk. It can also be whipped for toppings. You will also find evaporated "filled" milk, which has the same amount of fat as regular milk, but with soybean oil replacing the butterfat.

POSSIBLE CULPRITS
• Most canned soups and boxed soups are high in sodium.
• Canned fish or shellfish packed in oil are high in fat.
• Whole or 2 percent low-fat evaporated milk are also sources of fat calories.
• Beware: evaporated "filled" milk may contain coconut and/or palm oil even though the label proclaims "no cholesterol."

Aisle 8: Beverages

Fruit juices are your best choice in this aisle. They furnish a wealth of vitamins and minerals, and their natural sugars are far healthier than those used in carbonated beverages. (They are generally far less expensive, too.)

Look for those that contain 100 percent fruit juice and no added sugar. For variety, try unsweetened grapefruit juice, apple juice and cider, grape juice, pineapple juice, tropical fruit juices such as papaya and mango, prune juice, and any number of juice mixtures in addition to the ever popular orange juice.

Juice comes packed in a variety of containers and sizes. It comes vacuum packed in glass jars, canned, boxed, fresh refrigerated in jars or cartons in the produce and dairy departments, and in cans in the frozen-foods case. Container size ranges from 4- or 6-ounce individual servings in boxes, bottles, or cans to multiserving 1-gallon quantities.

Single-serving containers are convenient for keeping juice fresh and providing variety when quantity needs are small. With these, it's easy to take along nutritious beverages for school, meetings, or trips—no excuses for nutritionally poor choices.

Following the trend for "lighter" foods, several "lite" juices have appeared on the market. Some have added artificial sweeteners; all have added water. If this idea appeals to you, try buying 100 percent juice and make your own low-calorie drinks by adding sugar-free and low-sodium flavored seltzers.

One or two cups of regular coffee or tea is okay for most people. But decaffeinated coffees or teas are even better. Choose water-processed brands of decaf coffees such as Sanka, Taster's Choice, Nescafé, Folgers, and High Point. Decaffeinated teas processed with ethyl acetate are considered safe; herbal teas (except for Celestial Seasonings' Morning Thunder and Bigelow's Early Riser) are caffeine free.

Powdered milk is an excellent choice for drinking or cooking. A little extra skim-milk powder will make a richer-tasting product. Always mix ahead and refrigerate to allow the flavor to develop.

There are many skim-milk-based beverages that are great additions to our healthy-food-choice list. These include most of the regular and sugar-free cocoa mixes made by Alva, Carnation, Nestlé and Swiss Miss; flavored skim-milk "shakes" by Alba and Weight Watchers; and regular and sugar-free Carnation Instant Breakfast mixes.

POSSIBLE CULPRITS
- Carbonated soda drinks are not only worthless nutritionally, but a source of sugar and caffeine. Diet sodas contain practically nothing but artificial sugar substitutes, artificial colors, and artificial flavors. If you really like "fizz," consider substituting sugar-free, low-sodium sparkling waters and plain or flavored seltzers.

- "Juice drinks," "juice beverages," "juice cocktails," or powdered fruit-flavored beverages, found in the fruit juice section, are mostly colored and flavored sugar water, with a minimum of real juice (usually under 15 percent). If the label doesn't end with the word "juice," it isn't!
- Some regular teas come flavored with herbs and spices. Don't mistake these for decaffeinated herb-flavored teas or those made with only herbs and spices.
- Salted tomato or mixed vegetable juices (like V-8) contain 600 to 750 milligrams of sodium in 8 ounces (1 cup). That's too much sodium to get from your juice. Unsalted tomato or mixed-vegetable juice contains 40–50 milligrams of sodium. Cut the sodium in half by mixing equal portions of regular and unsalted juices, or use the unsalted versions plain or with only a dash of salt added.

Aisle 9: Condiments and Cooking Oils

This is a tricky aisle, so read the labels carefully. No vegetable oils contain cholesterol, which is found only in animal foods; but some vegetable oils do contain saturated fats, which can raise blood cholesterol. See what we mean by "tricky"? The product that claims "no cholesterol" is not necessarily the best choice.

Unsaturated fats include both polyunsaturated and monounsaturated fats. Some studies (see Chapter 2) have shown that polyunsaturated fats tend to lower both the undesirable (LDL) and desirable (HDL) cholesterol, while monounsaturated fats appear to lower the undesirable LDL cholesterol without lowering the beneficial HDL cholesterol. Saturated fats contribute to high blood cholesterol. It seems prudent to choose oils that are the lowest in saturated fats and highest in monounsaturated fats. Excellent choices are canola (rapeseed) oil and olive oil. Canola oil is the better choice for cooking at high temperatures (olive oil has a low smoke point and begins to smoke and break down at a lower temperature than canola oil); olive oil is the better choice when high temperatures are not necessary and the unique olive flavor is desired. Extra-virgin olive oil is made from the "first pressing" of ripe olives, without the chemical solvents used to produce lower grades.

Avocado oil is very low in saturated fats and an excellent source of monounsaturated fats and can withstand very high temperatures before reaching the smoke point. The problem is, it's not available everywhere and is expensive when you find it.

Oils low in saturated fat and high in total unsaturated fat content also are good choices. In order of preference, these include safflower, walnut, sunflower, corn, sesame, soybean, peanut, and wheat germ oils. (See the "Fats and Oils" chart, page 142.)

Use only fresh oils. Rancid oils have changed chemically; they lose their effectiveness and are potentially harmful. They also smell and taste bad. Avoid bottles that appear old. After opening, keep your oil in the refrigerator. Olive oil is semisolid at cold temperatures. For ease of use, keep a small amount of olive oil (that can be used within a week) in a small closed container at room temperature. When it's gone, thoroughly wash and dry the container before filling it with a new supply. Most other oils will stay liquid at refrigerated temperatures.

To keep the total percentage of fat calories low, use the smallest possible amount of oil, even the desirable kinds. One way to keep fats low in your foods is to coat cooking utensils with nonstick vegetable-oil sprays. Choose one made with an acceptable liquid oil. Currently, Mazola, Pam, Pam Butter-Flavored, and Weight Watchers Butter-Flavored Popcorn Spray are good choices. (Try plain popped corn sprayed lightly with a butter-flavored cooking spray and a few sprinkles of Molly McButter for a low-calorie, high-fiber treat.)

Mayonnaise is very high in fat—11 grams of fat and 100 calories per tablespoon—so use it sparingly. It nearly always contains a desirable unsaturated oil. The usual brands are made with soybean oil, but there are others (sometimes found in the special "dietetic" section) that contain safflower oil. Even with the presence of eggs, the cholesterol content is only 8 milligrams per tablespoon.

"Light" mayonnaise has about half the calories of the regular due to the presence of water. It's a good product to help you reduce your fat intake—if you don't use twice as much! It's possible to make your own "light" product by thinning regular mayonnaise with vinegar, lemon juice, water, or plain nonfat yogurt. Or come up with your own recipe, given your newfound knowledge! The recent no-fat, no-cholesterol mayonnaise offered by Kraft is another alternative.

Among salad dressings, choose those made with minimal

amounts of cream, cheese, and egg yolk. One recommendation is Old Dutch Sweet-Sour Dressing, which has no oil and no preservatives. Reduced-fat and low-calorie dressings are taking over the shelves. There are many excellent choices, ranging from almost no calories to one-third fewer than the regular product. Just read the labels so you know what you're getting. Estee makes salad dressing in single-serving packets that are quite low in calories and sodium. We like the Italian flavor best. Wishbone offers a Lite Classic Dijon Vinaigrette.

When you're making your own dressing, try reducing the amount of oil you add. Replace it with vinegar, lemon juice, tomato juice, or water. For a low-calorie alternative to commercial dressings, try lemon juice or flavored vinegars on your salads. Balsamic and tarragon vinegars are slightly sweet and flavorful, as is rice vinegar. They need little or no oil.

POSSIBLE CULPRITS

- Avoid coconut oil and palm oil, which are higher in saturated fat than lard. (See the "Fats and Oils" chart, page 142.) If you have the opportunity to smell an opened container of coconut oil, you'll probably recognize the odor, since the oil is widely used in many prepared products. It's solid at room temperature—even *looks* like it could clog arteries!
- Nonstick cooking sprays containing hydrogenated vegetable oil, palm, or coconut oil.
- Salad dressing with lots of cream, cheese, or eggs, such as blue cheese, Roquefort, and thousand island.
- Salad dressings and salad dressing mixes are often high in sodium. Read the labels. There are some low-sodium versions in the dietetic section.

Aisle 10: Sauces, Seasonings, and Spreads

Sauces, seasonings, and canned gravies are usually low in saturated fat and cholesterol, but their sodium content varies. Those low in fat and sodium include: flavorings, extracts, fruit sauces, herbs and spices, dry horseradish, lemon and lime juice, garlic and onion powder, dry mustard, liquid smoke (which can give the illusion of seasoning with cured meat but without the salt and calories),

Tabasco sauce, tomato paste, vinegar, and Mrs. Dash Steak Sauce. Try the many new salt-free herbal blends available from McCormick, Lawry, Mrs. Dash, and the American Heart Association.

Still low in fat, but with more sodium, are: prepared mustard, ketchup (there are "light" and unsalted versions), tomato sauce, and steak sauces, including Worcestershire sauce. Tomato sauces without salt added are made by Contadina, Del Monte, Hunt's, and Progresso. If you want to reduce your salt intake but don't need to go salt-free, why not mix your sauces—use one can of regular and one can of unsalted? You'll probably never miss the salt.

Spaghetti sauces vary in the amounts of salt and fat they contain. Generally, vegetable-flavored sauces are lower in fat than those containing meats. Prego makes a "Salt-to-Taste" sauce which allows you to add the amount of salt you want. It's not low in fat (6 grams, or 54 percent of the 100 calories, in ½ cup), but the type of fat is acceptable (corn or cottonseed oil—they don't tell you which). Ragú Chunky Gardenstyle or Slow-Cooked Homestyle Spaghetti Sauce is lower in fat than some of the other flavors this company makes. Enrico's No Salt Added All Natural Spaghetti Sauce contains a small amount of olive oil (1 gram of fat—15 percent of the 60 calories—in ½ cup).

Jams and jellies are available in regular or low-sugar versions, but for the difference in calories in an average serving, we're splitting hairs. If you make your own jams or jellies, we recommend the new "light" fruit pectins. The recipe uses less sugar, which produces a product with a more prominent fruit flavor. If you need a product without added sugar, try Slim Set Jelling Mix and the new all-fruit products.

In general, sugar used in moderation is preferable to sugar substitutes, unless you are a diabetic. Sugar contains only 16 calories per teaspoon. Again, think moderation! The safety of sugar substitutes is always controversial, and there have been reports that artificially sweetened products, especially those without calories and consumed without calorie-containing food, increase hunger later.

Natural peanut butters (the type where the oil separates) are a nutritious food consisting only of peanuts and a little salt. The oil in them is high in monounsaturated fats. As with all high-fat foods, use peanut butter sparingly. There are 95 calories in a level tablespoon, with 76 percent of them coming from fat.

To keep the oil mixed so the peanut butter stays soft and spreadable, it helps to turn the jar over every other day. This allows the oil to work its way back up through the peanut solids. Don't be tempted to pour off any oil that accumulates unless you want to try to spread a peanut brick on your bread or crackers.

POSSIBLE CULPRITS

- The culprits in this aisle are mainly those high in sodium. Soy sauce is highest—with 1,000 to 1,300 milligrams per tablespoon. Several companies make "lite" soy sauces—and it helps—but they generally still contain 600 milligrams of sodium per table-spoon. It's common for the label to give milligrams of sodium in a ½-teaspoon portion, which appears to be low. So pay attention!
- Other items that contain salt are barbecue sauces, bouillon, meat tenderizers, MSG (monosodium glutamate) flavor enhancer, pickles (Vlasic makes some with half the salt of its regular version), and olives. Tip: You can make your own low-salt, low-calorie pickles by marinating cucumber slices or chunks in your choice of vinegars plus garlic and dill. These make a zesty addition to salads too. Lemon peppers and some of the new regional seasoning mixtures (such as Cajun and Creole) contain salt.

Aisle 11: Snacks

The range in snacks is from healthy to nutritionally void. (See the "Snacks" chart, beginning on page 143.) Among crackers, chips, and "munchies," zero-fat choices include Finn Crisp, flatbread, matzo, rice cakes, and the Swedish crisp bread Wasa Brod. Low-fat products include Armenian cracker bread, bread sticks, melba toast and rounds, unseasoned Ry-Krisp, and Zwieback. All the above are also low or lacking in salt. Choices with moderate salt include oyster crackers, soda crackers, and saltines.

Low in fat but still higher in salt are pretzels and seasoned Ry-Krisp. Hain and Health Valley are two companies that make crackers with whole grain flours, unsaturated oils, and with or without salt. These and similar companies also make several kinds of "munchies" like potato chips, carrot chips, and corn curls that use only unsaturated oils and do not contain salt. They are not necessarily low in fat, but they have complete nutritional labels for your information. (The Lance Company removed all tropical oils from its products in 1989. Other companies are following its lead.)

Popcorn is nutritious and fat-free if air-popped—but popcorn packaged for microwaving is often made with coconut or palm oil, which by now you know are not good for you. Several kinds are now made with partially hydrogenated soybean oil, which is generally better than the tropical oils, but the labels don't tell us exactly how much unsaturated fat there is. Weight Watchers makes a microwave popcorn without added salt or fat. Now most companies offer microwave popcorn that's lower in salt and fat than their regular products. Try butter-flavored popcorn spray and Molly McButter on plain popcorn. Herbs and small amounts of Parmesan cheese also add variety.

Weight Watchers also makes several unsalted "munchie" snacks which are low in salt, fat, and calories. But check the labels.

If you go for cakes, your best choice is angel food. But, fortunately, your selection is getting broader every day. Entenmann's offers a variety of very low fat, low-cholesterol baked items. And Sara Lee's Free & Light frozen desserts includes selections like Cherry Streusel Pie (160 calories and 2 grams of fat), Apple Danish (130 calories and no fat), and fat-free muffins and cakes. One note of caution, however: nutrient data for these products are based on disappointingly small portion sizes.

If cookies are your passion, your better choices include Nabisco's Almost Home Fruit Sticks Family Style Cookies, Animal Crackers, Devil's Food Cakes (only one gram of fat in two cookies—13 percent of the 70 calories), Arrowroot biscuits, Famous Chocolate Wafers, Newtons (Apple, Blueberry, Cherry, or Fig), Nilla Wafers, Old Fashioned Ginger Snaps, and Social Tea Biscuits. All varieties of Health Valley's and Tree of Life's cookies and graham crackers are reasonable choices. Or try Sunshine Biscuit's Fig Chewies, Ginger Snaps, Golden Fruit Raisin Biscuits, Mallopuffs, Sprinkles, and Toy Cookies. Fat contributes less than 30 percent of the calories in the cookies listed above. These are not perfect choices. In some cases, very low fat cookies like animal crackers or graham crackers or Nabisco's Devil's Food Cakes contain a saturated fat, but the quantity is almost negligible. Health Valley and Tree of Life make cookies that use only highly unsaturated oils as a fat source and whole grain flours.

If you bake at home with mixes, choose those with acceptable fat ingredients. Angel food cake mixes, Betty Crocker's Sunkist Lemon Chiffon Cake, Nabisco's Dromedary Date Nut Roll and gingerbread mix, Pillsbury's gingerbread mix, all Estee mixes, and Fearn's carob and carrot cake mixes are all good choices. Look for mixes that allow you to add as many ingredients as possible, especially the fat, liquid, and eggs; then you have control over the amount and types you add. Several companies now include directions for making lower-fat, low-cholesterol variations on their products.

Here are some bread-product baking mixes that offer the goodness of whole grain flour and allow you to add the oil, eggs, and milk: Aunt Jemima Buckwheat Pancake & Waffle and Whole Wheat Pancake & Waffle mixes; Hodgson Mill's bran muffin mix, buttermilk biscuit mix, and cornbread and muffin mix; Jewel Evans's Original Recipe Pancake & Waffle mix; Jiffy's bran muffin mix with dates; Martha White's bran muffin mix. Use 1 or 2 egg whites and 1 teaspoon of oil for each whole egg; skim milk in place of whole; soft margarine for shortening—or use an unsaturated liquid oil.

Whole grain flours can form the basis of many nutritious baked products. Supermarkets seems to be carrying a larger selection now that there's more interest in nutrition. Choose from whole wheat, buckwheat, oat, rye, corn, and brown rice flours. And don't forget about barley—it makes a great addition to soups, or an interesting side dish.

Low-fat puddings and pudding mixes are healthy choices, especially when you prepare them with skim milk.

We are not recommending candies, due to their lack of nutrients. But if you must occasionally indulge, here's a list of some that do not have added fat: candy corn, divinity, fruit rolls, fruit jerky, hard candies, gummy candy shapes, gum drops, jelly beans, licorice, lollipops, marshmallows, hard mints (not creme), peppermint, and old-fashioned candy sticks.

POSSIBLE CULPRITS

- Many commercial crackers and the majority of cake mixes and cookies are made with animal-fat shortening or vegetable fat. Ask the store bake shop to make some baked products using oil or highly unsaturated margarine, egg whites, and skim milk.
- Dietetic cookies may be low in sugar and salt but high in saturated fat. Read the label.

• Chocolate-coated and chocolate candies, chocolate chips or tidbits, carob coatings or bits, and yogurt-coated fruits or candies are high in saturated fats, so look for better choices. As for the yogurt-covered fruit snacks, read labels carefully.

Now that we have toured the aisles together, we hope you feel more confident to make the right food choices for yourself and your family. The principle of substitution can work with food choices at the store as well as with ingredients that you cook with. So substitute pretzels (less fat and fewer calories) for potato chips, and exchange bagels (nearly no fat or sugar) for doughnuts. Use tub margarine, with less saturated fat, rather than stick margarine, and try nonfat dried milk (half the calories and no fat) instead of a nondairy creamer. Save 182 calories for each 6½-ounce can of tuna if you choose the water-packed versus the oil-packed variety. Have a tenfold calorie savings by choosing plain popcorn instead of a bag of peanuts.

The fundamentals of good nutrition can be translated into your food choices when dining out as well as in grocery shopping. We'll look at fast-food establishments and other restaurant dining experiences in the next two chapters.

Food Charts with Nutrient Listings

Lunch Meat

Product	Amount	Calories	Fat (gms)	% Fat Calories	Chol (mg)	Sodium (mg)
SLICED MEATS						
Butterball Fresh Deli Smoked Turkey Breast	⅓ oz	10	<1	—	—	70
Butterball Turkey Ham	1 oz	35	1	26	—	390
Eckrich Light Bologna	1 oz	70	6	77	15	250
Eckrich Light Cooked Ham	1 oz	25	1	36	15	360
Eckrich Light Oven Roasted Turkey Breast	1 oz	30	1	30	10	210
Eckrich Light Smoked Chicken Breast	1 oz	30	1	30	20	210
Eckrich Light Smoked Turkey Breast	1 oz	30	<1	<30	10	220
Hillshire Farm Deli Select (variety)	⅓ oz	10	<1	—	5	90–110
Hormel Light & Lean Ham, Boneless	2 oz	60	2	30	32	574
Kahn's Lite Sensations (variety)	⅓ oz	10	<1	—		80–100
Louis Rich Turkey Bologna	1 oz	60	5	75	20	230
Louis Rich Turkey Cotto Salami	1 oz	50	4	72	25	260
Louis Rich Turkey Ham	1 oz	35	0.3	8	15	285
Louis Rich Turkey Pastrami	1 oz	35	1	26	20	280
Louis Rich Turkey Salami	1 oz	50	4	72	25	245
Oscar Mayer Braunschweiger, Liver Sausage	1 oz	100	9	81	50	330
Oscar Mayer Cotto Salami	¾ oz	50	4	72	20	300
Oscar Mayer Ham and Cheese Loaf	1 oz	70	5	64	20	370
Oscar Mayer Head Cheese	1 oz	60	4	60	25	360
Oscar Mayer Lean Beef, Smoked	½ oz	14	<1	—	10	190
Oscar Mayer Lean Canadian-Style Bacon	¾ oz	30	<1	<30	10	300

Product	Amount	Calories	Fat (gms)	% Fat Calories	Chol (mg)	Sodium (mg)
Oscar Mayer Lean Chicken Breast, Roasted	1 oz	30	<1	<30	15	430
Oscar Mayer Lean Chicken Breast, Smoked	1 oz	25	<1	<36	15	410
Oscar Mayer Lean Corned Beef	½ oz	16	<1	—	10	210
Oscar Mayer Lean Ham, Baked	¾ oz	20	<1	—	10	250
Oscar Mayer Lean Ham, Boiled	¾ oz	25	<1	—	10	290
Oscar Mayer Lean Ham with Pepper	¾ oz	20	1	45	10	290
Oscar Mayer Lean Ham, Honey	¾ oz	25	1	36	10	280
Oscar Mayer Lean Ham, Lower Salt	¾ oz	25	1	36	10	170
Oscar Mayer Lean Ham, Smoked Cooked	¾ oz	20	<1	<45	10	280
Oscar Mayer Lean Honey Loaf	1 oz	35	1	26	15	390
Oscar Mayer Lean Pastrami	½ oz	16	<1	—	5	230
Oscar Mayer Lean Turkey Breast, Roasted	¾ oz	25	<1	<36	10	300
Oscar Mayer Lean Turkey Breast, Smoked	¾ oz	20	<1	<45	10	310
Oscar Mayer Liver Cheese, Pork Wrapped	1.3 oz	110	10	82	80	430
Oscar Mayer Luncheon Meat	1 oz	100	9	81	20	330
Oscar Mayer New England Brand Sausage	¾ oz	30	1	30	15	300
Oscar Mayer Old Fashioned Loaf	1 oz	60	4	60	15	350
Oscar Mayer Pickle and Pimiento Loaf	1 oz	60	4	60	15	410
Oscar Mayer Salami for Beer (Beef)	¾ oz	70	6	77	15	290
Oscar Mayer Salami, Hard	⅓ oz	35	3	77	10	180
Oscar Mayer Summer Sausage	¾ oz	70	6	77	20	340
Tyson Chicken Bologna	1 slice	44	4	82	—	185

Product	Amount	Calories	Fat (gms)	% Fat Calories	Chol (mg)	Sodium (mg)
Tyson Chicken Roll	1 slice	26	1	35	—	153
Tyson Hickory Smoked Breast	1 slice	26	0.8	28	—	195
Tyson Oven Roasted Breast	1 slice	25	0.8	29	—	185
Tyson Turkey Breast	1 slice	20	0.3	14	—	136
Tyson Turkey Ham	1 slice	23	1.0	39	—	182

SNACK PACK

Product	Amount	Calories	Fat (gms)	% Fat Calories	Chol (mg)	Sodium (mg)
Oscar Mayer Deluxe Beef & Ham	1 pkg	427	26	55	69	1,731
Oscar Mayer Turkey & Cheddar	1 pkg	361	22	55	62	1,446

SAUSAGES, WIENERS, FRANKS, AND BACON

Product	Amount	Calories	Fat (gms)	% Fat Calories	Chol (mg)	Sodium (mg)
Butterball Bun Size Turkey Franks	2 oz	120	10	75	—	620
Eckrich Light Bunsize Franks	1 frank	150	12	108	35	530
Eckrich Light Cheddar Smoked Sausage	1 link	190	16	76	70	820
Eckrich Light Franks	1 frank	120	10	75	25	430
Eckrich Light Polish Smoked Sausage	1 link	180	15	75	60	730
Eckrich Light Polska Kielbasa	1 oz	70	6	77	20	230
Eckrich Light Smok-Y-Links	2 links	120	10	75	25	470
Eckrich Light Smoked Bratwurst Links	1 link	190	17	81	60	870
Eckrich Light Smoked Sausage	1 link	150	13	78	35	600
Eckrich Light Smoked Sausage	1 oz	70	6	77	20	230
Eckrich Light Beef Smoked Sausage Links	1 link	200	16	72	60	360
Eckrich Light Smoked Sausage Links	1 link	200	17	77	60	560
Eckrich Sausage, Lite Cheddar Smoked	2.7 oz	190	16	76	70	820
Hormel Light & Lean Franks	1.6 oz	70	5	64	20	510
Hygrade's Ball Park Lite Franks	1 oz	140	12	77	—	525

Product	Amount	Calories	Fat (gms)	% Fat Calories	Chol (mg)	Sodium (mg)
Hygrade's Grillmaster Chicken Franks	2 oz	130	11	76	—	641
Louis Rich Turkey Bacon	⅓ oz	34	3	79	9	206
Louis Rich Turkey Franks	1.5 oz	105	9	77	—	490
Louis Rich Turkey Franks	2 oz	130	11	76	53	505
Louis Rich Turkey Polska Kielbasa	1 oz	40	2	45	19	246
Louis Rich Turkey Smoked Sausage	1 oz	43	2	42	18	239
Louis Rich Turkey Smoked Sausage with Cheese	1 oz	47	3	57	17	256
Oscar Mayer Bacon & Cheese Hot Dog	1.5 oz	135	12	80	30	500
Oscar Mayer Beef Franks	1.5 oz	140	13	84	30	470
Oscar Mayer Cheese Hot Dogs	1.5 oz	140	13	84	30	490
Oscar Mayer Franks, Beef Light	2 oz	130	11	76	25	600
Oscar Mayer Wieners, Light	2 oz	130	11	76	30	630

— = Data not available; < = Less than

Fish and Shellfish

Item	Calories	Fat (gms)	% Fat Calories	Cholesterol (mg)	Sodium (mg)
FINFISH, 3-ounce edible portions					
Cod, cooked, dry heat	89	0.7	7	47	66
Eel, cooked, dry heat	200	12.7	57	137	55
Fish sticks, frozen, reheated, 3 (4″ × 1″ × ½″)	228	10.3	41	93	489
Flounder or sole, cooked, dry heat	99	1.3	12	58	89
Grouper, cooked, dry heat	100	1.1	10	40	45
Haddock, cooked, dry heat	95	0.8	8	63	74

Item	Calories	Fat (gms)	% Fat Calories	Cholesterol (mg)	Sodium (mg)
Halibut, cooked, dry heat	119	2.5	19	35	59
Herring, cooked, dry heat	172	9.9	52	65	98
Mackerel, cooked, dry heat	223	15.1	61	64	71
Mackerel, jack, canned w/salt	133	5.4	37	67	322
Mullet, cooked, dry heat	127	4.0	28	54	61
Ocean perch, cooked, dry heat	123	1.8	16	46	82
Pike, northern, cooked, dry heat	96	0.8	8	43	42
Pollock, cooked, dry heat	96	1.0	9	82	98
Salmon, pink, canned w/bone, with salt	118	5.1	39	—	471
without salt					64
Salmon, sockeye, cooked, dry heat	183	9.3	46	74	56
Sardines, canned in oil	192	10.5	49	131	465
Smelt, cooked, dry heat	106	2.6	22	76	65
Snapper, cooked, dry heat	109	1.5	12	40	48
Surimi	84	0.8	9	25	122
Swordfish, cooked, dry heat	132	4.4	30	43	98
Trout, rainbow, cooked, dry heat	129	3.7	26	62	29
Tuna, bluefin, cooked, dry heat	157	5.3	30	42	43
Tuna, light, canned in oil, drained, with salt	169	7.0	37	15	301
without salt					43
Tuna, light, canned in water, with salt	111	0.4	3	—	303
without salt					43

SHELLFISH, 3-ounce edible portions

Item	Calories	Fat (gms)	% Fat Calories	Cholesterol (mg)	Sodium (mg)
Clam, cooked, moist heat	126	1.7	12	57	95
Crab, Alaska king, cooked, moist heat	82	1.3	14	45	911
Crab, blue, canned, drained	84	1.0	11	76	283
Crab, blue, cooked, moist heat	87	1.5	16	85	237
Crab, imitation from surimi	87	1.1	11	17	715
Crayfish, cooked, moist heat	97	1.2	11	151	58
Lobster, cooked, moist heat	83	0.5	5	61	323
Mussel, blue, cooked, moist heat	147	3.8	23	48	313
Oyster, cooked, moist heat	117	4.2	32	93	190

Item	Calories	Fat (gms)	% Fat Calories	Cholesterol (mg)	Sodium (mg)
Oyster, Eastern, raw (6 medium)	58	2.1	33	46	94
Scallops, cooked, breaded, fried (5–6 large)	183	9.3	46	52	395
Shrimp, canned, drained	102	1.7	15	143	147
Shrimp, cooked, moist heat	84	0.9	10	166	190
Shrimp, imitation from surimi	86	1.3	14	31	599
Squid, cooked, fried	149	6.4	39	221	260

Note: "Cooked, dry heat" includes baking, broiling, and microwaving without added fat, salt, or seasonings. "Cooked, moist heat" includes procedures involving added liquid, such as boiling, poaching, and steaming.
Chart based on data from Agriculture Handbook No. 8–15, USDA Composition of Foods, Finfish and Shellfish Products.

Milk

Type of Milk (per cup)	Calories	Fat (gms)	% Fat Calories	Cholesterol (mg)	Calcium (mg)
Skim milk, < 0.5% fat	86	0.4	4	4	302
Buttermilk, cultured	99	2.2	20	9	285
Low-fat milk, 1% fat	102	2.6	23	10	300
Low-fat milk, 2% fat	121	4.7	35	18	297
Whole milk, 3.3% fat	150	8.2	49	33	291
Chocolate milk, 1% fat	158	2.5	14	7	287
Chocolate milk, whole	208	8.5	37	30	280
Evaporated skim, canned	198	0.5	2	10	738
Evaporated whole, canned	338	19.1	51	74	658
Sweetened condensed, canned	982	26.6	24	104	868

Note: Milk labeled "low-fat" can have a fat content of 0.5%, 1%, 1.5%, or 2%. The calcium, protein, and carbohydrate content of whole milk and skim milk is approximately the same. The sodium content of buttermilk (257 mg per cup) is more than twice that of regular milks.
Chart based on data from Agriculture Handbook, No. 8–1, USDA Composition of Foods, Dairy and Egg Products.

Cheese

Item	Calories	Fat (gms)	% Fat Calories	Cholesterol (mg)	Sodium (mg)	Calcium (mg)
AMERICAN (1 ounce)						
Alpine Lace Free, Lean	35	<0.5	1	5	290	200
Borden Lite-line	50	2	36	10	410	200
Borden Lite-line Reduced-Sodium Singles	70	4	51	8	90	200
Cheese Smart Singles	50	2	36	10	400	200
Kraft Free Singles Nonfat	45	0	0	5	430	200
Kraft Light n' Lively	70	4	51	15	410	200
Traditional, pasteur-ized process	106	9	76	27	406	175
Weight Watchers	50	2	40	5	400	200
BLUE (1 ounce)						
Traditional	100	8	72	21	396	150
BRIE (1 ounce)						
Traditional	95	8	76	28	178	52
CAMEMBERT (1 ounce)						
Traditional	85	7	74	20	239	110
CHEDDAR (1 ounce)						
Alpine Lace Free n' Lean	35	<0.5	<13	5	290	200
Dorman's Low Sodium Reduced Fat	80	5	56	20	140	—
Kraft Light Naturals	84	5	54	18	210	215
Lifetime 50%	65	3	42	9	65	400
Lorraine Lites Reduced Fat	90	6	60	20	140	200
Traditional	114	9	71	30	176	204
Weight Watchers 40% Less Fat	80	5	56	28	150	200

Item	Calories	Fat (gms)	% Fat Calories	Cholesterol (mg)	Sodium (mg)	Calcium (mg)
CHEESE FOOD (1 ounce)						
Alpine Lace Free n' Lean Singles	35	<0.5	<13	5	290	200
Churny Delicia Hickory Smoked American Cheese Substitute	80	6	68	0	470	200
Traditional cold pack	95	7	66	18	275	140
Kraft Cracker Barrel (variety)	90	7	70	—	270	120
Kraft Singles	90	7	70	25	390	150
Kraft Velveeta	100	7	63	20–25	410–420	150
Kuakana Lite Cold Pack	70	4	51	15	200–230	—
Land O Lakes (variety)	90	7	70	20	430	150
Traditional, pasteurized process	93	7	68	18	337	163
Shedd's Country Crock Cheddar	70	4	51	15	190	200
Shedd's Country Crock Neufchâtel	70	7	90	20	190	20
Shedd's Country Crock Swiss	70	4	51	15	220	200
CHEESE SPREAD (1 ounce)						
Hernke Lite Spread	70	4	51	—	135	—
Kraft Cheese Whiz (variety)	80	6	68	20	370–470	80–120
Kraft Squeez-a-Snack	90	7	70	20	280–320	120
Traditional pasteurized process	82	6	66	18	380	160
COLBY (1 ounce)						
Alpine Lace Colbi-Lo	80	5	56	20	85	280
Alpine Lace Low-Sodium	85	5	53	19	85	200

Item	Calories	Fat (gms)	% Fat Calories	Cholesterol (mg)	Sodium (mg)	Calcium (mg)
Churny Lite Reduced-Fat	80	5	56	20	160	160
Churny Delicia Colby Longhorn Imitation	80	6	68	0	500	30
Kraft Light Naturals	80	5	56	20	150	224
Lorraine Lites Reduced Fat	90	6	60	20	140	—
Traditional	112	9	72	27	171	195
COTTAGE CHEESE (4 ounces—about ½ cup)						
Creamed, 4.5%	117	5	38	17	457	68
Dry curd, 0.5%, uncreamed	96	0.5	1	8	14	36
Low-fat, 1%	82	1	11	5	459	69
Low-fat, 2%	101	2	18	9	459	77
EDAM (1 ounce)						
Traditional	101	8	72	25	274	207
FARMER (1 ounce)						
Holland Farm	81	5	56	18	—	217
May-Bud	90	7	70	29	210	—
FETA (1 ounce)						
Churny Natural	90	7	70	22	388	110
Traditional	75	6	72	25	316	140
FONTINA (1 ounce)						
Traditional	110	9	74	33	290	156
GOUDA (1 ounce)						
Traditional	101	8	71	32	232	198
GRUYERE (1 ounce)						
Traditional	117	9	69	31	95	287

Item	Calories	Fat (gms)	% Fat Calories	Cholesterol (mg)	Sodium (mg)	Calcium (mg)
JARLSBERG (1 ounce)						
Traditional	100	7	63	16	130	160
LIMBURGER (1 ounce)						
Traditional	93	8	77	26	227	141
MONTEREY JACK (1 ounce)						
Alpine Lace	80	4	45	14	—	195
Alpine Lace Low Sodium	80	4	45	14	75	195
Alpine Lace Monti-Jack-Lo	80	5	56	15	75	212
Dorman's Low Sodium Reduced Fat	80	5	56	18	140	—
Kraft Light Natural	84	5.5	59	19	160	217
Lorraine Lites Reduced Fat	90	6	60	20	140	200
Borden Lite-line, process	50	2	36	10	470	200
Churny Lite Reduced Fat, process	80	5	56	20	180	160
Weight Watchers, process	80	5	56	28	150	160
Traditional	106	9	76	—	152	212
MOZZARELLA (1 ounce)						
Alpine Lace Free n' Lean	35	0.5	13	5	290	—
Alpine Lace Low Sodium	72	4	50	15	65	—
Dorman's Low Sodium Reduced Fat	80	4	45	—	140	—
Kraft Light Natural	80	5	56	15	90	175
Lifetime 50% Less	60	2	30	7	50	350
Lorraine Lites Reduced Fat	80	5	56	15	140	200

Item	Calories	Fat (gms)	% Fat Calories	Cholesterol (mg)	Sodium (mg)	Calcium (mg)
Sargento Preferred Light	60	3	45	10	150	200
Traditional, part skim	72	5	63	16	132	183
Traditional, part skim, low moisture	79	5	57	15	150	207
Traditional, whole milk, low moisture	90	7	70	25	118	163
Weight Watchers Natural	70	4	51	28	—	250
MUENSTER (1 ounce)						
Dorman's Lo-Chol	100	7	63	<5	140	200
Borden Lite-line, process	50	2	36	10	—	200
Ryster Part Skim	85	5	53	14	—	200
Traditional	104	8	69	27	178	203
NEUFCHATEL (1 ounce)						
Light Philadelphia	80	7	79	25	115	40
Traditional	74	7	85	22	113	21
PARMESAN (1 ounce)						
Traditional	111	7	57	19	454	336
PROVOLONE (1 ounce)						
Alpine Lace Provo-Lo Lightly Smoked	70	5	64	15	85	280
Dorman's Low Sodium Reduced Fat	80	4	45	17	140	200
Lorraine Lites Reduced Fat	80	5	56	15	140	200
Traditional	100	8	72	20	248	214
RICOTTA (4 ounces)						
Frigo, part skim	180	12	60	40	160	240
Frigo, whole milk	200	16	72	60	—	240
Frigo Low Fat	80	4	45	20	—	240

Item	Calories	Fat (gms)	% Fat Calories	Cholesterol (mg)	Sodium (mg)	Calcium (mg)
Sargento, part skim	120	8	60	40	160	120
Sargento, whole milk	200	16	72	65	140	250
Sargento Lite	92	4	39	56	—	136
Traditional, part skim	170	10	53	38	155	337
Traditional, whole milk	215	15	63	63	104	257

ROMANO (1 ounce)

Item	Calories	Fat (gms)	% Fat Calories	Cholesterol (mg)	Sodium (mg)	Calcium (mg)
Traditional	110	8	65	29	340	302

SAPSAGO (1 ounce)

Item	Calories	Fat (gms)	% Fat Calories	Cholesterol (mg)	Sodium (mg)	Calcium (mg)
Traditional	68	2	26	9	510	—

STRING/STRIP CHEESES (1 ounce)

Item	Calories	Fat (gms)	% Fat Calories	Cholesterol (mg)	Sodium (mg)	Calcium (mg)
Dorman Strip, Low Sodium	70	4	51	12	—	200
Kraft, low moisture, part skim	80	5	56	15	190	200
Sargento	80	5	56	15	150	200
Traditional	85	6	64	12	125	200

SWISS (1 ounce)

Item	Calories	Fat (gms)	% Fat Calories	Cholesterol (mg)	Sodium (mg)	Calcium (mg)
Alpine Lace Swiss-Lo	100	7	63	20	35	250
Churny Lite Reduced Fat	90	5	50	20	45	—
Deli-Light No Salt Added	100	8	72	26	8	—
Dorman's Low Sodium Reduced Fat	90	5	50	17	60	250
Kraft Light n' Lively	79	4	46	15	350	200
Kraft Light Natural	90	5	50	20	55	326
Lifetime 50% Less	60	3	45	9	39	350
Lorraine Lites Reduced Fat	90	5	50	20	80	250
Borden Lite-line, process	50	2	36	10	380	200
Swiss Valley Farms	80	6	68	20	—	400

Item	Calories	Fat (gms)	% Fat Calories	Cholesterol (mg)	Sodium (mg)	Calcium (mg)
Traditional	107	8	67	26	74	275
Weight Watchers	50	2	36	5	370	200

— = Data not available; < = Less than
Chart based on data from Agriculture Handbook No. 8–1, USDA Composition of
Foods, Dairy and Egg Products, processors' data, and label information.

Dietary Fiber per Serving of Commonly Eaten Foods

Food	Portion	Fiber (gms)	Calories
BREAKFAST CEREALS			
Kellogg's All-Bran	⅓ cup (1 oz)	8.5	71
General Mills Cheerios	1¼ cups (1 oz)	1.1	111
Kellogg's Corn flakes	1¼ cups (1 oz)	0.6	110
Post Grape-nuts	¼ cup (1 oz)	1.4	110
Quaker Oatmeal	¾ cup (1 oz dry)	2.7	100
Post Raisin Bran	¾ cup (1 oz)	4.0	115
Nabisco Shredded Wheat	⅔ cup (1 oz)	3.0	110
BREAD, PASTA, AND RICE			
Bagel	1	1.1	163
Bran muffin	1	2.5	112
Bread, white	1 slice	0.7	67
Bread, whole wheat	1 slice	2.8	61
Bread, pumpernickel	1 slice	1.9	81
Rice, brown	½ cup	1.7	105
Rice, white	½ cup	1.1	132
Spaghetti, regular	1 cup	2.2	155
Spaghetti, whole wheat	1 cup	3.9	155
FRUITS			
Apple with skin	1 average	3.0	81
Banana	1 average	1.8	105
Cantaloupe	¼ melon	1.0	30

Food	Portion	Fiber (gms)	Calories
Grapefruit	½ average	1.6	38
Grapes	½ cup	0.6	30
Orange	1 average	3.1	62
Prunes	3	1.8	60
Raisins	¼ cup	2.0	108
Strawberries	1 cup	3.9	45
LEGUMES			
Baked beans, tomato sauce	½ cup	9.8	118
Kidney beans, cooked	½ cup	6.3	115
Lima beans, cooked	½ cup	4.2	85
Navy beans, cooked	½ cup	4.7	113
VEGETABLES, COOKED			
Broccoli	½ cup	3.6	6
Carrots	½ cup	3.0	35
Corn, canned	½ cup	1.7	67
Green beans	½ cup	1.1	18
Potato with skin	1 average (5 oz)	3.4	154
VEGETABLES, RAW			
Cucumber with peel	1 average	1.0	14
Lettuce, iceberg	1 cup	0.6	7
Tomato	1 average	1.6	24
Spinach	1 cup	1.5	12

Fiber Sources and Benefits

Type	Food Sources	Possible Health Benefits and Actions
WATER INSOLUBLE		
Cellulose Lignin Some hemicellulose	Fruits, vegetables, cereals, whole wheat, wheat bran, wheat germ, legumes, nuts, seeds	Helps prevent and relieve constipation. Absorbs water, increases bulk, softens stool, reduces time it takes

Type	Food Sources	Possible Health Benefits and Actions
		food to move through bowels. Binds bile acids, reduces problems of diverticulosis, constipation, hemorrhoids. May reduce risk of developing colon cancer. Excesses may cause loss of trace minerals.

WATER SOLUBLE

Type	Food Sources	Possible Health Benefits and Actions
Pectin Mucilages Gums Some hemicellulose	Fruits, vegetables, oats, oat bran, barley, rice bran, legumes, beans, psyllium	Delays absorption of sugar. Decreases serum cholesterol. Decreases serum triglycerides. Delays stomach emptying. May bind bile acids, causing decreased fat absorption. May protect against colon cancer.

Healthier Choices for Shelf-Stable, Refrigerated, and Frozen Dinners/Entrees

Prepared dinners and entrees are convenient but often contain too much fat, salt, and sugar. The following is a representative listing of more than 160 shelf-stable, refrigerated, and frozen entrees and dinners that provide less than 30% fat calories. These dinners provide less than 1,000 mg of sodium; entrees, less than 800 mg. There are others.

These products are not necessarily free of ingredients that might raise cholesterol, but many are. Some low-fat entrees and dinners have small amounts of butter or chicken fat added for flavor, but they may provide an acceptable occasional choice when the total fat is low.

Manufacturers change the composition of their products periodically—sometimes substantially. Many are much lower in salt and fat than just two years ago. A few are higher. It isn't always obvious when manufacturers change the composition of their products, especially when the change is not positive. The change occasionally results in higher fat or sodium content, so use label information to keep informed.

Product	Calories	Fat (gms)	% Fat Calories	Cholesterol (mg)	Sodium (mg)
ARMOUR CLASSIC LITES					
Baby Bay Shrimp in Sherried Cream Sauce	220	6	25	105	890
Beef Pepper Steak	220	4	16	35	970
Beef Stroganoff	250	6	22	55	510
Chicken à la King	290	7	22	55	630
Chicken Burgundy	210	2	9	45	780
Chicken Marsala	250	7	25	80	930
Chicken Oriental	180	1	5	35	660
Shrimp Creole	260	2	7	45	900
Steak Diane	290	9	28	80	440
Sweet and Sour Chicken	240	2	8	35	820
ARMOUR DINNER CLASSICS					
Chicken & Noodles	230	7	27	50	660
Sirloin Roast	190	4	19	55	970
Sirloin Tips	230	7	27	70	820
BUDGET GOURMET LIGHT AND HEALTHY DINNERS					
Stuffed Turkey Breast	230	6	23	40	520
BUDGET GOURMET REGULAR ENTREES					
Pepper Steak with Rice	320	9	25	30	590
BUDGET GOURMET LIGHT ENTREES					
Glazed Turkey	270	5	17	40	760
Mandarin Chicken	300	7	21	40	670
BUDGET GOURMET THREE DISH DINNERS					
Scallops & Shrimp Mariner	320	9	25	70	690

Product	Calories	Fat (gms)	% Fat Calories	Cholesterol (mg)	Sodium (mg)
DINING LITE DINNERS					
Beef Teriyaki with Vegetables and Rice	270	5	17	45	850
Cheese Cannelloni with Tomato Sauce	310	9	26	70	650
Cheese Lasagna	260	6	21	30	800
Chicken à La King with Rice	240	7	26	40	780
Chicken Chow Mein	180	2	10	30	650
Chicken with Noodles	240	7	26	50	570
Glazed Chicken	220	4	16	45	680
Lasagna with Meat Sauce	240	5	19	25	800
HEALTHY CHOICE DINNERS					
Beef Pepper Steak	290	6	19	65	530
Breast of Turkey	290	5	16	45	420
Chicken Oriental	220	2	8	55	460
Chicken & Pasta Divan	310	4	12	60	510
Chicken Parmigiana	280	3	10	60	310
Herb Roasted Chicken	260	3	10	40	300
Mesquite Chicken	310	2	6	45	270
Salisbury Steak	300	7	21	50	480
Shrimp Creole	210	1	4	65	560
Shrimp Marinara	220	1	4	50	320
Sirloin Tips	290	6	19	70	350
Sole Au Gratin	270	5	17	55	470
Sweet & Sour Chicken	280	2	6	50	260
Yankee Pot Roast	260	4	14	45	310
HEALTHY CHOICE ENTREES					
Beef Pepper Steak	250	4	14	40	340
Chicken à l'Orange	260	2	7	45	90
Chicken Chow Mein	220	3	12	45	440
Fettucini Alfredo	240	7	26	45	370
Glazed Chicken	220	3	12	50	390
Lasagna with Meat Sauce	260	5	17	20	420
Linguini with Shrimp	230	2	8	55	390

Product	Calories	Fat (gms)	% Fat Calories	Cholesterol (mg)	Sodium (mg)
Seafood Newburg	200	3	14	55	440
Sole with Lemon Butter Sauce	230	4	16	45	390
Spaghetti with Meat Sauce	310	6	17	15	440

HEALTH VALLEY FAST MENU DINNERS

Product	Calories	Fat (gms)	% Fat Calories	Cholesterol (mg)	Sodium (mg)
Amaranth with Garden Vegetables	140	3	19	0	140
Hearthy Lentil & Garden Vegetables	150	4	24	0	200
Honey Baked Organic Beans with Tofu Wieners	140	4	26	0	140
Oat Bran Pilaf with Garden Vegetables	210	7	30	0	330
Organic Black Beans with Tofu Wieners	150	1	6	0	170
Organic Lentils with Tofu Wieners	170	5	26	0	260
Western Black Bean with Garden Vegetables	160	5	28	0	250

HORMEL: CHICKEN BY GEORGE

Product	Calories	Fat (gms)	% Fat Calories	Cholesterol (mg)	Sodium (mg)
Caribbean Grill	180	4	20	—	—
Hickory Barbecue	170	4	21	55	600
Italian Style Parmesan	160	5	28	65	510
Lemon Herb	150	4	24	70	480
Lemon Pepper	160	4	23	60	680
Mesquite Barbecue	170	4	21	70	680
Teriyaki	180	4	20	65	340

HORMEL: TOP SHELF ENTREES

Product	Calories	Fat (gms)	% Fat Calories	Cholesterol (mg)	Sodium (mg)
Cheese Tortellini in Marinara Sauce	210	4	17	30	660
Chicken Cacciatore	190	2	9	40	680
Sweet & Sour Chicken	260	2	7	55	750

KID CUISINE

Product	Calories	Fat (gms)	% Fat Calories	Cholesterol (mg)	Sodium (mg)
Cheese Pizza	240	4	15	20	390
Mini-Cheese Ravioli	250	2	7	20	730

Product	Calories	Fat (gms)	% Fat Calories	Cholesterol (mg)	Sodium (mg)
LE MENU HEALTHY DINNERS (LightStyle)					
Cheese Tortellini	230	6	23	15	460
Glazed Chicken Breast	230	3	12	55	480
Herb Roasted Chicken	240	7	26	70	400
Salisbury Steak	280	9	29	35	400
Sliced Turkey	210	5	21	30	540
3-Cheese Stuffed Shells	280	8	26	25	690
Turkey Divan	260	7	24	60	420
Veal Marsala	230	3	12	75	700
LE MENU HEALTHY ENTREES (LightStyle)					
Chicken à la King	240	5	19	30	670
Chicken Dijon	240	7	26	40	500
Chicken Enchiladas	280	8	26	35	530
Empress Chicken	210	5	21	30	690
Garden Vegetables Lasagna	260	8	28	25	500
Glazed Turkey	260	6	21	35	720
Herb Roasted Chicken	260	6	21	45	500
Lasagna with Meat Sauce	290	8	25	30	510
Meat Sauce & Cheese Tortellini	250	8	29	15	480
Spaghetti with Beef Sauce and Mushrooms	280	6	19	15	450
Swedish Meatballs	260	8	28	40	700
Traditional Turkey	200	5	23	25	610
LIGHT BALANCE MICROWAVEABLE MEALS ENTREE					
Beef Americana	170	3	16	15	700
Beef & Pasta Bordeaux	180	1	5	25	660
Chicken Cacciatore	200	1	5	25	730
Chicken Fiesta	210	3	13	15	640
Pasta & Garden Vegetables	190	1	5	0	650

Product	Calories	Fat (gms)	% Fat Calories	Cholesterol (mg)	Sodium (mg)
MRS. PAUL'S LIGHT SEAFOOD ENTREES					
Fish Dijon	200	5	23	60	650
Seafood Lasagna	290	8	25	57	750
Seafood Rotini	240	6	23	25	570
Shrimp and Clams with Linguini	240	5	19	40	750
STOUFFER'S LEAN CUISINE					
Breast of Chicken Marsala with Vegetables	190	5	24	80	400
Breast of Chicken Parmesan	260	8	28	80	870
Chicken à l'Orange with Almond Rice	260	5	17	55	430
Chicken and Vegetables with Vermicelli	270	8	27	45	980
Chicken Cacciatore with Vermicelli	250	7	25	45	860
Chicken Chow Mein with Rice	250	5	18	35	980
Chicken Enchiladas	270	9	30	65	850
Chicken Oriental	230	6	23	100	790
Fiesta Chicken	250	6	22	45	880
Filet of Fish Divan	260	7	24	85	750
Glazed Chicken with Vegetable Rice	270	8	27	55	810
Lasagna with Meat Sauce	270	8	27	60	970
Linguini with Clam Sauce	270	7	23	30	890
Oriental Beef with Vegetables and Rice	250	7	25	45	900
Sliced Turkey Breast in Mushroom Sauce	240	7	26	50	790
Spaghetti with Beef and Mushroom Sauce	280	7	23	25	940
Zucchini Lasagna	260	7	24	25	950
STOUFFER'S LEAN CUISINE FRENCH BREAD PIZZAS					
Cheese French Bread Pizza	310	10	29	15	750

Product	Calories	Fat (gms)	% Fat Calories	Cholesterol (mg)	Sodium (mg)
STOUFFER'S RIGHT COURSE ENTREES					
Beef Dijon with Pasta & Vegetables	290	9	28	40	580
Beef Ragout with Rice Pilaf	300	8	24	50	550
Chicken Italiano with Fettucini & Vegetables	280	8	26	45	560
Chicken Tenderloins in Barbecue Sauce	270	6	20	40	590
Chicken Tenderloins in Peanut Sauce	330	10	27	50	570
Fiesta Beef with Corn Pasta	270	7	23	30	590
Homestyle Pot Roast	220	7	29	35	550
Sesame Chicken	320	9	25	50	590
Shrimp Primavera	240	7	26	50	590
Sliced Turkey in Curry Sauce with Rice Pilaf	320	8	23	50	570
Vegetarian Chili	280	7	23	0	590
SWANSON HOMESTYLE ENTREES					
Sirloin Tips in Burgundy Sauce	160	5	28	—	550
TOMBSTONE LIGHT PIZZAS					
Sausage Pizza (½ package)	250	8	29	10	570
Vegetable Cheese Pizza (½ package)	250	8	29	10	500
TYSON ENTREES					
Grilled Chicken Sandwich	203	5	22	30	500
Microwave BBQ Chicken Sandwich	208	4	17	50	600
TYSON GOURMET SELECTION DINNERS					
Chicken à l'Orange	300	8	24	—	670
Chicken Mesquite	320	10	28	—	700

Product	Calories	Fat (gms)	% Fat Calories	Cholesterol (mg)	Sodium (mg)
TYSON LOONEY TUNES MEALS					
Daffy Duck™ Spaghetti & Meatballs	300	8	24	—	820
Road Runner™ Chicken Sandwich	320	11	31	—	610
Tweety™ Macaroni & Cheese	280	8	26	—	630
TYSON MARINATED CHICKEN BREASTS					
Barbecue	120	3	23	—	400
Italian	130	2	14	—	430
Lemon Pepper	120	2	15	—	210
Teriyaki	130	2	14	—	290
ULTRA SLIM-FAST DINNERS					
Chicken & Vegetables	290	3	9	30	850
Country-Style Vegetables & Beef Tips	230	5	20	45	960
Mesquite Chicken	360	1	3	65	300
Roasted Chicken in Mushroom Sauce	280	6	19	55	830
Shrimp Marinara	290	3	9	70	880
Spaghetti with Beef & Mushroom Sauce	370	10	24	25	990
Turkey Medallions/Herb Sauce & Rice Pilaf	280	6	19	40	950
WEIGHT WATCHERS					
Angel Hair Pasta with Italian Style Sauce	210	5	21	20	420
Beef Fajitas	270	7	23	30	720
Broccoli and Cheese and Baked Potato	290	8	25	25	600
Cheese Pizza	300	7	21	35	630
Cheese Tortellini	310	6	17	15	570
Chicken Fajitas	230	5	20	30	590
Chicken Fettucini	280	9	29	40	590
Deluxe Combination Pizza	330	10	27	25	650

Product	Calories	Fat (gms)	% Fat Calories	Cholesterol (mg)	Sodium (mg)
Fillet of Fish Au Gratin	200	6	27	60	700
Garden Lasagna	290	7	22	20	670
Homestyle Turkey Baked Potato	300	6	18	60	670
London Broil in Mushroom Sauce	140	3	19	40	510
Spaghetti with Meat Sauce	280	7	23	25	610
Sweet 'n Sour Chicken Tenders	240	3	11	35	640

— = Data not available.
Chart based on manufacturer's data and label information, updated 3/91.

Frozen Desserts

Product	Amount	Calories	Fat (gms)	% Fat Calories	Cholesterol (mg)	Sodium (mg)
Dove Bar	4-oz bar	318	16	45	—	40
Welch's No Sugar Added Fruit Juice Bar	1 bar	25	0	0	0	0
Dole Fruit 'N Juice Bar	1 bar	60	<1	0	0	5
Dole Raspberry Sorbet	4 oz	100	<9	<8	0	10
Häagen-Dazs Fruit Ice	4 oz	100	0	0	0	20
Häagen-Dazs Ice Cream with nuts	4 oz	340	24	64	—	180
Pepperidge Farm Dessert Light Strawberry Shortcake	1 pkg	170	5	26	—	50
Klondike Lite Sugar Free Frozen Dessert Bar	2.5 fl oz	110	7	57	5	70
Life Savers Flavor Pop	1 bar	40	0	0	0	5
Jell-O Pudding Pop	1 bar	80	2	23	10	55
Bordon Orange Sherbet	½ cup	110	1	8	5	40

Product	Amount	Calories	Fat (gms)	% Fat Calories	Cholesterol (mg)	Sodium (mg)
Eskimo Pie, Sugar-Free with Crisped Rice	1 bar	150	11	66	—	40
Tofutti Lite, Strawberry	4 oz	90	<1	<10	0	155
Tofutti	4 oz	200	11	50	0	90
Sara Lee Classic Cheesecake	1 cake	200	14	63	—	150
Sara Lee Lights, Strawberry French Cheesecake	3.5 oz	150	2	12	5	65
Sara Lee Deluxe Carrot Cake	1 cake	180	7	35	—	200
Sara Lee Lights, Carrot Cake	1 cake	170	6	32	10	135
Sweet 'N Low LowFat Frozen Dessert	4 fl oz	90	2	20	0	40
Vanilla ice cream (16% fat)	½ cup	175	12	62	44	54
Weight Watchers Chocolate Treat	1 bar	100	1	9	0	75
Sealtest Free Red Raspberry Nonfat Frozen Yogurt	½ cup	100	<0.5	<5	<2	40
Sealtest Fat Free Chocolate Nonfat Frozen Dairy Dessert	4 fl oz	100	0	0	0	55
Edy's or Breyer's American Dream Nonfat Frozen Dairy Dessert, Rocky Road	3 fl oz	110	1	8	0	45

— = Data not available.

Chart based on data from manufacturers or the U.S. Department of Agriculture, updated 3/91.

Fats and Oils

Fat or Oil	Polyunsaturated fat (%)	Monounsaturated fat (%)	Saturated fat (%)	Cholesterol (milligrams) per tbsp
Canola oil	35	58	7	0
Hazelnut oil	11	82	8	0
Almond oil	18	73	8	0
Walnut oil	67	24	9	0
Safflower oil	78	13	9	0
Sunflower oil	68	21	11	0
Corn oil	62	25	13	0
Olive oil	9	77	14	0
Sesame oil	44	41	15	0
Soybean oil	60	25	15	0
Peanut oil	34	48	18	0
Wheat germ oil	64	16	20	0
Cottonseed oil	55	18	27	0
Goose fat	11	60	29	13
Chicken fat	22	47	31	11
Turkey fat	24	45	31	13
Duck fat	14	51	35	13
Pork fat (lard)	11	48	41	12
Mutton tallow	8	42	50	13
Palm oil	10	38	52	0
Beef tallow	4	43	53	14
Cocoa butter	3	35	62	0
Butter	5	31	64	33
Palm kernel oil	1	12	87	0
Coconut oil	2	6	92	0

NOTE: Fats are arranged from lowest to highest in saturated fat.

Not all of the fats listed above are readily available separate from the foods in which they are found. These have been included to illustrate the nature of the fats in the nuts, seeds, and animal products containing them.

Chart based on data from Agriculture Handbook No. 8–4, USDA Composition of Foods, Fats and Oils.

Snacks

Item	Amount	Calories	Fat (gms)	% Fat Calories	Cholesterol (mg)	Sodium (mg)
BEVERAGES						
Beer, regular	12 oz	144	0	0	0	24
light	12 oz	96	0	0	0	12
Moussy (non-alcoholic)	10 oz	50	0	0	0	5
Club soda	12 oz	0	0	0	0	72
Cola-type soda	12 oz	147	0	0	0	12
Cranberry juice, regular	1 cup	147	0	0	0	10
low-calorie	1 cup	40	0	0	0	8
Diet soft drink	12 oz	0	0	0	0	24
Fruit beverage (10% juice)	1 cup	120	0	0	0	50
Grape juice, un-sweetened	1 cup	128	0	0	0	9
Grapefruit juice, un-sweetened	1 cup	93	0	0	0	3
Milk, 3.3% fat	1 cup	150	8	48	33	120
Milk, skim	1 cup	86	0.4	4	4	126
Milk shake, vanilla	12 oz	350	10	26	37	299
Mineral water	8 oz	0	0	0	0	3
Orange juice, un-sweetened	1 cup	112	0	0	0	2
Tomato juice, regular	1 cup	42	0.1	2	0	882
unsalted	1 cup	42	0.1	2	0	24
Vegetable juice cock-tail, regular	1 cup	49	0	0	0	819
unsalted	1 cup	49	0	0	0	58

Item	Amount	Calories	Fat (gms)	% Fat Calories	Cholesterol (mg)	Sodium (mg)
CHEESE, MEAT, AND FISH						
Cheese spread	1 oz	82	6	66	16	381
Cheese, Alpine Lace	1 oz	100	8	72	26	35
Cheese, cheddar	1 oz	114	9	71	30	176
Cheese, cottage, low-fat, 1%	½ cup	82	1	11	5	459
Cheese, cream	1 oz	99	10	91	31	84
Cheese, light, processed	1 oz	70	4	51	15	410
Cheese, mozzarella, part skim	1 oz	72	5	63	16	132
Cheese, natural, reduced fat	1 oz	84	5–6	54–64	18–21	53–205
Frank, beef (1)	1.6 oz	145	13	81	30	460
Frank, turkey (1)	1.6 oz	106	9	76	40	490
Ham, lean	1 oz	44	1.6	33	15	350
Hamburger, Micro-Magic	1	350	18	46	55	500
Salami, hard	1 oz	116	10	78	23	640
Sardines, canned in oil, 3″ × 1″ × ½″	2	50	3	54	34	121
Tombstone Light Vegetable Cheese Pizza	½ pkg	250	8	29	10	500
Tuna, in water, single-serving can	3.25 oz	98	0.4	4	0	406
Turkey breast cold cuts	1 oz	30	0.6	18	10	290
Turkey breast slices, fresh	1 oz	45	1	20	15	30
Turkey pastrami	1 oz	40	1	23	17	383
Wieners, little cocktail, 1 link	⅓ oz	30	3	90	5	90

Item	Amount	Calories	Fat (gms)	% Fat Calories	Cholesterol (mg)	Sodium (mg)
CRUNCHIES/MUNCHIES						
Bagel, plain	1	163	1.4	8	0	198
Cheese puffs	1 oz	160	10	56	0	368
Chips, apple, Tastee	1 oz	130	6	42	0	10
Chips, carrot, Knudsen	1 oz	121	4	30	0	—
Chips, corn	1 oz	155	9	52	0	164
Chips, potato	1 oz	150	10	60	0	130–200
Chips, tortilla cheese	1 oz	141	7	45	0	182
Corn nuts	1 oz	120	4	30	0	200
Crackers, Cracklebred	2 slices	33	0	0	0	1
Crackers, Pepperidge Farm Goldfish	45 pcs	140	6	39	0	160–250
Crackers, Hain Stoneground Wheat Crackers, no salt	11 each (1 oz)	130	6	42	0	5
Crackers, Sesame Ry-Krisp	2 triple crackers	50	2	36	0	160
Crackers, Toastchee, Lance peanut butter/ cheese	1 pkg (1.4 oz)	190	10	47	5	310
Crackers, Town House Low Salt	4	70	4	51	0	60
Crackers, whole wheat, thin, low salt	8 pcs	70	3	39	0	35
Croissant, Sara Lee	1 each	170	9	48	—	310
French Fries, Micro-Magic	3 oz pkg	290	13	40	0	30

Item	Amount	Calories	Fat (gms)	% Fat Calories	Cholesterol (mg)	Sodium (mg)
French Fries, Ore Ida Lites	3 oz	90	2	20	0	35
Muffin, hearty fruit	1 each	230	9	35	—	310
Multi Bran Chex, dry, ⅔ cup	1 oz	90	0	0	0	200
Popcorn, caramel microwave	2½ cups	240	14	53	0	90
Popcorn, popped, with oil and salt	4 cups	160	8	45	0	696
Popcorn, popped plain	4 cups	100	0	0	0	0
Pretzel thin sticks or twists	1 oz	113	1	8	0	456
Pretzels with cheddar cheese filling	1.8-oz pkg	240	9	34	—	580
Rice cake, Chico-San, sodium free	1 cake	35	0	0	0	0
Snack Mix, Ralston Chex, ⅔ cup	1 oz	120	5	38	0	320

FRUITS AND VEGETABLES

Item	Amount	Calories	Fat (gms)	% Fat Calories	Cholesterol (mg)	Sodium (mg)
Apple, raw	1 medium	81	0.5	6	0	1
Applesauce, cinnamon, unsweetened, single serving	4 oz	50	0	0	0	0
Banana, raw	1 small	105	0.6	5	0	1
Carrot, cut into slices	1 whole	31	0.1	3	0	25
Celery, raw	1 stalk	6	0	0	0	35
Fruit bar, Nature's Choice	1 bar	50	<1	<18	0	0
Fruit cup, canned in juice	4½ oz	80	0	0	0	0
Fruit leather, rolled	½ oz	50	<1	<18	0	10

Item	Amount	Calories	Fat (gms)	% Fat Calories	Cholesterol (mg)	Sodium (mg)
Fruit mix, dried orchard	1 pouch	70	0	0	0	10
Fruit mix, dried tropical	1 pouch	90	1	10	0	15
Sunkist Fun Fruit	1 pouch	100	1	9	0	10
Fruit snacks, yogurt-covered	1 pouch	120	5	38	0	25
Orange, raw	1 medium	62	0.2	3	0	0
Raisins, seedless	1 oz	85	0.1	1	0	3

NUTS

Item	Amount	Calories	Fat (gms)	% Fat Calories	Cholesterol (mg)	Sodium (mg)
Cashews, oil or dry roasted	1 oz	163	13	72	0	177
unsalted	1 oz	163	13	72	0	5
Coconut meat, raw, 2″ × 2″ × ½″	1 pc	159	15	85	0	0.5
Filberts, dried, unblanched	1 oz	179	18	91	0	1
Macadamia nuts, oil or dry roasted	1 oz	204	22	97	0	74
Peanut butter	2 tbsp	190	16	76	0	150
Peanuts, honey roasted	1 oz	170	12	64	0	135
Peanuts, oil or dry roasted	1 oz	162	14	78	0	122–250
unsalted	1 oz	162	14	78	0	4
Pecans, dried	1 oz	190	19	90	0	0
Pistachio nuts, dry roasted	1 oz	172	15	78	0	221
Walnuts, English	1 oz	182	18	89	0	3

SWEETS

Item	Amount	Calories	Fat (gms)	% Fat Calories	Cholesterol (mg)	Sodium (mg)
Almost Home Fruit Sticks	1 stick	70	1–2	13–26	—	30–100
Angel food cake	2-oz slice	150	0.1	1	0	145
Cherry snack pie	1 each	416	20	43	19	410

Item	Amount	Calories	Fat (gms)	% Fat Calories	Cholesterol (mg)	Sodium (mg)
Chocolate-chip cookie, 2"	⅓ oz	46	3	59	5	21
Chocolate covered peanuts (14)	1 oz	160	9	51	0	15
Entenmann's Raspberry Twist	1.1 oz	90	0	0	0	75
Gingerbread cake, 1 slice	2 oz	175	4	21	1	90
Graham crackers, 2 squares	½ oz	60	1	15	0	90
Health Valley Honey Jumbos Cookies	1 each	60	2	30	0	35
Hostess Li'l Angels	1 oz	90	2	20	2	95
Hostess Twinkies	1 cake	143	4	25	21	189
Hostess Twinkies Lights	1 cake	110	2	16	0	160
Jelly beans (10)	1 oz	67	0	0	0	3
Little Debbie Oatmeal Creme cookie	1 each	170	6	32	—	125
Nabisco Devil's Food Cakes (1)	1 oz	110	1	8	0	70
Newtons, fruit bars (1–2)	1 oz	110	2	16	0	45
Oreo Big Stuff chocolate sandwich cookie (1)	1.7 oz	250	12	43	0	220
Oreo sandwich cookie (1)	⅓ oz	47	2	38	0	63
Pudding cup	5 oz	180	5	25	—	310
Snickers candy bar (1)	2.16 oz	290	14	43	0	170
Teddy Grahams (honey, cinnamon, chocolate)	11 each (½ oz)	60	2	30	0	90

Item	Amount	Calories	Fat (gms)	% Fat Calories	Cholesterol (mg)	Sodium (mg)
Toaster pastry (1)	1-¾ oz	196	6	28	0	230
Yogurt, fruit, nonfat with Aspartame	8 oz	100	0	0	5	115

— = Data not available.

Chart based on data from manufacturers or the U.S. Department of Agriculture, updated 3/91.

Charts on pages 118–149 are compiled by Linda J. Bethel, M.S., R.D., L.D., C.D.E., Bethel Nutrition Services, 1526 Nuremberg Blvd., Punta Gorda, Fla. 33983, based on manufacturers' and label data.

6

Fast Food and the Fast Track:
A Likely Pair

Of the following three choices, which is the most nutritional fast-food lunch—six chicken nuggets with hot mustard sauce, a chef salad with one ounce of ranch dressing, or a small, plain hamburger? If you answer the chef salad or chicken nuggets, you're bound to find a great deal of enlightening information in this chapter. The small hamburger is actually the best choice, with 260 calories, 33 percent of them coming from fat, and 36 milligrams of cholesterol.[1] Next are the chicken nuggets, with 58 percent of their 266 calories coming from fat and with 61 milligrams of cholesterol.[2] The hot mustard sauce brings the total up to 336 calories, 56 percent from fat, and 61 milligrams of cholesterol. Last choice

[1]Average of Wendy's Junior hamburger, McDonald's hamburger, and Burger King's hamburger.
[2]Average of McDonald's 6-piece Chicken McNuggets and Burger King's Chicken Tenders, Wendy's Crispy Chicken Nuggets, Kentucky Fried Chicken's Kentucky Nuggets, 6 each. The hot mustard sauce is available only at McDonald's.

is the chef salad. With its turkey, ham, cheese, egg toppings, and rich ranch dressing, it provides 122 milligrams of cholesterol and 317 calories, 85 percent of them from fat.[3]

Fast food blends with today's accelerated life-style but in many ways contradicts today's increasingly health-conscious attitudes. Medical and nutritional professionals continue to be concerned about the effect of fast foods on our health. The dietary guidelines that we discussed in Chapter 4 are often at odds with the staples served by most fast-food establishments. But the industry in general is responding to more healthful life-style trends by diversifying its menus to include more nutritional food choices.

Born in the mid–twentieth century as hamburger joints or ice cream stands, fast-food restaurants have evolved into international chains with thousands of outlets. Until 1980, the fast-food chains stuck with their staple items. If you were a hamburger chain, for example, all you had to do was sell hamburgers, fries, and soft drinks. But competition drove the different chains to diversify their menus, and with diversification came more choices, both good and bad, from a nutritional standpoint.

We know that if you're a fast food enthusiast, it is unrealistic to expect you to deny yourself a Big Mac, a Whopper, or any other of your fast-food favorites. But it would make nutritional sense to balance each fast-food meal you eat that is higher in fat, sodium, and/or calories with the other foods you eat that day. Here is where you can put the concept of trade-offs that we discussed in Chapter 3 to good use. (The concept is getting what you need—not too much and not too little.) So on a day when you have your Big Mac, french fries, and milk shake for dinner, try whole wheat toast, fruits, and low-fat milk or yogurt for breakfast and a light salad with a low-calorie dressing and an assortment of vegetables for lunch.

In this chapter, you will learn about the nutritional value of fast foods, from the good to the not-so-good choices. Whether you avoid or frequent fast-food chains, you may be in for some surprises.

---

[3]Average of chef salads from McDonald's, Hardees, Burger King, and Wendy's without dressing. Regular ranch dressing from Burger King.

Fast Food Is Here to Stay

Ray A. Kroc opened the doors of the first McDonald's restaurant—McDonald's Speedee Service Drive-In—in Des Plaines, Illinois, on April 15, 1955. In 1960, only 250 McDonald's dotted the landscape, and Americans chose fast-food restaurants only one in twenty times when they ate out. By 1990, the company boasted 8,300 restaurants in the United States and a total of 11,200 worldwide.

Every second, an estimated two hundred people in the United States order one or more hamburgers. The U.S. National Restaurant Association estimates that on a typical day, 45.8 million people (a fifth of the American population) are served at fast-food restaurants. Americans spend more than $70 billion a year on fast food. Each year advertising dollars spent by the fast-food industry is in the billions.

And fast-food chains are springing up on college campuses, in the suburbs, at museums, in hospitals, at department stores, in military installations and zoos, floating on the Mississippi River, and even in the Soviet Union. A McDonald's in Taiwan does twice as much business as the average United States restaurant. Domino's is now delivering in London. In France, wine is served with fast food, while Germany serves beer with its burgers.

It is not difficult to understand the phenomenal success of the fast-food industry. We can eat quickly—drive-through windows are now the norm. We can eat whenever we're hungry—twenty-four-hour or late-hour service is often available. We don't have to make a lot of decisions, since fast-food menus and recipes are uniform from one outlet to another. For the hurried, harried, and overworked, it's eat and run at reasonable prices.

The fast-food restaurant is most alluring to working parents with small children. Children are among the most frequent customers of the fast-food chains, and the major fast-food chains have been pulling out everything from video cartoons to stuffed bears to gain the youngsters' loyalty. Survey after survey indicates that parents let their children make restaurant choices. McDonald's and Burger King offer playlands for kids because they found that restaurants with playgrounds tend to bring in the whole family. Special packages have been designed for children, like McDonald's "Happy Meal," Hardee's "Action Meal," and Arby's "Adventure Meal." Ronald McDonald, with the help of advertising dollars and

Saturday-morning television, has become as well known to children as Santa Claus. And roughly one-third of McDonald's 20
million customers each week are children.

Some of the people you met earlier in this book are very opinion-
ated about fast food, generally in a negative way. Some of them
may share your views.

Carole Gerber, a freelance writer who often lunches at her desk,
eats pizza from Pizza Hut twice a week, and she occasionally eats at
Wendy's salad bar when she gets out. But her general response to
other kinds of fast foods is negative: "I can't eat fast foods because
they make me sick. I don't like the taste, and I find the food too
salty." Judy Markey, a syndicated columnist who doesn't describe
herself as health conscious, concurs, describing fast foods as "too
heavy."

Jane Hartley, a working mother who lives in Manhattan, fre-
quents a McDonald's on the Upper East Side once a week with her
daughter. The restaurant is conveniently located near the child's
school, and the small merry-go-round is certainly an attraction for
children. Jane orders a chocolate-chip cookie with milk because
she says she's "afraid to order the other stuff."

Barry Nash, aware of fats in his diet and consciously trying to cut
down on them, lunches almost weekly on a fast-food hamburger,
fries, and a Coke to save time during a hectic work day. Pritikin-
follower Herb Glimcher, who also avoids fats in his diet, occasionally eats fast food, but his choice is a careful one. He orders a
grilled-chicken sandwich (without the skin) with lettuce and tomato and no sauces or mayonnaise on the bread.

New York executive Burt Staniar has stayed away from fast
foods for several years, part of a general change toward a healthier
life-style as he approached forty. He attributes his decision to "the
fat content—and I can't stand the taste anymore."

The Positives and Negatives of Fast Foods

But where does all this lead us in terms of our nutrition? Many
before us have asked whether a lifetime of fast foods could place
our nation's children at greater risk of developing chronic diseases
such as atherosclerosis, cancer, and obesity and deficiencies in vitamins and other nutrients.

Earlier, we discussed dietary recommendations made by prestigious organizations that are based on a wealth of scientific evidence. Americans are told to reduce their intake of total fat, saturated fat, cholesterol, sodium, and sugar. We are told to increase our intake of foods rich in fiber and calcium, to get the recommended levels of vitamins and minerals, to eat only moderate levels of protein, especially animal protein, and to maintain our body weight through a proper balance of calorie intake and physical activity. Let's look at how fast foods fit in with these recommendations.

In general, the majority of fast-food meals tend to be high in calories. And most of the high-calorie foods are also high in saturated fat. Choice is the key to calorie control, and fast-food menus today are sufficiently varied to permit that control if you are informed and careful. The total calories from a fast-food meal can range from 300 to nearly 1,500. And the number of calories in typical fast-food meals is often out of proportion to the amount of nutrients.

A high proportion of calories in most fast-food meals comes from fat—between 40 and 55 percent, or more. In fact, you'll be hard pressed to find many low-fat foods on fast-food menus. Fat tastes good, and taste is certainly a factor equal to convenience when considering the success of the fast-food industry. Fried food tastes good. So if the food isn't high in fat to begin with—and much of it is—it is drenched in fat (sometimes beef fat) and deep fried or fried on a grill before you buy it.

The perfect example is chicken nuggets, introduced by McDonald's in 1983. In its natural state, chicken is much lower in saturated fat and total fat than red meats. But after being deep fried, the fat content of six chicken nuggets surpasses that of a single hamburger. (Fat composes 32 to 59 percent of the calories in a fast-food hamburger.) Deep-frying more than triples the calories supplied by fat. For example, Kentucky Fried Chicken's Extra Crispy version is 45 percent more fatty than its Original Recipe (also fried), which is high in fat to begin with.

In addition, chicken nuggets and chicken-patty sandwiches are often made with processed chicken and ground-up chicken skin, high in fat. Chicken Tenders at Burger King (236 calories, 50 percent fat), made from whole pieces of chicken and fried in vegetable oil, contain fewer calories and less fat than McDonald's Chicken McNuggets (270 calories, 50 percent fat), Wendy's Crispy Chicken

Nuggets (280 calories, 64 percent fat), or Kentucky Fried Chicken's Kentucky Nuggets (276 calories, 59 percent fat).

Usually, the sandwiches are loaded with mayonnaise as well, adding even more fat. Burger King's Specialty Chicken Sandwich has one of the highest fat contents of all chicken products made by fast-food chains (40 grams of fat, with 53 percent of its 685 calories coming from fat). But if you order it without mayonnaise, you cut the fat by half (along with 200 calories). Taco Bell's Taco Salad, despite the word "salad," drums up 58 percent of its 941 calories from fat. With the cheese, sour cream, and guacamole piled on top of the lettuce and tomato, that shouldn't be too much of a surprise. Remember that fat has more than twice as many calories per gram as do carbohydrates and protein, so fatty foods are generally high-calorie foods.

Try to limit your family's consumption to only one fried food per meal (or trade off by reducing the amount of fat contained in other meals eaten throughout the day). In other words, don't have fried chicken and french fries at one meal. Instead of french fries, try baked potatoes without butter, cheese sauce, or sour cream. An 8-ounce baked potato has 250 calories, while 4 ounces of french fries provides more than 300 calories—less food at a greater caloric cost. Remove the skin from fried chicken and order large pieces of fish or chicken if they've been fried. Tidbits like clams and nuggets have more grease in proportion to the meat.

Many fast-food restaurants advertise that their products contain 100 percent vegetable oil. This is not necessarily positive—it depends on what *kind* of vegetable oil is used. Palm and coconut oils are vegetable oils, so they don't contain cholesterol; but they are highly saturated, even more saturated than beef fat. Other vegetable oils, which are naturally highly unsaturated, become more saturated when they are repeatedly subjected to the high cooking temperatures used in frying foods.

A typical fast-food sandwich contains between 700 and 900 milligrams of sodium (salt), sometimes higher. The National Research Council recommends a 2,400-milligram-a-day sodium limit, and the federally recommended daily allowance of sodium is 1,100 to 3,300 milligrams; but the human requirement for sodium is less than 200 milligrams per day. Specialty items such as triple cheeseburgers, roast beef sandwiches with cheese, and cheeseburgers with bacon can contain a day's supply of sodium. Ham, sausage, and bacon add a lot of sodium to food. Hardee's Big Country Breakfast (Country Ham) offers a walloping 1,780 milligrams of sodium, and its Big Country Breakfast (Sausage) racks up 1,980 milligrams. Other big sodium suppliers include Arby's Bac'n Cheddar Deluxe (1,672) and its Sub Deluxe (1,530); Taco Bell's Taco Salad with Salsa (1,662); Wendy's Bacon and Cheese Potato (1,460); Hardee's Hot Ham 'n Cheese (1,420) and Three Pancakes with 1 Sausage Pattie (1,290); Burger King's Chicken Specialty Sandwich (1,417 milligrams) and Double Whopper with Cheese (1,245); and McDonald's Biscuit with Sausage (1,040). French fries, ketchup, a milk shake, or a pastry will raise the sodium content of a meal as well.

Surprisingly, Arby's and Hardee's chocolate shakes, with around 340 milligrams of sodium, surpass a strip of Wendy's bacon (100 milligrams) and McDonald's large french fries (200 milligrams). French fries are at the lower end for sodium content of the fast foods offered. Wendy's regular french fries have 145 milligrams of sodium; McDonald's have 110 milligrams; and Burger King, which says that you can ask for french fries without the salt, adds 241 milligrams of sodium to its medium-size fries. Fried foods can spell double trouble, though, because it's tempting to add a little extra salt to greasy foods. Finding a fast-food entree that is appropriate for a salt-restricted diet is difficult. Stick with the baked potato and salad bar (minus the bacon bits, cheese, croutons, or Chinese noodles) and limit your salad dressing if you're watching your sodium intake.

Fast-food meals tend to be low in dietary fiber. Sources of fiber—fruits, vegetables, and whole-grain cereals—have not been traditional fast-food offerings. But since the late 1970s, high-fiber foods have been available at salad bars, especially those offering kidney or garbanzo beans and fruit. (McDonald's also now offers Wheaties, Cheerios, and fat-free apple bran and blueberry bran muffins at many of its outlets.) The trend toward salad bars is a positive one, from a nutritional standpoint. But for the majority of fast-food chains, set up to sell only preassembled items, salad bars require high maintenance and are less profitable.

Along with soluble fiber, salads are good sources of vitamins A and C, nutrients that are limited in other fast-food items and are among those most commonly lacking in American diets. Sources for vitamin A include dark-green leafy vegetables and bright-orange fruits and vegetables. Vitamin C is found in abundance in citrus fruits as well as in red and green peppers, tomatoes, and dark, leafy greens.

You need to be selective and use restraint at salad bars, sticking with fresh fruits and vegetables and going easy on high-fat items such as meats, cheese, nuts, seeds, and dressings. Salads can be low in calories, sodium, and fat, provided reduced-calorie salad dressings are used and selections exclude such items as macaroni and potato salads, croutons, bacon bits, and cheese. Just a tablespoon of sunflower seeds adds 50 calories and 4 grams of fat to a salad. The same amount of cheese or bacon bits contributes 25 to 30 calories and 2 grams of fat. Keep in mind that most people use multiple-tablespoon helpings of these toppings. Regular salad dressings contain approximately 70 calories per tablespoon, and a typical salad-bar ladle can hold up to four tablespoons (about 280 calories) of salad dressing! Half a cup of potato salad can add 250 calories to your meal.

While the salad bar provides many foods rich in vitamin C, the daily requirement for this nutrient (60 milligrams) can be obtained by drinking just four ounces of orange juice, an item offered by many fast-food restaurants today. The oversized baked potato contains more than half of the daily vitamin C allowance—even more if the potato is topped with broccoli.

Iron is also a nutrient in abundance, particularly in meat-oriented fast-food outlets. A typical roast beef or large hamburger sandwich contains about 25 percent of the U.S. RDA for this mineral. Most of the iron-rich foods are typically high in fat and calories. McDonald's Big Mac, Hardee's Big Twin, and Burger King's double burgers get 50–60 percent of their calories from fat and provide 20–25 percent of the U.S. RDA of iron. Lean roast beef sandwiches without creamy sauces are the better bet. Only 30–40 percent of their calories come from fat. Additional iron can be found at the salad bar in garbanzo beans, broccoli, cauliflower, spinach, and raisins.

Calcium is a mineral in short supply in the typical fast-food meal. We talked about the danger of low-calcium diets in Chapter 2. To offset low calcium levels in the meal you order, accompany your meal with low-fat milk or a milk shake (the latter is high in sugar and calories) instead of soda or coffee—both are available at most fast-food restaurants. The milk-based beverages are also good sources of vitamins A and D. And there's good news for pizza fans: one slice provides 33 percent of the daily recommended intake for calcium, which is 800 milligrams.

The virtues of protein are typically promoted by fast-food chains, since much of their foods have an abundance of it. Protein in fast-food meals does provide iron, thiamine, niacin, and zinc. A typical meal contains high-quality protein that meets between 50 and 100 percent of the daily recommended amount of protein for your body size and age. So if some protein is good, more must be better, right?

Not really. The dietary guidelines discussed in Chapter 4 advised you to maintain protein at moderate levels—12 to 15 percent of your daily calories. An excess of protein promotes calcium excretion and could lead to osteoporosis. Other studies suggest a link between high-protein diets and loss of renal function in later adulthood. While the possible adverse effects of too much protein are still speculative, they should be considered. Furthermore, too many calories all end up in the same place, whether they're fat, carbohydrate, or protein calories.

Which brings us to sugar. Sugary beverages and desserts are a common component of the fast-food meal. Dairy Queen, with its variety of desserts and beverages, offers more high-sugar foods than other fast-food chains, although it is now possible to get non-fat frozen yogurt at a DQ. Again, the major problem with sugar-laden foods is that they contribute too many calories and too few nutrients. All the calories in regular soft drinks come from sugar— more than 5 teaspoons are contained in the average 8-ounce drink, 8 teaspoons in 12 ounces. A fast-food shake may contain as many as 14 teaspoons of sugar. Nonetheless, a milk shake is still a better beverage choice than a soft drink, since most are made from dried-milk products and supply significant amounts of protein, calcium, riboflavin, and niacin. One of the least caloric and least fatty desserts we found was McDonald's Strawberry Lowfat Frozen Yogurt Sundae, with 210 calories and 1 gram of fat (4 percent fat calories) in a 6-ounce serving. McDonald's also offers low-fat cones and shakes, which are great choices. In sum, drink low-fat milk or fruit juice instead of the sugary beverages, and if you have a sweet tooth, try some fresh fruit, sorbet, or frozen yogurt (if available) instead of a pastry, cookie, or sundae.

Unfortunately, sugar is often added to fast foods for taste or appearance. The french fries have a sugar coating that browns when it hits hot grease. The batter coatings on many foods contain sugar as well.

Healthful Fast-Food Trends: An Appeal to the Nutrition-Minded Customer

Most fast-food restaurants have responded to the concern of many Americans toward lighter eating. Innovations have been made over the last decade at various restaurants in both the way food is prepared and the variety of new foods offered. Before 1980, fast food had no interest in new products. Now the chains are rushing to catch up with their customers: adding dishes that are grilled or broiled, not fried; cooking fries in vegetable oil instead of beef fat. Even the chain whose middle name is Fried— Kentucky Fried Chicken—is experimenting with broiled chicken, now offers Lite 'n Crispy skinless fried chicken, and has switched its logo to simply say "KFC."

It is important to note here that some of the changes made at fast-food chains to improve the nutritional quality of their food have been met in the past less than enthusiastically by the fast-food customer, so change has taken time and experimentation. People said they wanted less fat, but when Wendy's began cooking its french fries in vegetable oil instead of beef fat in the late 1980s, customers backed off. "People want lower sodium, lower fat, and less cholesterol," said Wendy's spokesperson Dennis Lynch, "but it must taste good or they won't buy it. It's an ongoing challenge for the fast-food industry to find food that is nutritionally balanced and has taste appeal."

To meet that challenge and address other trends, Wendy's developed the salad bar in 1979. Since Wendy's is set up to prepare many of its foods on the restaurant's premises each day, the salad bar was a successful way to address the growing national interest in more nutritional foods, as well as the trends of working women, two-income families, and rising beef prices. Rax, a chain predominantly in the Midwest, offers a Mexican bar and a selection of puddings alongside its salad bar. McDonald's experimented with salad bars as far back as 1974 but rejected them because they were often messy and expensive to operate; so it countered its competition in 1987 with prepackaged salads, with costs it could control. The best selections are a garden salad, shrimp salad, or chunky chicken salad, all with the low-cal dressing. The chef salad includes ham and cheese, which raise fat and sodium contents.

As we have seen, a problem with salad bars is that they can offer a great selection of fatty foods, such as macaroni and potato salads, rich salad dressings, and appetizing toppings. But the fresh fruits and vegetables provide fiber, vitamins, and minerals and are low in fat and calories. And many chains offer low-calorie dressings.

Meanwhile, some fast-food restaurants have introduced baked potatoes, following Wendy's lead. A plain baked potato is fine, since it is only 250 calories. But if you add bacon and cheese (it's really a cheese sauce or an imitation cheese topping), the calories add up as well, to the tune of 520, along with large doses of fat and cholesterol.

Wendy's test-marketed a "Light Menu" in 1985 which included the plain baked potato, the salad bar and the side salad, diet soft drinks, and the multi-grain bun. While only 20 percent of Wendy's sandwiches were sold on the multi-grain bun in 1985, the company had high hopes, predicting these bun sales would increase to 80 percent by 1990. Instead, after a full year of advertising, customer response was still not good, and the bun was phased out in 1988–89. Wendy's still offers the baked potato and has built the salad bar into a three-section, fifty-item "SuperBar," an all-you-can-eat hot-and-cold-food bar that includes an enhanced salad section of thirty items, including fresh fruits and vegetables rotated according to season and two to five reduced-calorie dressings, an Italian section, and Mexican fare.

Several other chains test-marketed items considered to be more nutritional. Others advertised their nutritional assets. In 1988, Burger King went so far as to pour $200 million into an advertising campaign touting broiled over fried burgers, as a direct attack on McDonald's.

The switch from animal fats to vegetable oils was also made visible to consumers through advertising. In 1986, reacting to consumer concerns and criticism for its use of a cholesterol-rich blend of animal and vegetable oil to deep-fry its Chicken McNuggets and Filet-O-Fish, McDonald's switched to pure vegetable shortening for those products as well as its hot pies. Hardee's, since June 1988, had been the only chain of the top five using all-vegetable oil for its french fries. The others used beef tallow blended with a little vegetable oil because they found that customers preferred the taste of the animal-fat blend. (Beef tallow contains cholesterol and is high in saturated fat, while vegetable oil has no cholesterol and tends to be high in unsaturated fat, considered better for the heart. But let's face facts here—french fries are still a fatty food.) Suddenly, in late July of 1990, Burger King, Wendy's, and McDonald's vowed to start cooking french fries in 100 percent vegetable oil by year's end. Just two months earlier, in May 1990, Rax restaurants, which specialize in roast beef, became one of the first fast-food chains to use a name-brand vegetable oil. It began cooking its french fries and other deep-fried foods in Crisco oil as part of a venture with Procter and Gamble to move the fast-food industry away from animal fats.

Actually, Rax has long been an innovator in this area. In 1984, the chain contacted the American Heart Association in order to assess what items on its menu fit the AHA's guidelines in regard to dietary fat and cholesterol, calories, and sodium. Rax became the first chain to name those menu items meeting the dietary guidelines of the AHA so customers could know which foods were considered healthy choices. The regular roast beef sandwich, the large roast beef sandwich with only lettuce and tomato, and certain salad-bar items at Rax were among those that made the AHA list. Arby's and other chains later followed Rax's lead.

Chicken and fish sandwiches are offered by most hamburger chains, but they also may be deep-fried in beef fat. However, more and more chains are offering baked fish and grilled, skinless chicken breast on their menus. Since 1986, the purveyors of fast food have been slimming down their offerings. Burger King, Wendy's, Hardee's, and Rax now offer a grilled-chicken sandwich. Add fresh vegetables and ask for any added sauces on the side so you can control the amounts.

Even Kentucky Fried Chicken has been test-marketing broiled chicken in cities like Louisville, Las Vegas, and Canberra, Australia. Grilled chicken will be Kentucky Fried Chicken's first fundamental menu change since the company was founded in 1955 by Harland Sanders, known as the Colonel. Propelled by sagging earnings, Kentucky Fried Chicken sees its middle name as a liability at a time when more Americans are turning away from anything fried as their concern about fat and cholesterol mounts. In fact, an economist with the National Broiler Council, a Washington trade group for chicken producers, recently predicted, "Over the next two or three years, the proportion of chicken grilled, baked, or broiled could easily double. There are a lot of people out there—nobody knows how many—who say, 'I love chicken, but I just won't eat it fried.' "

While not on anyone's nutritional A-list, the Egg McMuffin began the breakfast trend at fast-food restaurants. In 1972, McDonald's put an egg, cheese, and Canadian bacon in the middle of an English muffin and began selling the product in selected markets. It was formally introduced in 1973, and by 1976 Egg McMuffin was a national product and breakfast was a fast-food phenomenon. Unfortunately, the Egg McMuffin offered a day's supply of cholesterol, 740 milligrams of sodium, and nearly half of its 293 calories from fat calories. A trimmer Egg McMuffin now provides 280 calories (35 percent from fat) and 710 milligrams of sodium. And the Egg McMuffin opened the door to the development of other, lower-fat breakfast foods, such as pancakes, English muffins, and fruit juices, offered by many of the fast-food chains today. McDonald's has added to its breakfast menu low-fat milk (1 percent), and, as we mentioned earlier, Wheaties, Cheerios, and fat-free muffins.

Pizza has been the fastest-growing fast food and is one of the best nutritional bets, if you choose wisely. While traditional toppings such as pepperoni, ground beef, and sausage add hefty amounts of fat and salt, one slice of plain cheese pizza (or a cheese pizza with vegetable toppings), contains 9 grams of fat, about half saturated and half unsaturated. About 33 percent of the calories come from fat (close to the recommended 30 percent range). The tomato sauce contains vitamin A; the cheese provides protein and calcium; and both the cheese and the crust contain B vitamins.

Pizza Hut, with 6,300 domestic outlets, is the largest of the pizza chains; Domino's is second with 4,800. Both chains now provide home delivery service. In 1990 Pizza Hut tested a Light Pizza with a one-third reduction in fat in its outlets in Columbus, Ohio, and San Diego. That product is back in development due to customer dissatisfaction. Since July 1989 McDonald's has been testing McPizza in a half-dozen test markets, such as Evansville, Indiana; Fresno, California; and Hartford, Connecticut. McDonald's developed and patented an oven that bakes the pizza in five and a half minutes with superheated air. National introduction is uncertain. The company is known for lengthy test-marketing of new products before national introduction—it spent seven years testing salads before rolling them out nationally.

No new product has made the McDonald's menu faster than the McLean Deluxe, McDonald's low-fat hamburger which hit the market in April 1991, five years after it was proposed and only five months after it began test marketing. The fat in the ground beef is replaced with another substance that retains moisture called carrageenan. McDonald's says the process yields a burger that contains 10 grams of fat and 320 calories versus the 20.7 grams of fat and 410 calories of a Quarter Pounder. The McLean Deluxe was developed by Auburn University in conjunction with the Beef Industry Council.

In response to the demands for information, more and more fast-food chains have contracted for direct analyses of the nutrient composition of their food and beverage items. Some fast-food chains, however, are reluctant to release data because menu and recipe changes have made many of them outdated. Others have not yet analyzed their foods, in part because composition and trace-mineral analyses are quite costly. Some chains have determined nutrient values of their foods by using recipe contents and nutrient-composition data, thus avoiding the costs of direct chemical analyses.

McDonald's became the first chain to consent to a government agency's request to make ingredient information available to patrons in its company-owned outlets in New York State in 1986. McDonald's also has a nutritional information number: (708) 575-6198. Other large chains also offer information, typically through their consumer affairs departments. Today, both ingredient and nutrition information is available in booklet form upon request at most fast-food restaurants. McDonald's began to post this information in its restaurants in the United States in the summer of 1990. And if recommendations from a September 1990 report from the Institute of Medicine (part of the National Academy of Sciences) are adopted, ingredient and nutrition information will be required by *all* fast-food restaurants in the future.

Some chains have even attempted to make nutrition their main focus. In 1981, Atlanta-based D'Lites was opened by a former health-club owner and Wendy's franchisee. It offered a multi-grain bun, "lite" mayonnaise on its sandwiches, and lower-calorie versions of many traditional fish and chicken items. In August of 1986, D'Lites cut back from 100 to 10 outlets, all in Atlanta, when financial stresses forced the chain to reorganize under bankruptcy law. Apparently, the public wasn't willing to eat "healthy" fast food.

Nutritional fast food, a 1980s trend, didn't change the system significantly. But it may have stimulated established fast-food operators to introduce low-calorie, low-fat, low-sodium, and low-sugar alternatives to traditional fast food.

So for overall healthful eating tips at fast-food chains, remember that special sauces, ketchup, tartar sauce, and mayonnaise all add up. Order items plain, or scrape off the sauces. Ordering fish without tartar sauce at Long John Silver's, for example, saves more than 120 calories—the seafood sauce has only 35 calories and no fat. McDonald's Filet-O-Fish minus tartar sauce saves a third of the calories and almost two-thirds of the fat. A Burger King Whopper without mayonnaise saves almost 150 calories and 16 grams of fat; a BK Broiler minus the sauce saves 90 calories and more than half the fat. An ounce of McDonald's barbecue sauce contains more than 300 milligrams of sodium, almost three times as much as in a regular order of fries. Arby's Horsey Sauce gets nearly half its calories from fat—a 1-ounce serving yields 120 calories.

Also limit cheeseburgers, which add extra fat. One slice of cheese adds more than 80 calories to McDonald's Quarter Pounder.

Order potatoes plain or with vegetables, and cut out the cheese topping and sour cream. At salad bars, load up on fresh vegetables and fruit, without sauces or dressings, and use low-fat salad dressings, or vinegar with just a little oil. Avoid processed meats such as bacon, pepperoni, and sausage—they're high in sodium and fat. Each of the handy packets of croutons or chow mein noodles adds 50 calories to a salad.

To cut your salt intake, hold the pickles, mustard, ketchup, and special sauce. Leave out the cheese and avoid ordering processed meats such as bacon, ham, sausage, and hot dogs. If you're a pizza lover, stick with cheese (in lesser amounts if possible, but mozzarella is a low-fat cheese) and choose toppings like peppers and onions rather than sausage, pepperoni, salami, ham, anchovies, or olives. That way you'll add flavor without adding sodium, fat, and calories.

To get fiber, choose from the salad bar or prepackaged salads.

Fresh fruits and fruits canned in their own juice, not in syrup, are good sources of fiber without added calories. Choose items that are not coated with any form of dressing. Beans, like kidney and garbanzo beans, tend to be high in fiber and protein. Cereals and bran muffins are also good sources of fiber.

Avoid the biscuits, croissants, bacon, ham, eggs, and sausage syndrome at breakfast. The Sausage-and-Egg Croissant at Arby's contains 645 milligrams of cholesterol—more than twice the total daily dose recommended by the American Heart Association. An Egg McMuffin at McDonald's contains the equivalent of four tea-spoonsful of fat. Even scrambled eggs, scrambled on a greasy grill, tend to have higher percentages of fat than the hamburger and roast beef sandwiches.

Fish and chicken items can pose the biggest trap for the nutrition-conscious but underinformed. Many people just assume that chicken and fish are "better for you" than beef and tell themselves that they're "watching themselves" by ordering a chicken or fish sandwich at a fast-food restaurant. Unfortunately, many of these restaurants deep-fry their chicken and fish and leave on the fatty skin. And since many restaurants use saturated fats for frying, the fish and chicken may contain even more fat than a hamburger. McDonald's Filet-O-Fish provides 44 percent of its 370 calories from fat. Kentucky Fried Chicken's Original Recipe Drumstick, Chicken Little Sandwich, and Colonel's Chicken Sandwich all derive more than 50 percent of their calories from fat. At Arby's, the Regular Roast Beef Sandwich has less than half the fat and no more saturated fat than a Roast Chicken Club or Chicken Cordon Bleu.

In sum, when you do order deep-fried foods, discard the breading and batter and avoid the "extra crispy" versions. Be wary of words such as "grande" and "deluxe" as they refer to burgers (or pizza or any sandwiches, for that matter) or those terms will soon apply to your body. Cut toppings and sauces, for the most part. And, most important, be aware of what you're ordering!

Fast-Food Chart

Here's how the top five fast-food chains—McDonald's, Burger King, Kentucky Fried Chicken, Wendy's, and Hardee's—stack up nutritionally.

NUTRIENT ABBREVIATIONS USED AT THE TOP OF THE FAST-FOOD TABLES

WT = Weight (grams)
CAL = Calories
CARB = Carbohydrate (grams)
PRO = Protein (grams)
FAT = Fat (grams)
FAT % Cal = Fat (% of Calories)
   OR % Fat Calories
SAT = Saturated fat (grams)
CHOL = Cholesterol (milligrams)

SOD = Sodium (milligrams)
POT = Potassium (milligrams)
A = Vitamin A
C = Vitamin C
THIA = Thiamine
RIBO = Riboflavin
NIA = Niacin
CA = Calcium
IRON = Iron

Nutrients in Fast Foods

McDONALD'S

BREAKFAST

Menu Item	WT (g)	CAL	CARB (g)	PRO (g)	FAT (g)	FAT % Cal	SAT (g)	CHOL (mg)	SOD (mg)	POT (mg)	A	C	THIA	RIBO	NIA	CA	IRON
											Percentage of U.S. RDA						
Egg McMuffin®	135	280	28	18	11	35	4.0	224	710	—	10	*	30	20	20	25	15
Hotcakes with Margarine & Syrup	174	410	74	8	9	20	1.5	8	640	—	4	*	20	20	15	10	10
Scrambled Eggs (2)	100	140	1	12	10	64	3.0	399	290	—	10	*	4	15	*	6	10
Sausage	43	160	0	7	15	84	5.0	43	310	—	*	*	15	6	10	*	4
English Muffin	58	170	26	5	5	26	0.8	0	230	—	2	*	20	8	10	15	8
Hash Brown Potatoes	53	130	15	1	7	48	1.0	0	330	—	*	2	4	*	4	*	*
Biscuit with Biscuit Spread	75	260	32	5	13	45	3.4	1	730	—	*	*	15	6	8	8	8
Biscuit with Sausage	118	420	32	12	28	60	8.0	44	1040	—	*	*	30	10	20	8	10

Menu Item	WT (g)	CAL	CARB (g)	PRO (g)	FAT (g)	FAT % Cal	SAT (g)	CHOL (mg)	SOD (mg)	POT (mg)	A	C	THIA	RIBO	NIA	CA	IRON
														Percentage of U.S. RDA			
Biscuit with Sausage & Egg	175	500	33	19	33	59	10.0	270	1210	—	6	*	30	20	20	10	20
Biscuit with Bacon, Egg & Cheese	153	430	33	15	26	54	8.0	248	1190	—	10	*	25	20	10	20	15
Sausage McMuffin®	109	345	27	15	20	52	7.0	57	770	—	4	*	35	15	25	20	15
Sausage McMuffin with Egg®	159	415	27	21	25	54	8.0	256	915	—	10	*	35	25	25	25	20
Cheerios®, ¾ cup	19	80	14	3	1	11	0.2	0	210	—	15	15	15	15	15	2	30
Wheaties®, ¾ cup	23	90	19	2	1	10	0.1	0	220	—	20	20	20	20	20	2	20

MUFFINS AND DANISH

Menu Item	WT (g)	CAL	CARB (g)	PRO (g)	FAT (g)	FAT % Cal	SAT (g)	CHOL (mg)	SOD (mg)	POT (mg)	A	C	THIA	RIBO	NIA	CA	IRON
Fat-Free Apple Bran Muffin	75	170	39	4	0	0	0	0	200	—	*	*	6	6	2	2	4
Fat-Free Blueberry Muffin	75	170	40	3	0	0	0	0	220	—	*	*	6	6	4	8	4
Apple Danish	115	390	51	6	17	39	4.0	25	370	—	*	25	20	10	10	*	8
Iced Cheese Danish	110	390	42	7	21	48	6.0	47	420	—	4	*	20	15	10	4	8

SANDWICHES AND FRENCH FRIES

Raspberry Danish	117	410	62	6	16	35	3.0	26	310	—	*	6	20	10	10	*	8
Cinnamon Raisin Danish	110	440	58	6	21	43	5.0	34	430	—	*	6	20	15	15	4	10
Hamburger	102	250	29	10	9	32	3.0	37	490	—	4	4	20	10	20	10	15
Cheeseburger	114	300	29	15	12	36	4.0	50	710	—	8	4	20	15	20	20	15
Quarter Pounder®	164	410	34	23	20	44	8.0	85	650	—	4	6	25	15	35	15	20
Quarter Pounder® with Cheese	189	490	33	28	26	48	10.0	114	1090	—	15	6	25	20	35	30	20
Big Mac	212	500	42	25	26	47	9.0	100	930	—	6	2	30	25	35	25	20
McLean Deluxe	206	320	35	22	10	28	4.0	60	670	—	10	10	25	20	35	15	20
McLean Deluxe with Cheese	219	370	35	24	14	34	5.0	75	890	—	15	10	25	20	35	20	20
McD.L.T.®	229	510	35	26	30	53	10.0	106	960	—	15	10	25	20	35	20	20
Filet-O-Fish®	141	370	38	14	18	44	4.0	50	1020	—	2	*	20	8	15	15	10

Menu Item	WT (g)	CAL	CARB (g)	PRO (g)	FAT (g)	FAT % Cal	SAT (g)	CHOL (mg)	SOD (mg)	POT (mg)	A	C	THIA	RIBO	NIA	CA	IRON
											Percentage of U.S. RDA						
McChicken®	187	415	39	19	20	43	4.0	42	770	—	2	4	60	10	45	15	15
Small French Fries	68	220	26	3	12	49	2.5	0	110	—	*	15	10	*	10	*	2
Medium French Fries	97	320	36	4	17	48	3.5	0	150	—	*	20	15	*	15	*	4
Large French Fries	122	400	46	6	22	50	4.5	0	200	—	*	25	15	*	15	*	6

CHICKEN MCNUGGETS® AND SAUCES

Menu Item	WT (g)	CAL	CARB (g)	PRO (g)	FAT (g)	FAT % Cal	SAT (g)	CHOL (mg)	SOD (mg)	POT (mg)	A	C	THIA	RIBO	NIA	CA	IRON
Chicken McNuggets®, 6 pieces	109	270	17	20	15	50	3.5	56	580	—	*	*	8	8	40	*	6
Hot Mustard Sauce, 1.05 oz	30	70	8	0	4	51	0.5	5	250	—	*	*	*	*	*	2	*
Barbecue Sauce, 1.12 oz	32	50	12	0	0.5	9	0.1	0	340	—	4	4	*	*	*	*	2
Sweet 'N Sour Sauce, 1.12 oz	32	60	14	0	0.2	3	0	0	190	—	6	*	*	*	*	*	*
Honey, ½ oz	14	45	12	0	0	0	0	0	0	—	*	*	*	*	*	*	*

SALADS AND SALAD DRESSINGS

Chef Salad	265	170	8	17	9	48	3.6	111	400	—	100	35	20	15	20	15	8
Garden Salad	189	50	6	4	2	36	0.6	65	70	—	90	35	6	6	2	4	8
Chunky Chicken Salad	255	150	7	25	4	24	1.0	78	230	—	170	45	15	10	45	4	6
Side Salad	106	30	4	2	1	30	0.3	33	35	—	80	20	4	4	*	2	4
Croutons	11	50	7	1	2	36	0.5	0	140	—	*	*	4	*	2	*	*
Bacon Bits	3	15	0	1	1	60	0.5	1	95	—	*	*	*	*	*	*	*
Bleu Cheese Dressing, 1 tbsp (5/packet)	14	70	1	0	7	90	1.2	6	150	—	*	*	*	*	*	*	*
Ranch Reduced Calorie Dressing, 1 tbsp (4/packet)	14	55	1	0	5	82	1.0	5	130	—	*	*	*	*	*	*	*
1000 Island Dressing, 1 tbsp (5/packet)	14	78	2	0	8	92	1.0	8	100	—	*	*	*	*	*	*	*
Lite Vinaigrette Dressing, 1 tbsp (4/packet)	14	15	2	0	0.5	30	0.1	0	60	—	*	*	*	*	*	*	*

Menu Item	WT (g)	CAL	CARB (g)	PRO (g)	FAT (g)	FAT % Cal	SAT (g)	CHOL (mg)	SOD (mg)	POT (mg)	A	C	THIA	RIBO	NIA	CA	IRON
													Percentage of U.S. RDA				
Red French Reduced Calorie Dressing, 1 tbsp (4/packet)	14	40	5	0	2	45	0.3	0	115	—	*	*	*	*	*	*	*

DESSERTS AND MILK SHAKES

Menu Item	WT (g)	CAL	CARB (g)	PRO (g)	FAT (g)	FAT % Cal	SAT (g)	CHOL (mg)	SOD (mg)	POT (mg)	A	C	THIA	RIBO	NIA	CA	IRON
Vanilla Lowfat Frozen Yogurt Cone, 3 oz	80	105	22	4	1	9	0.4	3	80	—	2	*	2	10	2	10	*
Strawberry Lowfat Frozen Yogurt Sundae, 6 oz	171	210	49	6	1	4	0.6	5	95	—	4	2	4	20	*	20	*
Hot Fudge Lowfat Frozen Yogurt Sundae, 6 oz	169	240	50	7	3	11	2.3	6	170	—	4	*	6	20	*	25	2
Hot Caramel Lowfat Frozen Yogurt Sundae, 6 oz	174	270	59	7	3	10	1.5	13	180	—	6	*	6	20	*	20	*

Apple Pie, 3 oz	83	260	30	2	15	52	4.8	6	240	—	*	20	4	*	*	*	4
Vanilla Lowfat Milk Shake, 10.4 oz	293	290	60	11	1	3	0.6	10	170	—	6	*	8	30	*	35	*
Chocolate Lowfat Milk Shake, 10.4 oz	293	320	66	11	2	6	0.7	10	240	—	6	*	8	30	2	35	*
Strawberry Lowfat Milk Shake, 10.4 oz	293	320	67	11	1	3	0.6	10	170	—	6	*	8	30	2	35	*
McDonaldland Cookies, 2 oz	56	290	47	4	9	28	1.9	0	300	—	*	*	15	10	10	*	10
Chocolaty Chip Cookies, 2 oz	56	330	42	4	16	44	5.0	4	280	—	*	*	10	10	10	2	10

BEVERAGES

1% Lowfat Milk, 8 fluid oz	244	110	12	9	2	16	1.6	10	130	—	10	4	8	30	*	30	*
Orange Juice, 6 fluid oz	183	80	19	1	0	0	0	0	0	—	*	120	10	*	*	*	*
Grapefruit Juice, 6 fluid oz	183	80	19	1	0	0	0	0	0	—	*	100	4	2	2	*	*
Apple Juice, 6 fluid oz	183	91	23	0	0	0	0	0	5	—	*	2	2	*	*	*	4

Menu Item	WT (g)	CAL	CARB (g)	PRO (g)	FAT (g)	FAT % Cal	SAT (g)	CHOL (mg)	SOD (mg)	POT (mg)	A	C	THIA	RIBO	NIA	CA	IRON
											\		Percentage of U.S. RDA				
Coca-Cola Classic®, 16 fluid oz (medium with ice)	454	190	50	0	0	0	0	0	20	—	*	*	*	*	*	*	*
Diet Coke®, 16 fluid oz (medium with ice)	454	1	1	0	0	0	0	0	40	—	*	*	*	*	*	*	*
Sprite®, 16 fluid oz (medium with ice)	454	190	48	0	0	0	0	0	20	—	*	*	*	*	*	*	*
Orange Drink, 16 fluid oz (medium with ice)	454	180	44	0	0	0	0	0	15	—	*	*	*	*	*	*	*

* = Less than 2% U.S. RDA; — = Data not available.

Chart based on data provided by the McDonald's Nutrition Information Center, McDonald's Corporation, Oak Brook, Ill. 60521. Values are based on March 1991 national menu data and represent analyses from Hazleton Laboratories America, Inc., Madison, Wis., combined with data from the U.S. Department of Agriculture and suppliers.

BURGER KING

Menu Item	WT (g)	CAL	CARB (g)	PRO (g)	FAT (g)	FAT % Cal	SAT (g)	CHOL (mg)	SOD (mg)	POT (mg)	A	C	THIA	RIBO	NIA	CA	IRON
														Percentage of U.S. RDA			
BREAKFAST																	
Croissan'wich™ with Egg & Cheese	110	315	19	13	20	57	7	222	607	—	10	*	16	22	8	14	10
Croissan'wich™ with Bacon, Egg & Cheese	118	361	19	15	24	60	8	227	719	—	10	*	20	23	10	14	10
Croissan'wich™ with Sausage, Egg & Cheese	159	534	22	21	40	67	13	268	985	—	10	*	24	25	22	15	16
Croissan'wich™ with Ham, Egg & Cheese	144	346	19	19	21	55	7	241	962	—	10	*	32	24	16	15	11
Croissant	41	180	18	4	10	50	2	4	285	—	*	*	14	6	8	3	6
Bagel Sandwich with Egg & Cheese	161	407	46	19	16	35	5	247	759	—	10	*	18	30	11	13	16

Menu Item	WT (g)	CAL	CARB (g)	PRO (g)	FAT (g)	FAT % Cal	SAT (g)	CHOL (mg)	SOD (mg)	POT (mg)	A	C	THIA	RIBO	NIA	CA	IRON
													Percentage of U.S. RDA				
Bagel Sandwich with Bacon, Egg & Cheese	169	453	46	21	20	40	7	252	872	—	10	*	22	31	13	13	16
Bagel Sandwich with Sausage, Egg & Cheese	210	626	49	27	36	52	12	293	1137	—	10	*	26	33	25	14	22
Bagel Sandwich with Ham, Egg & Cheese	196	438	46	25	17	35	6	266	1114	—	10	*	34	33	19	13	17
Bagel with Cream Cheese	120	370	45	12	16	39	6	58	523	—	7	*	17	16	11	4	12
Bagel	92	272	44	10	6	20	1	29	438	—	*	*	17	14	11	*	12
Biscuit with Bacon	102	378	42	8	20	48	5	8	867	—	*	*	24	15	18	19	*
Biscuit with Sausage	127	478	44	11	29	55	8	33	1007	—	*	*	26	16	24	19	4
Biscuit with Bacon & Egg	158	467	43	14	27	52	7	213	1033	—	8	*	26	29	18	23	5
Biscuit with Sausage & Egg	183	568	45	17	36	57	10	238	1172	—	8	*	28	30	25	24	8
Biscuit	94	332	42	5	17	46	3	2	754	—	*	*	21	14	15	19	15

Scrambled Egg Platter	211	549	44	17	34	56	9	365	893	—	22	9	25	34	19	11	16
Scrambled Egg Platter with Bacon	221	610	44	21	39	58	11	373	1043	—	22	9	29	36	22	11	16
Scrambled Egg Platter with Sausage	260	768	47	26	53	62	15	412	1271	—	22	9	32	37	32	12	21
French Toast Sticks	141	538	53	10	32	54	5	80	537	—	*	*	16	16	18	8	16
Hash Browns	71	213	25	2	12	51	3	3	318	—	12	9	7	4	10	*	2
Danish (typical)	71	500	40	5	36	65	23	6	288	—	—	—	18	12	16	9	9

BURGERS MENU

Whopper® Sandwich	270	614	45	27	36	53	12	90	865	—	11	20	24	24	34	8	27
Whopper® with Cheese Sandwich	294	706	47	32	44	56	16	115	1177	—	19	20	24	28	34	22	27
Double Whopper® Sandwich	351	844	45	46	53	57	19	169	933	—	11	20	25	33	52	9	40
Double Whopper® with Cheese Sandwich	375	935	47	51	61	59	24	194	1245	—	19	20	25	37	52	24	40

Menu Item	WT (g)	CAL	CARB (g)	PRO (g)	FAT (g)	FAT % Cal	SAT (g)	CHOL (mg)	SOD (mg)	POT (mg)	A	C	THIA	RIBO	NIA	CA	IRON
													Percentage of U.S. RDA				
Cheeseburger	121	318	28	17	15	42	7	50	661	—	7	5	15	17	19	11	15
Cheeseburger Deluxe	151	390	29	18	23	53	8	56	652	—	10	9	15	17	19	11	15
Hamburger	108	272	28	15	11	36	4	37	505	—	3	5	15	15	19	4	15
Hamburger Deluxe	138	344	28	15	19	50	6	43	496	—	5	9	15	15	19	4	15
Bacon Double Cheeseburger	160	515	26	32	31	54	14	105	748	—	8	*	20	25	31	18	21
Bacon Double Cheeseburger Deluxe	195	592	28	33	39	59	16	111	804	—	12	5	20	25	32	18	21
Barbecue Bacon Double Cheeseburger	174	536	31	32	31	52	14	105	795	—	10	*	20	25	32	18	22
Mushroom Swiss Double Cheeseburger	176	473	27	31	27	51	12	95	746	—	5	113	20	28	32	24	23
Double Cheeseburger	172	483	29	30	27	50	13	100	851	—	11	5	16	24	29	18	21

SANDWICH/SIDE ORDER																	
BK Broiler Chicken Sandwich	168	379	31	24	18	43	3	53	764	—	7	9	30	13	51	6	13
Chicken Sandwich	229	685	56	26	40	53	8	82	1417	—	3	*	32	18	49	8	19
Ocean Catch Fish Fillet	194	495	49	20	25	45	4	57	879	—	*	4	31	13	18	6	14
Chicken Tenders™	90	236	14	16	13	50	3	46	541	—	*	*	7	5	40	*	4
Fish Tenders	99	267	18	12	16	54	3	28	870	—	*	*	5	5	7	3	5
Chef Salad (no dressing)	273	178	7	17	9	46	4	103	568	—	95	25	18	15	20	16	9
Chunky Chicken Salad (no dressing)	258	142	8	20	4	25	1	49	443	—	92	34	10	10	47	4	7
Garden Salad (no dressing)	223	95	8	6	5	47	3	15	125	—	100	58	5	6	4	15	6
Side Salad (no dressing)	135	25	5	1	0	0	0	0	27	—	88	20	3	*	3	3	3
French Fries, medium, salted	111	341	36	4	20	53	10	21	241	—	*	26	10	27	11	2	4

| | | | | | | FAT | | CHOL | SOD | POT | A | C | THIA | RIBO | NIA | CA | IRON |
Menu Item	WT (g)	CAL	CARB (g)	PRO (g)	FAT (g)	% Cal	SAT (g)	(mg)	(mg)	(mg)	Percentage of U.S. RDA						
Onion Rings	86	302	34	4	17	51	4	3	559	—	13	*	9	5	11	10	3
Apple Pie	125	311	44	3	14	41	4	4	412	—	*	8	18	9	3	*	7

SANDWICH CONDIMENTS AND TOPPINGS

Menu Item	WT (g)	CAL	CARB (g)	PRO (g)	FAT (g)	FAT % Cal	SAT (g)	CHOL (mg)	SOD (mg)	POT (mg)	A	C	THIA	RIBO	NIA	CA	IRON
Processed American Cheese	25	92	1	5	7	68	5	25	312	—	8	*	*	5	*	14	*
Processed Swiss Cheese	25	82	1	6	6	66	4	20	352	—	4	*	*	4	*	20	2
Cream Cheese	28	98	1	2	10	92	5	28	86	—	7	*	*	3	*	2	*
Lettuce	21	3	0	0	0	0	0	0	2	—	*	*	*	*	*	*	*
Tomato	28	6	1	0	0	0	0	0	3	—	4	9	*	*	*	*	*
Onion	14	5	1	0	0	0	0	0	0	—	*	*	*	*	*	*	*
Pickles	14	1	0	0	0	0	0	0	119	—	*	*	*	*	*	*	*
Ketchup	14	17	4	0	0	0	0	0	183	—	5	8	*	*	*	*	*
Mustard	3	2	0	0	0	0	0	0	34	—	*	*	*	*	*	*	*
Mayonnaise	28	194	2	0	21	97	4	16	142	—	*	*	*	*	*	*	*

Item																	
Tartar Sauce	28	134	2	0	14	94	2	20	202	—	*	*	*	*	*	*	*
BK Broiler Sauce	14	90	0	0	10	100	1	7	95	—	*	*	*	*	*	*	*
Bull's Eye® Barbecue Sauce	14	22	5	0	0	0	0	0	47	—	*	*	*	*	*	*	*
Mushroom Topping	23	13	1	1	1	69	tr	0	70	—	*	113	*	3	5	3	*
Bacon Bits	3	16	0	1	1	56	tr	5	tr	—	*	*	*	*	*	*	*
Croutons	7	31	5	1	1	29	tr	tr	90	—	*	*	*	*	*	*	*
SALAD DRESSINGS																	
Thousand Island Dressing	63	290	15	1	26	81	5	36	403	—	64	*	*	*	*	*	*
French Dressing	64	290	23	0	22	68	3	0	400	—	31	*	*	*	*	*	*
Ranch Dressing	57	350	4	1	37	95	7	20	316	—	*	*	*	*	*	*	*
Bleu Cheese Dressing	59	300	2	3	32	96	7	58	512	—	*	*	*	*	*	*	*
Olive Oil & Vinegar Dressing	56	310	2	0	33	96	5	0	214	—	*	*	*	*	*	*	*
Reduced Calorie Light Italian Dressing	59	170	3	0	18	95	3	0	762	—	*	*	*	*	*	*	*

Menu Item	WT (g)	CAL	CARB (g)	PRO (g)	FAT (g)	FAT % Cal	SAT (g)	CHOL (mg)	SOD (mg)	POT (mg)	A	C	THIA	RIBO	NIA	CA	IRON
											*Percentage of U.S. RDA						

DIPPING SAUCES

Menu Item	WT (g)	CAL	CARB (g)	PRO (g)	FAT (g)	FAT % Cal	SAT (g)	CHOL (mg)	SOD (mg)	POT (mg)	A	C	THIA	RIBO	NIA	CA	IRON
Burger King A.M. Express Dip	28	84	21	0	0	0	0	0	18	—	*	*	*	*	*	*	*
Honey Dipping Sauce	28	91	23	0	0	0	0	0	12	—	*	*	*	*	*	*	*
Ranch Dipping Sauce	28	171	2	0	18	95	3	0	208	—	*	*	*	*	*	*	*
Barbecue Dipping Sauce	28	36	9	0	0	0	0	0	397	—	3	4	*	*	*	*	*
Sweet & Sour Dipping Sauce	28	45	11	0	0	0	0	0	52	—	*	*	*	*	*	*	*
Tartar Dipping Sauce	28	174	3	0	18	93	3	16	302	—	*	*	*	*	*	*	*

DRINKS

Menu Item	WT (g)	CAL	CARB (g)	PRO (g)	FAT (g)	FAT % Cal	SAT (g)	CHOL (mg)	SOD (mg)	POT (mg)	A	C	THIA	RIBO	NIA	CA	IRON
Vanilla Shake	284	334	51	9	10	27	6	33	213	—	*	*	7	35	*	31	*
Chocolate Shake	284	326	49	9	10	28	6	31	198	—	7	4	6	28	*	31	4

Chocolate Shake (syrup added)	312	409	68	10	11	24	6	33	248	—	*	*	7	35	*	31	*
Strawberry Shake (syrup added)	312	394	66	9	10	23	6	33	230	—	*	*	7	35	*	31	*
Pepsi® Cola (medium)	444	193	47	0	0	0	0	0	V	—	*	*	*	*	*	*	*
Diet Pepsi® (medium)	444	1	0	0	0	0	0	0	V	—	*	*	*	*	*	*	*
7-Up® (medium)	444	175	46	0	0	0	0	0	V	—	*	*	*	*	*	*	*
Orange Juice	183	82	20	1	0	0	0	0	2	—	3	119	10	*	*	*	*
Coffee	244	2	0	0	0	0	0	0	2	—	*	*	*	*	4	*	*
Milk, 2% Low Fat	244	121	12	8	5	37	3	18	122	—	10	4	6	24	*	30	*
Milk, Whole	244	157	11	8	9	52	6	35	119	—	7	6	6	23	*	29	*

* = Less than 2% U.S. RDA; — = Data not available; V = Varies with local water supply; tr = Trace.
Chart based on data released August 1990 for standard menu items by the Burger King Corporation, 17777 Old Cutler Road, Miami, Fla. 33157. Values are based on analytical data from the Pillsbury Company, Hazleton Laboratories, Inc., Silliker Laboratories, and ABC Research Corporation, combined with representative values from the United States Department of Agriculture and suppliers.

KENTUCKY FRIED CHICKEN

Menu Item	WT (g)	CAL	CARB (g)	PRO (g)	FAT (g)	FAT % Cal	SAT (g)	CHOL (mg)	SOD (mg)	POT (mg)	A	C	THIA	RIBO	NIA	CA	IRON
													Percentage of U.S. RDA				
ORIGINAL RECIPE® CHICKEN																	
Wing (1.9 oz)	55	178	6	12	12	61	3.0	64	372	—	*	*	2	5	19	5	7
Side Breast (3.2 oz)	90	267	11	19	17	57	4.2	77	735	—	*	*	4	8	35	7	7
Center Breast (4.1 oz)	115	283	9	28	15	48	3.8	93	672	—	*	*	6	10	58	4	5
Drumstick (2 oz)	57	146	4	13	9	55	2.2	67	275	—	*	*	3	7	16	2	6
Thigh (3.7 oz)	104	294	11	18	20	61	5.3	123	619	—	2	*	6	18	27	7	7
EXTRA TASTY CRISPY™ CHICKEN																	
Wing (2.3 oz)	65	254	9	12	19	67	4.4	67	422	—	*	*	3	4	17	2	4
Side Breast (3.9 oz)	110	343	14	22	22	58	5.5	81	748	—	*	*	6	7	42	3	5

Center Breast (4.8 oz)	135	342	12	33	20	53	4.8	114	790	—	*	*	7	8	65	3	5
Drumstick (2.4 oz)	69	204	6	14	14	62	3.4	71	324	—	*	*	4	7	19	1	4
Thigh (4.2 oz)	119	406	14	20	30	67	7.7	129	688	—	3	*	6	13	33	5	7

KENTUCKY NUGGETS® AND SAUCE

Kentucky Nuggets® (1 = 0.6 oz)	16	46	2	3	3	59	0.7	12	140	—	*	*	*	*	5	*	*
Barbecue (1 oz)	28	35	7	0.3	0.6	15	0.1	<1	450	—	7	*	*	*	*	*	*
Sweet 'n Sour (1 oz)	28	58	13	0.1	0.6	9	0.1	<1	148	—	*	*	*	*	*	*	*
Honey (0.5 oz)	14	49	12	0	tr	0	tr	<1	<15	—	*	*	*	*	*	*	*
Mustard (1 oz)	28	36	6	1	1	25	0.1	<1	346	—	*	*	*	*	*	*	*

KFC® LITE 'N CRISPY

Side Breast (2.7 oz)	75	204	—	—	12	53	3.2	53	417	—	—	—	—	—	—	—	—
Center Breast (3 oz)	86	220	—	—	12	49	2.9	57	416	—	—	—	—	—	—	—	—
Drumstick (1.7 oz)	47	121	—	—	7	52	1.7	51	196	—	—	—	—	—	—	—	—
Thigh (2.8 oz)	79	246	—	—	17	62	4.3	80	386	—	—	—	—	—	—	—	—

OTHER ITEMS

Menu Item	WT (g)	CAL	CARB (g)	PRO (g)	FAT (g)	FAT % Cal	SAT (g)	CHOL (mg)	SOD (mg)	POT (mg)	Percentage of U.S. RDA						
											A	C	THIA	RIBO	NIA	CA	IRON
Hot Wings, six pieces (4.2 oz)	119	376	—	22	24	57	5.3	148	677	—	—	—	—	—	—	—	—
Chicken Littles™ Sandwich (1.7 oz)	47	169	14	6	10	53	2.0	18	331	—	*	*	11	7	11	2	10
Buttermilk Biscuits, one (2.3 oz)	65	235	28	5	12	46	3.2	1	655	—	*	*	16	11	13	10	9
Mashed Potatoes & Gravy (3.5 oz)	98	71	12	2	2	25	0.4	<1	339	—	*	*	*	2	6	2	2
French Fries (2.7 oz)	77	244	31	3	12	44	2.6	2	139	—	*	26	10	3	10	3	3
Corn-on-the-Cob (5 oz)	143	176	32	5	3	15	0.5	<1	<21	—	5	4	10	7	9	*	4
Cole Slaw (3.2 oz)	91	119	13	2	7	53	1.0	5	197	—	6	36	2	*	*	3	*
Colonel's™ Chicken Sandwich (5.9 oz)	166	482	39	21	27	50	5.7	47	1060	—	*	26	26	16	56	5	7

* = Less than 2% U.S. RDA; — = Data not available; < = Less than.
Chart based on data received December 1990 for standard menu items from Kentucky Fried Chicken Corporation, P.O. Box 32070, Louisville, Ky. 40232. Values determined by Hazleton Laboratories America, Inc., Madison, Wisconsin, from representative samples and may vary for specific items.

WENDY'S

Menu Item	WT (g)	CAL	CARB (g)	PRO (g)	FAT (g)	FAT % Cal	SAT (g)	CHOL (mg)	SOD (mg)	POT (mg)	A	C	THIA	RIBO	NIA	CA	IRON
													Percentage of U.S. RDA				
SANDWICHES																	
Hamburger Patty (¼ lb)	74	180	<1	19	12	60	5.0	65	210	210	*	*	4	*	20	*	20
Plain Single	126	340	30	24	15	40	5.7	65	500	275	*	*	25	20	30	10	30
Single with Everything	210	420	35	25	21	45	5.7	70	890	430	5	15	25	20	30	10	30
Wendy's® Big Classic	260	570	47	27	33	52	5.9	90	1085	525	10	20	30	25	35	15	35
Jr. Hamburger	111	260	33	15	9	31	3.3	34	570	215	2	4	25	20	20	10	20
Jr. Cheeseburger	125	310	33	18	13	38	3.2	34	770	215	2	4	25	50	20	10	20
Jr. Bacon Cheeseburger	155	430	32	22	25	52	5.5	50	835	290	2	15	30	50	25	10	20
Jr. Swiss Deluxe	163	360	34	18	18	45	3.3	40	765	290	4	10	25	60	20	20	20
Kids' Meal Hamburger	104	260	32	15	9	31	3.3	35	570	205	2	2	25	20	20	10	20

Menu Item	WT (g)	CAL	CARB (g)	PRO (g)	FAT (g)	FAT % Cal	SAT (g)	CHOL (mg)	SOD (mg)	POT (mg)	A	C	THIA	RIBO	NIA	CA	IRON
											* Percentage of U.S. RDA						
Kids' Meal Cheeseburger	116	300	33	18	13	39	3.3	35	770	205	2	2	25	50	20	10	20
Grilled Chicken Fillet	70	100	<1	18	3	27	0.6	55	330	210	*	*	4	4	35	*	6
Grilled Chicken Sandwich	175	340	36	24	13	34	2.5	60	815	340	2	8	30	25	50	10	20
Chicken Breast Fillet	99	220	11	21	10	41	2.0	55	400	270	*	*	8	8	60	*	70
Chicken Sandwich	219	430	41	26	19	40	2.8	60	725	390	2	8	30	25	70	10	80
Chicken Club Sandwich	205	506	42	30	25	44	5.0	70	930	450	2	15	35	30	80	10	80
Fish Fillet Sandwich	170	460	42	18	25	49	5.0	55	780	320	2	2	40	35	20	10	15
Kaiser Bun	65	200	37	6	3	14	1.0	10	350	70	*	*	25	20	10	10	10
White Bun	56	160	30	5	3	17	1.0	tr	290	60	*	*	20	20	10	10	10
Sandwich Toppings																	
American Cheese Slice	18	70	<1	4	6	77	3.5	15	260	30	6	*	*	4	*	12	*
Bacon	6	30	<1	2	3	90	1.0	5	100	30	*	4	4	2	*	*	*

Ketchup	14	17	4	<1	<1	—	—	—	145	50	4	4	*	*	*	*	*	*
Lettuce	10	1	<1	<1	<1	—	0	0	tr	15	*	*	*	*	*	*	*	*
Mayonnaise	13	90	<1	<1	10	100	1.6	10	60	tr	*	*	*	*	*	*	*	*
Mustard	5	4	<1	<1	<1	—	tr	0	45	5	*	*	*	*	*	*	*	*
Onion	10	4	<1	<1	<1	—	<1	0	tr	15	*	*	*	*	*	*	*	*
Pickles	14	2	<1	<1	<1	—	tr	0	200	30	*	*	*	*	*	*	*	*
Tomatoes	21	4	<1	<1	<1	—	tr	0	tr	45	*	6	*	*	*	*	*	*
Honey Mustard	14	71	4	<1	6	76	1.0	5	170	—	*	*	*	*	*	*	*	*
Tartar Sauce	21	120	<1	<1	—	—	2.1	15	115	10	*	*	10	15	*	*	*	*

POTATOES, CHILI, AND NUGGETS

French Fries, small (3.2 oz)	91	240	33	3	12	45	2.5	0	145	510	*	10	10	10	2	10	*	4
French Fries, large (4.2 oz)	118	312	43	4	16	45	3.3	0	189	663	—	13	13	13	3	13	—	5
French Fries, Biggie (6 oz)	170	449	62	8	22	45	4.7	0	271	954	—	19	19	19	4	19	—	8
Chili, regular (9 oz)	255	220	23	21	7	29	2.6	45	750	495	15	15	8	8	10	10	8	35

Menu Item	WT (g)	CAL	CARB (g)	PRO (g)	FAT (g)	FAT % Cal	SAT (g)	CHOL (mg)	SOD (mg)	POT (mg)	A	C	THIA	RIBO	NIA	CA	IRON
											Percentage of U.S. RDA						
Chili, large (13.5 oz)	383	330	35	32	11	30	4	68	1125	743	23	23	12	15	15	12	53
Cheddar Cheese, shredded	28	110	1	7	10	82	6.0	30	175	30	10	*	*	6	*	20	*
Sour Cream	28	60	1	1	6	90	3.6	10	15	40	6	*	*	2	*	4	*
Crispy Chicken Nuggets (6)	93	280	12	14	20	64	4.5	50	600	200	*	*	6	6	30	4	4
Crispy Chicken Nuggets (9)	140	420	18	21	30	64	6.8	75	900	300	—	—	9	9	45	6	6
Crispy Chicken Nuggets (20)	307	924	40	46	66	64	14.9	165	2970	990	—	—	20	20	99	13	13
Nugget Sauces																	
Barbecue	28	50	11	<1	<1	—	tr	0	100	95	6	*	*	*	*	*	4
Honey	14	45	12	<1	<1	—	tr	0	tr	tr	*	*	*	*	*	*	*
Sweet & Sour	28	45	11	<1	<1	—	tr	0	55	40	*	*	*	*	*	*	2
Sweet Mustard	28	50	9	<1	1	18	<1	0	140	30	*	*	*	*	*	*	*
Hot Stuffed Baked Potatoes																	
Plain	250	270	63	6	<1	—	tr	0	20	1045	*	50	20	6	20	2	20

Bacon & Cheese	362	520	70	20	18	31	5.1	20	1460	1350	10	60	35	15	35	8	24
Broccoli & Cheese	350	400	58	8	16	36	2.9	tr	455	1530	14	60	20	10	20	10	15
Cheese	318	420	66	8	15	32	4.0	10	310	1080	10	50	20	100	20	6	20
Chili & Cheese	403	500	71	15	18	32	4.0	25	630	1270	15	60	20	100	25	8	28
Sour Cream & Chives	323	500	67	8	23	41	9.3	25	135	1185	50	75	20	10	20	10	20

SALAD/SUPER BAR

Salad Dressings: One full ladle contains 2 tbsp; one packet contains approximately 4 tbsp.

Blue Cheese, 1 tbsp	15	90	<1	<1	10	100	1.9	10	105	10	*	*	*	*	*	*	*
Blue Cheese, 1 packet (2 oz calculated)	54	324	<1	<1	36	100	6.8	36	378	36	—	—	—	*	—	*	—
Celery Seed, 1 tbsp	15	70	3	<1	6	77	0.9	5	65	10	*	*	*	*	*	*	*
French, 1 tbsp	15	60	4	<1	6	90	0.9	0	178	20	*	*	*	*	*	*	*
French, 1 packet (2 oz calculated)	54	216	14	<1	22	92	3.2	0	641	72	—	—	—	—	—	*	—
French, Sweet Red, 1 tbsp	15	70	5	<1	6	77	0.8	0	125	15	*	*	*	*	*	*	*

Menu Item	WT (g)	CAL	CARB (g)	PRO (g)	FAT (g)	FAT % Cal	SAT (g)	CHOL (mg)	SOD (mg)	POT (mg)	Percentage of U.S. RDA						
											A	C	THIA	RIBO	NIA	CA	IRON
Hidden Valley Ranch™, 1 tbsp	15	50	<1	<1	6	—	1.0	5	95	15	*	*	*	*	*	*	*
Hidden Valley Ranch™, 1 packet (2 oz calculated)	54	180	—	—	22	—	3.6	18	342	54	—	—	—	—	—	—	—
Italian Caesar, 1 tbsp	15	80	<1	<1	9	100	1.4	5	140	5	*	*	*	*	*	*	*
Italian, Golden, 1 tbsp	15	45	3	<1	4	80	0.5	0	250	10	*	*	*	*	*	*	*
Salad Oil, 1 tbsp	14	125	0	0	14	100	2.1	0	0	0	*	*	*	*	*	*	*
Thousand Island, 1 tbsp	15	70	2	<1	7	90	1.1	5	105	15	*	*	*	*	*	*	*
Thousand Island, 1 packet (2 oz calculated)	54	252	7	—	25	90	4.0	18	378	54	—	—	—	—	—	—	—
Wine Vinegar, 1 tbsp	15	2	<1	<1	0	0	0	0	5	10	*	*	*	*	*	*	*
Reduced Calorie Bacon & Tomato, 1 tbsp	15	45	3	<1	4	80	0.6	<1	190	15	*	*	*	*	*	*	*

Reduced Calorie Italian, 1 tbsp	15	25	2	<1	2	72	0.3	0	185	10	*	*	*	*	*	*	*	*

Prepared Salads (without dressing)

Chef Salad	331	180	10	15	9	45	—	120	140	590	110	110	15	25	6	6	25	15
Garden Salad	277	102	9	7	5	44	—	0	110	560	110	110	10	20	6	6	20	10
Taco Salad	791	660	46	40	37	50	—	35	1110	1330	80	80	30	45	25	80	80	35

SuperBar—Mexican Fiesta

Cheese Sauce	56	39	5	1	2	46	1.0	tr	305	75	*	*	*	*	*	*	6	*
Picante Sauce	56	18	4	<1	<1	—	<1	—	5	155	10	30	2	2	2	*	*	2
Refried Beans	56	70	10	4	3	39	0.9	tr	215	210	*	*	4	2	2	2	2	6
Rice, Spanish	56	70	13	2	1	13	0.2	tr	440	130	6	*	45	*	8	8	4	10
Taco Chips	40	260	40	4	10	35	0.7	0	20	0	*	*	2	4	2	*	8	4
Taco Meat	56	110	4	10	7	57	1.7	25	300	240	*	*	8	6	10	8	4	10
Taco Sauce	28	16	3	<1	<1	—	tr	tr	140	90	4	2	*	*	*	*	*	*
Taco Shells	11	45	6	<1	3	60	0.7	0	45	25	*	*	*	*	*	*	*	*
Tortilla, Flour	37	110	19	3	3	25	0.4	—	220	—	*	*	4	2	2	8	8	2

Menu Item	WT (g)	CAL	CARB (g)	PRO (g)	FAT (g)	FAT % Cal	SAT (g)	CHOL (mg)	SOD (mg)	POT (mg)	A	C	THIA	RIBO	NIA	CA	IRON
													Percentage of U.S. RDA				
SuperBar—Pasta																	
Alfredo Sauce	56	35	5	1	1	26	0.8	tr	300	70	*	*	*	*	*	6	*
Fettucini	56	190	27	4	3	14	0.6	10	3	15	*	*	10	6	6	2	6
Garlic Toast	18	70	9	2	3	39	0.6	tr	65	20	4	*	6	2	2	2	2
Pasta Medley	56	60	9	2	2	30	0.3	tr	5	60	6	15	6	4	4	*	4
Rotini	56	90	15	3	2	20	0.3	tr	tr	10	*	*	6	6	6	*	4
Spaghetti Sauce	56	28	7	<1	tr	tr	tr	tr	345	95	*	*	*	*	*	*	*
Spaghetti Meat Sauce	56	60	8	4	2	30	0.7	10	315	125	4	4	2	4	4	*	4
Garden Spot™ Salad Bar																	
Alfalfa Sprouts	28	8	1	1	0	0	0	0	tr	15	*	4	*	2	*	*	*
Applesauce, Chunky	28	22	6	<1	<1	—	tr	0	tr	15	*	*	*	*	*	*	*
Bacon Bits	14	40	<1	5	2	45	0.7	10	400	90	*	2	6	4	6	*	2
Bananas	28	26	7	<1	<1	—	tr	0	tr	110	*	4	*	2	*	*	*
Breadsticks	8	30	5	1	1	30	<1	0	30	15	*	*	2	2	2	2	2
Broccoli	43	12	2	1	0	0	0	0	10	140	6	65	2	2	*	2	2

Cantaloupe	57	20	5	<1	0	0	0	0	5	175	20	30	*	*	*	*	*
Carrots	27	12	2	<1	0	0	0	0	10	90	80	4	2	2	2	*	*
Cauliflower	57	14	3	1	0	0	0	0	10	200	*	70	4	2	2	2	2
Cheddar Chips	28	160	12	3	12	68	—	5	445	50	*	*	2	*	4	6	2
Cheese, shredded (imitation)	28	90	1	6	6	60	4.0	tr	125	0	4	*	*	15	*	20	*
Chicken Salad	56	120	4	7	8	60	1.5	tr	215	60	*	4	*	4	6	*	2
Chives	28	71	18	6	1	13	0.2	0	20	850	195	313	15	25	8	25	30
Chow Mein Noodles	14	74	8	1	4	49	0.6	0	60	15	*	*	6	4	4	*	4
Cole Slaw	57	70	8	<1	5	64	0.9	5	130	90	4	25	*	*	*	*	*
Cottage Cheese	105	108	3	13	4	33	3.0	15	425	90	6	*	*	10	6	*	*
Croutons	14	60	8	2	3	45	—	—	155	30	*	*	4	4	4	*	4
Cucumbers	14	2	<1	<1	0	0	0	0	tr	20	*	*	*	*	*	*	*
Eggs, hard cooked	20	30	<1	3	2	60	0.7	90	25	25	4	*	*	6	*	*	*
Garbanzo Beans	28	46	8	3	1	20	0.1	0	5	85	*	*	2	*	2	*	6
Green Peas	28	21	4	1	0	0	0	0	30	40	4	8	6	2	6	*	2
Green Peppers	37	10	2	<1	0	0	0	0	tr	65	2	60	2	*	2	*	*
Honeydew Melon	57	20	5	<1	0	0	0	0	5	155	*	25	2	2	2	*	*

Menu Item	WT (g)	CAL	CARB (g)	PRO (g)	FAT (g)	FAT % Cal	SAT (g)	CHOL (mg)	SOD (mg)	POT (mg)	A	C	THIA	RIBO	NIA	CA	IRON
														Percentage of U.S. RDA			
Jalapeño Peppers	14	2	<1	<1	0	0	0	0	190	10	*	*	*	*	*	*	*
Lettuce, Iceberg	55	8	1	<1	0	0	0	0	5	85	2	4	2	*	*	*	2
Lettuce, Romaine	55	9	1	1	0	0	0	0	5	160	15	20	4	4	*	2	4
Mushrooms	17	4	<1	<1	0	0	0	0	tr	65	*	*	*	4	4	*	*
Olives, Black	28	35	2	<1	3	77	0.4	0	245	5	*	*	*	*	*	2	4
Oranges	56	26	7	<1	0	0	0	0	0	100	*	50	4	*	*	2	*
Parmesan Cheese	28	130	1	12	9	62	5.4	20	525	30	6	*	*	6	*	40	*
Parmesan Cheese, imitation	28	80	4	9	3	34	3.0	tr	410	95	20	*	*	*	*	50	*
Pasta Salad	57	35	6	2	<1	—	—	0	120	—	*	*	*	2	2	*	2
Peaches	57	31	8	<1	0	0	0	0	5	55	2	2	*	*	2	*	*
Pepperoni, sliced	28	140	2	5	12	77	4.5	35	435	55	*	*	160	4	10	*	2
Pineapple Chunks	100	60	16	<1	0	0	0	0	tr	120	*	15	6	*	*	*	2
Potato Salad	57	125	6	<1	11	79	0.8	10	90	135	*	10	2	*	2	2	2
Pudding, Butter-scotch	57	90	11	1	4	40	—	tr	85	—	*	*	*	*	*	6	2
Pudding, Chocolate	57	90	12	<1	4	40	—	tr	70	—	*	2	2	2	*	15	2

Red Onions	9	2	<1	<1	0	0	0	0	tr	15	*	*	*	*	*	*	*
Red Peppers, crushed	28	120	15	5	4	30	—	0	5	40	200	15	10	15	20	2	15
Seafood Salad	56	110	7	4	7	57	0.2	tr	455	95	*	*	*	2	*	20	2
Strawberries	56	17	4	<1	0	0	0	0	tr	45	*	50	2	2	2	*	*
Sour Topping	28	58	2	<1	5	78	5.0	0	30	45	*	*	*	*	*	*	10
Sunflower Seeds & Raisins	28	140	6	5	10	64	7.4	0	5	240	*	*	30	4	6	2	10
Three Bean Salad	57	60	13	1	<1	—	tr	—	15	55	4	*	*	*	*	*	2
Tomatoes	28	6	1	<1	0	0	0	0	5	65	2	10	*	*	*	*	2
Tuna Salad	56	100	4	8	6	54	0.9	15	290	90	*	4	*	4	25	*	4
Turkey Ham	28	35	<1	5	1	26	0.5	15	275	80	*	*	*	4	6	*	4
Watermelon	57	18	4	<1	0	0	0	0	tr	65	2	10	4	*	*	*	*
DESSERTS, BEVERAGES																	
Frosty Dairy Dessert, small (8 oz)	243	400	59	8	14	32	4.8	50	220	585	10	*	8	30	2	30	6
Frosty Dairy Dessert, medium (10.5 oz)	316	520	77	10	18	32	6.2	65	286	761	13	—	10	39	3	39	8

Menu Item	WT (g)	CAL	CARB (g)	PRO (g)	FAT (g)	FAT % Cal	SAT (g)	CHOL (mg)	SOD (mg)	POT (mg)	A	C	THIA	RIBO	NIA	CA	IRON
											Percentage of U.S. RDA						
Frosty Dairy Dessert, large (14 oz)	413	680	100	14	24	32	8.2	85	374	995	17	—	14	51	3	51	10
Chocolate Chip Cookie	64	275	40	3	13	43	4.2	15	256	70	2	*	8	8	6	2	8
Cola, small (8 fluid oz)	246	100	25	0	0	0	0	0	10	tr	*	*	*	*	*	*	*
Cola, medium (12 fluid oz)	369	150	38	0	0	0	0	0	15	tr	—	—	—	—	—	—	—
Cola, large (16 fluid oz)	492	200	50	0	0	0	0	0	20	tr	—	—	—	—	—	—	—
Cola, Biggie (28 fluid oz)	861	350	88	0	0	0	0	0	35	tr	—	—	—	—	—	—	—
Diet Cola, small (8 fluid oz)	246	1	<1	0	0	0	0	0	20	tr	*	*	*	*	*	*	*
Lemon-Lime Soft Drink, small (8 fluid oz)	246	100	24	0	0	0	0	0	20	tr	*	*	*	*	*	*	*

Coffee (6 fluid oz)	177	2	<1	0	0	0	0	5	90	*	*	*	*	*	*	*
Decaffeinated Coffee (6 fluid oz)	177	2	<1	0	0	0	0	tr	125	*	*	*	*	*	*	*
Hot Chocolate (6 fluid oz)	188	110	22	2	1	8	1.0	tr	115	210	*	*	*	8	6	2
Lemonade (8 fluid oz)	248	90	24	0	0	0	0	tr	35	*	15	*	*	4	*	2
Milk, Chocolate (8 fluid oz)	250	160	24	7	5	28	2.8	15	140	385	15	4	6	20	25	4
Milk, 2% (8 fluid oz)	244	110	11	8	4	33	2.7	20	115	350	10	4	6	20	30	*
Tea, Hot or Iced (6 fluid oz)	178	1	0	0	0	0	0	5	65	*	*	*	*	*	*	*

* = Less than 2% U.S. RDA; — = Data not available; tr = Trace; < = Less than.
Chart based on data received January 1991 for standard menu items from Wendy's International, Inc., P.O. Box 256, Dublin, Ohio 43017. Values obtained through one of the following sources: analysis by Hazleton, Wisconsin, Food Processor II, Nutrition and Diet Analysis Software, United States Department of Agriculture and suppliers.

HARDEE'S

Menu Item	WT (g)	CAL	CARB (g)	PRO (g)	FAT (g)	FAT % Cal	SAT (g)	CHOL (mg)	SOD (mg)	POT (mg)	A	C	THIA	RIBO	NIA	CA	IRON
													Percentage of U.S. RDA				
BREAKFAST																	
Rise 'N' Shine™ Biscuit	83	320	34	5	18	51	3	0	740	80	—	—	—	—	—	10	10
Cinnamon 'N' Raisin™	80	320	37	4	17	48	5	0	510	80	—	—	—	—	—	10	10
Sausage Biscuit	118	440	34	13	28	57	7	25	1100	190	—	—	—	—	—	15	15
Sausage & Egg Biscuit	150	490	35	18	31	57	8	170	1150	240	—	—	—	—	—	15	20
Bacon Biscuit	93	360	34	10	21	53	4	10	950	140	—	—	—	—	—	10	10
Bacon & Egg Biscuit	124	410	35	15	24	53	5	155	990	180	—	—	—	—	—	15	20
Bacon, Egg & Cheese Biscuit	137	460	35	17	28	55	8	165	1220	200	—	—	—	—	—	20	20
Ham Biscuit	106	320	34	10	16	45	2	15	1000	170	—	—	—	—	—	10	10
Ham & Egg Biscuit	138	370	35	15	19	46	4	160	1050	210	—	—	—	—	—	15	20

Item															
Ham, Egg & Cheese Biscuit	151	420	35	18	23	49	6	170	1270	230	—	—	—	20	20
Country Ham Biscuit	108	350	35	11	18	46	3	25	1550	210	—	—	—	10	15
Country Ham & Egg Biscuit	139	400	35	16	22	50	4	175	1600	260	—	—	—	15	20
Canadian Rise 'N' Shine™ Biscuit	161	470	35	22	27	52	8	180	1550	280	—	—	—	20	20
Steak Biscuit	148	500	46	15	29	52	7	30	1320	240	—	—	—	15	20
Steak & Egg Biscuit	179	550	47	20	32	52	8	175	1370	280	—	—	—	15	25
Chicken Biscuit	146	430	42	17	22	46	4	45	1330	260	—	—	—	15	10
Big Country Breakfast™ (Sausage)	274	850	51	33	57	60	16	340	1980	670	—	—	—	20	35
Big Country Breakfast™ (Bacon)	217	660	51	24	40	55	10	305	1540	530	—	—	—	15	30
Big Country Breakfast™ (Ham)	251	620	51	28	33	48	7	325	1780	620	—	—	—	15	30

Menu Item	WT (g)	CAL	CARB (g)	PRO (g)	FAT (g)	FAT % Cal	SAT (g)	CHOL (mg)	SOD (mg)	POT (mg)	A	C	THIA	RIBO	NIA	CA	IRON
											Percentage of U.S. RDA						
Big Country Breakfast™ (Country Ham)	254	670	52	29	38	51	9	345	2870	710	—	—	—	—	—	15	35
Hash Rounds™	79	230	24	3	14	55	3	0	560	400	—	—	—	—	—	*	6
Biscuit 'N' Gravy™	221	440	45	9	24	49	6	15	1250	210	—	—	—	—	—	15	10
Three Pancakes	137	280	56	8	2	6	1	15	890	240	—	—	—	—	—	6	20
Three Pancakes with 1 Sausage Pattie	176	430	56	16	16	33	6	40	1290	350	—	—	—	—	—	8	20
Three Pancakes with 2 Bacon Strips	150	350	56	13	9	23	3	25	1110	290	—	—	—	—	—	6	20
Syrup	43	120	31	<1	<1	<8	<1	0	25	10	—	—	—	—	—	*	4
Margarine/Butter Blend	5	35	0	0	4	100	<1	5	40	1	—	—	—	—	—	*	*
Blueberry Muffin	106	400	51	6	19	43	4	80	320	160	—	—	—	—	—	4	6
Oat-Bran Raisin Muffin	122	440	62	8	18	41	3	55	350	300	—	—	—	—	—	8	25

Hamburger	110	270	33	13	10	33	4	20	490	200	—	—	—	—	10	15
Cheeseburger	122	320	33	16	14	39	7	30	710	210	—	—	—	—	20	20
Quarter-Pound Cheeseburger	182	500	34	29	29	52	14	70	1060	350	—	—	—	—	25	30
Big Deluxe™ Burger	216	500	32	27	30	54	12	70	760	390	—	—	—	—	20	30
Bacon Cheeseburger	219	610	31	34	39	58	16	80	1030	460	—	—	—	—	20	30
Mushroom 'N' Swiss™ Burger	186	490	33	30	27	50	13	70	940	370	—	—	—	—	30	30
Big Twin™	173	450	34	23	25	50	11	55	580	280	—	—	—	—	20	20
Regular Roast Beef	114	260	31	15	9	31	4	35	730	260	—	—	—	—	10	20
Big Roast Beef™	134	300	32	18	11	33	5	45	880	320	—	—	—	—	10	25
Hot Ham 'N' Cheese™	149	330	32	23	12	33	5	65	1420	300	—	—	—	—	30	15
Turkey Club™	208	390	32	29	16	37	4	70	1280	460	—	—	—	—	15	15

Menu Item	WT (g)	CAL	CARB (g)	PRO (g)	FAT (g)	FAT % Cal	SAT (g)	CHOL (mg)	SOD (mg)	POT (mg)	A	C	THIA	RIBO	NIA	CA	IRON
											Percentage of U.S. RDA						
Fisherman's Fillet™	207	500	49	23	24	43	6	70	1030	410	–	–	–	–	–	20	20
Chicken Fillet™	173	370	44	19	13	32	2	55	1060	290	–	–	–	–	–	10	15
Grilled Chicken Sandwich	192	310	34	24	9	26	1	60	890	410	–	–	–	–	–	15	15
All Beef Hot Dog	120	300	25	11	17	51	8	25	710	180	–	–	–	–	–	8	15

SALADS AND SPECIAL ITEMS

Menu Item	WT (g)	CAL	CARB (g)	PRO (g)	FAT (g)	FAT % Cal	SAT (g)	CHOL (mg)	SOD (mg)	POT (mg)	A	C	THIA	RIBO	NIA	CA	IRON
Side Salad	112	20	1	2	<1	<45	<1	0	15	170	–	–	–	–	–	2	2
Garden Salad	241	210	3	14	14	60	8	105	270	430	–	–	–	–	–	30	6
Chef Salad	294	240	5	22	15	56	9	115	930	590	–	–	–	–	–	30	10
Chicken 'N' Pasta Salad	414	230	23	27	3	12	1	55	380	620	–	–	–	–	–	8	50
Chicken Stix™ (6 pieces)	100	210	13	19	9	39	2	35	680	260	–	–	–	–	–	2	4
Chicken Stix™ (9 pieces)	150	310	20	28	14	41	3	55	1020	390	–	–	–	–	–	2	6
Regular French Fries (2.5 oz)	71	230	30	3	11	43	2	0	85	350	–	–	–	–	–	*	6

Large French Fries (4 oz)	113	360	48	4	17	43	3	0	135	560	—	—	—	—	*	8
Big Fry (5.5 oz)	156	500	66	6	23	41	5	0	180	770	—	—	—	—	2	10
Crispy Curls™	85	300	36	4	16	48	3	0	840	370	—	—	—	—	2	6

SHAKES AND DESSERTS
(Shakes and cones contain milk)

Vanilla Shake	341	400	66	13	9	20	6	50	320	470	—	—	—	—	50	*
Chocolate Shake	341	460	85	11	8	16	5	45	340	520	—	—	—	—	50	6
Strawberry Shake	341	440	82	11	8	16	5	40	300	380	—	—	—	—	50	*
Cool Twist™ Cone, Vanilla	119	190	28	5	6	28	4	15	100	105	—	—	—	—	10	*
Cool Twist™ Cone, Chocolate	119	200	31	4	6	27	4	20	65	220	—	—	—	—	10	10
Cool Twist™ Cone, Vanilla/Chocolate	119	190	29	4	6	28	4	20	80	180	—	—	—	—	10	10
Cool Twist™ Sundae, Hot Fudge	168	320	45	7	12	34	6	25	270	280	—	—	—	—	20	6
Cool Twist™ Sundae, Caramel	169	330	54	6	10	27	5	20	290	220	—	—	—	—	20	4

Menu Item	WT (g)	CAL	CARB (g)	PRO (g)	FAT (g)	FAT % Cal	SAT (g)	CHOL (mg)	SOD (mg)	POT (mg)	A	C	THIA	RIBO	NIA	CA	IRON
											Percentage of U.S. RDA						
Cool Twist™ Sundae, Strawberry	166	260	43	5	8	28	5	15	115	150	—	—	—	—	—	15	4
Apple Turnover	91	270	38	3	12	40	4	0	250	75	—	—	—	—	—	*	4
Big Cookie™	49	250	31	3	13	47	4	5	240	45	—	—	—	—	—	*	4

* = Less than 2% U.S. RDA; — = Data not available; < = Less than.
Chart based on data provided January, 1991 by Hardee's Research and Development Department, 1233 Hardee's Boulevard, Rocky Mount, N.C. 27804–2815. Nutritional analysis was conducted by Southern Testing and Research Laboratories, Inc., an independent testing laboratory.

Charts on pages 167–206 are compiled by Linda J. Bethel, M.S., R.D., L.D., C.D.E., Bethel Nutrition Services, 1526 Nuremberg Blvd., Punta Gorda, Fla. 33983.

The Real Life Checklist for Fast-Food Eating

Here's what we recommend as good nutritional choices at each of the top five fast-food chains for breakfast, lunch, and dinner:

MCDONALD'S

Apple Bran Muffin (170 calories with no fat or cholesterol, 200 milligrams sodium)

Blueberry Muffin (170 calories with no fat or cholesterol, 220 milligrams sodium)

English Muffin with Honey (215 calories, 5 grams/21 percent fat, no cholesterol, 230 milligrams sodium)

Cheerios (80 calories, 1 gram/11 percent fat, no cholesterol, 210 grams sodium)

Wheaties (90 calories, 1 gram/10 percent fat, no cholesterol, 220 milligrams sodium)

Hotcakes *without* **margarine or syrup** (estimated at 240 calories, trace of fat, 8 milligrams cholesterol, 531 milligrams sodium)

Hotcakes with margarine and syrup (410 calories, 9 grams/20 percent fat, 8 milligrams cholesterol, 640 milligrams sodium)

Hamburger (250 calories, 9 grams/32 percent fat, 37 milligrams cholesterol, 490 milligrams sodium)

McLean Deluxe (320 calories, 10 grams/28 percent fat, 60 milligrams cholesterol, 670 milligrams sodium)

McLean Deluxe with Cheese (370 calories, 14 grams/34 percent fat, 75 milligrams cholesterol, 890 milligrams sodium)

Cheeseburger (300 calories, 12 grams/36 percent fat, 50 milligrams cholesterol, 710 milligrams sodium)

Chunky Chicken Salad (150 calories, 4 grams/24 percent fat, 78 milligrams cholesterol, 230 milligrams sodium)

Side Salad with Lite Vinaigrette Dressing (45 calories, 1.5 grams/30 percent fat, 33 milligrams cholesterol, 95 milligrams sodium)

Orange or Grapefruit Juice, 6 fluid ounces (80 calories, no fat, cholesterol, or sodium)

Apple Juice, 6 fluid ounces (91 calories, no fat or cholesterol, 5 milligrams sodium)

1% Lowfat Milk, 8 fluid ounces (110 calories, 2 grams/16 percent fat, 10 milligrams cholesterol, 130 milligrams sodium)

Vanilla Lowfat Frozen Yogurt Cone (105 calories, 1 gram/9 percent fat, 3 milligrams cholesterol, 80 milligrams sodium)

Strawberry Lowfat Frozen Yogurt Sundae (210 calories, 1 gram/4 percent fat, 5 milligrams cholesterol, 95 milligrams sodium)

BURGER KING

Plain Bagel (272 calories, 6 grams/20 percent fat, 29 milligrams cholesterol, 438 milligrams sodium)

Bagel with 1 tablespoon cream cheese (½ container) (321 calories, 11 grams/31 percent fat, 43 milligrams cholesterol, 481 milligrams sodium)

BK Broiler Sandwich *without* **sauce** (289 calories, 8 grams/25 percent fat, 46 milligrams cholesterol, 669 milligrams sodium)

Hamburger (272 calories, 11 grams/36 percent fat, 37 milligrams cholesterol, 505 milligrams sodium)

Chunky Chicken Salad with 1 tablespoon Reduced-Calorie Italian Dressing (185 calories, 9 grams/44 percent fat, 49 milligrams cholesterol, 634 milligrams sodium)

Garden Salad with 1 tablespoon Reduced-Calorie Italian Dressing (138 calories, 10 grams/65 percent fat, 15 milligrams cholesterol, 316 milligrams sodium)

Side Salad with 1 tablespoon Reduced-Calorie Italian Dressing (68 calories, 5 grams/66 percent fat, no cholesterol, 218 milligrams sodium)

Milk, 2% Lowfat, 8 fluid ounces (121 calories, 5 grams/37 percent fat, 18 milligrams cholesterol, 122 milligrams sodium)

Orange Juice, 6 fluid ounces (82 calories, no fat or cholesterol, 2 milligrams sodium)

KENTUCKY FRIED CHICKEN

Original Recipe Center Breast without the skin (Peeling away the breading and skin cuts calories in half and fat by two-thirds. Estimate 140 calories, 5 grams/32 percent fat)

Lite 'N Crispy Center Breast (220 calories, 12 grams/49 percent fat, 57 milligrams cholesterol, 415 milligrams sodium. Remove most of the breading to reduce fat and calories)

Chicken Littles™ Sandwich (169 calories, 10 grams/53 percent fat, 18 milligrams cholesterol, 331 milligrams sodium)

Mashed Potatoes and Gravy (71 calories, 2 grams/25 percent fat, less than 1 gram cholesterol, 339 milligrams sodium)

Corn-on-the-Cob (176 calories, 3 grams/15 percent fat, less than 1 gram cholesterol, less than 21 milligrams sodium)

Cole Slaw (119 calories, 7 grams/53 percent fat, 5 milligrams cholesterol, 197 milligrams sodium)

WENDY'S

Jr. or Kids' Meal Hamburger (260 calories, 9 grams/31 percent fat, 34 milligrams cholesterol, 570 milligrams sodium)

Jr. or Kids' Meal Cheeseburger (310 calories, 13 grams/38 percent fat, 34 milligrams cholesterol, 770 milligrams sodium)

Grilled Chicken Fillet (100 calories, 3 grams/27 percent fat, 55 milligrams cholesterol, 330 milligrams sodium)

Grilled Chicken Fillet Sandwich (340 calories, 13 grams/34 percent fat, 60 milligrams cholesterol, 815 milligrams sodium; even less fat, calories, and sodium without the sauce)

Regular Chili (220 calories, 7 grams/29 percent fat, 45 milligrams cholesterol, 750 milligrams sodium)

Plain Baked Potato (270 calories, trace of fat, no cholesterol, 20 milligrams sodium; consider topping with vegetables or a small amount of sauce from the salad bar)

Plain Baked Potato with 1 tablespoon sour cream and sprinkle of pepper (310 calories, 3 grams/9 percent fat, 10 milligrams cholesterol, 35 milligrams sodium)

Chef Salad with 2 tablespoons Reduced Calorie Italian Dressing (230 calories, 13 grams/51 percent fat, 120 milligrams cholesterol, 510 milligrams sodium)

Garden Salad with 1 tablespoon Reduced Calorie Italian Dressing (127 calories, 7 grams/50 percent fat, no cholesterol, 295 milligrams sodium)

Salad Bar including any fresh fruits and vegetables (alfalfa sprouts, blueberries, broccoli, cabbage, cantaloupe, carrots, cauliflower, celery, cherry peppers, cucumbers, garbanzo beans, grapes, green peas, kidney beans, lettuce, mushrooms, oranges, red onions, romaine, spinach, strawberries, tomatoes, and watermelon), with reduced-calorie salad dressing (lower in calories, fat, and cholesterol) or, better yet, wine vinegar and a little oil.

Other good choices include ½ cup cottage cheese (108 calories, 4 grams/33 percent fat, 15 milligrams cholesterol, 425 milligrams sodium); **¼ cup Cole Slaw** (70 calories, 5 grams/64 percent fat, 5 milligrams cholesterol, 130 milligrams sodium); **½ cup Three Bean Salad** (120 calories, with a trace of fat, no cholesterol, 30 milligrams sodium); **¼ cup Taco Meat in a Flour Tortilla** (220 calories, 10 grams/41 percent fat, 25 milligrams cholesterol, 520 milligrams sodium); **½ cup Spanish Rice** (140 calories, 2 grams/13 percent fat, trace of cholesterol, 880 milligrams sodium); **½ cup Fettucini with ¼ cup Spaghetti Sauce** (225 calories, 4 grams/16 percent fat, 10 milligrams cholesterol, 303 milligrams sodium); **1 piece Garlic Toast** (70 calories, 3 grams/39 percent fat, trace of cholesterol, 65 milligrams sodium); **½ cup Pasta Medley** (60 calories, 2 grams fat, trace of cholesterol, 5 milligrams sodium); **½ cup Rotini with ¼ cup Spaghetti Meat Sauce** (150 calories, 4 grams/24 percent fat, 10 milligrams cholesterol, 315 milligrams sodium).

The trick is to choose a balanced meal with moderate portions—avoid the temptation to have all of the above at a single meal!

Milk, 2% Lowfat, 8 fluid ounces (110 calories, 4 grams/33 percent fat, 20 milligrams cholesterol, 115 milligrams sodium).

HARDEE'S

Three Pancakes (plain) 280 calories, 2 grams/6 percent fat, 15 milligrams cholesterol, 890 milligrams sodium; **with a serving of syrup and a teaspoon of butter blend,** *add* 155 calories, 5 grams/30 percent fat, 5 milligrams cholesterol, 65 milligrams sodium)

Regular Hamburger (270 calories, 10 grams/33 percent fat, 20 milligrams cholesterol, 490 milligrams sodium)

Regular Roast Beef (260 calories, 9 grams/31 percent fat, 35 milligrams cholesterol, 730 milligrams sodium)

Grilled Chicken Sandwich (310 calories, 9 grams/26 percent fat, 60 milligrams cholesterol, 890 milligrams sodium)

Chicken 'N' Pasta Salad (230 calories, 3 grams/12 percent fat, 55 milligrams cholesterol, 380 milligrams sodium)

Chicken Stix™ (6 pieces) 210 calories, 9 grams/39 percent fat, 35 milligrams cholesterol, 680 milligrams sodium)

Side Salad (20 calories, trace of fat, no cholesterol, 15 milligrams sodium—add a reduced-calorie salad dressing)

Cool Twist™ Cone, any flavor (200 calories, 6 grams/27 percent fat, 20 milligrams cholesterol, 65 milligrams sodium)

Dining Out and
Eating Right

Dining out, whether for business or for pleasure, is an activity that is on the rise. According to the National Restaurant Association, Americans eat out an average of nearly four times a week, spending about forty to forty-five cents of every food dollar on fare prepared away from home. That's nearly twice as much as we spent in the 1950s. In 1990 alone, Americans spent $156 billion on restaurant food.

The problem of not eating right can occur whether you eat fast food or haute cuisine. It's the sauces and condiments; the butter on the bread; the oil and mayonnaise in the salad dressing; the cream, butter, and cheese in the pasta sauce; the shortening in the pie crust. Rich flavor doesn't have a price tag—it only has a lot of fat. And chefs who are trained in classical techniques generally cook with a lot of saturated fat and butter-laden sauces. As chefs Robert Briggs and Tracy Ritter emphasized in Chapter 3, it takes a different kind of skill to add flavor without fat.

But it's incorrect to assume that you can't eat healthfully when you eat out. Just like the fast-food chains, other restaurants nationwide, from family places to the finest dining establishments, are taking steps to improve the nutritional content of their menus. For careful and informed customers, there is a broad range of choices for nutritious meals. Almost all restaurants will serve salad dressing on the side; many cook with unsaturated fat and will broil or bake instead of fry; and most will alter food preparation upon request. Many table-service (as opposed to fast-food) restaurants are offering a few menu items modified to provide less fat or cholesterol or sodium or fewer calories, or all of the above. When the National Restaurant Association did a survey in 1986, only about a quarter to a third of the surveyed restaurants featured modified menu items. The same survey in September 1988 found that almost 40 percent were offering these kinds of menu items for nutrition-conscious consumers.

Consumers also can get some help in dining out nutritiously from the American Heart Association's "Eating Away from Home" program, a pilot program in which participating restaurants offer diners a limited but appealing selection of dishes that promote a healthy heart. A variety of names, such as "Dine à la Heart," "Creative Cuisine," or "Dine to Your Heart's Content," are given to the basic program by various state affiliates of the AHA, in such cities as Los Angeles and Minneapolis. Watch for the name American Heart Association on restaurant menus where meal options approved by the AHA can sometimes be found.

The AHA also offers a free guide to restaurant dining called "Dining Out." The brochure features nutrition tips, information about cooking procedures and portion control, and examples of healthful American and ethnic foods. Copies are available by calling your local American Heart Association office. In addition, many of these local chapters have developed guides that list area restaurants and the accommodations these restaurants are willing to make.

While nutritious food choices do claim space on restaurant menus, diners are mostly on their own in putting together healthful meals. Research by the National Restaurant Association shows that six out of ten consumers say they are very interested in nutritional menu items at table-service restaurants. However, another survey, by *Nation's Restaurant News*, a trade journal, reported that only one out of three Americans says that nutrition plays a role in determining where to eat. It seems that people might like the idea of eating nutritiously, but it doesn't play a major role in determining where to eat. Let's look at three of the people we met earlier in the book and see how dining out affects their eating habits.

He's on the Road Four Days a Week

Remember Barry Nash? He's a partner in a small Dallas consulting firm specializing in marketing television news and training people for on-camera performance. In his early thirties, married, with two young daughters, Barry needs to watch his fats and cholesterol due to a strong family history of heart disease.

But Barry's work schedule is, he admits, a hectic one. He travels 60 percent of the week, and his in-town workdays usually require quick and convenient (as in fast-food) meals. If he's out of the office, he'll drive through a McDonald's and get a small cheeseburger with an iced tea, although sometimes, he confesses, he gets a chocolate milk shake. If he orders in a sandwich, his control tends to break down when faced with the prospect of a peanut butter–chocolate chip cookie to end his meal. But during his business lunches out, he orders a pasta, with water or iced tea.

While traveling, Barry may have a business meeting at breakfast, lunch, and dinner. "I generally stay away from the breakfast buffet, and I don't order eggs very often," he says. He tends to veer toward sauceless or light meals but finds that to be a challenge when dining out. "I may be working until 7:00 p.m. and my clients decide to go to dinner at 8:00. So I'm at a restaurant in the later evening, often a really nice restaurant with very rich food and large portions." Barry generally tries to order some kind of fish or chicken, but has a hard time cutting out the fat- and calorie-rich desserts.

He's Not Shy About Asking a Restaurant to Make Some Modifications

Herb Glimcher has undergone several open heart surgeries and is a religious Pritikin follower. Chairman of the national real estate company that bears his name, Herb works everywhere in the country and has certainly had many occasions to dine out for both business and pleasure. In fact, he has dinner out three or four out of seven days, usually with his wife and some friends. While he doesn't dine out frequently for business, when he does it is usually in a major city.

Herb's approach is an assertive one. The local *nouvelle* restaurants that he chooses will accommodate his special dining requests. They prepare him plain broiled chicken or fish or pasta with a light marinara sauce. Salads always come with dressing—a low-fat variation—on the side. His out-of-town engagements don't cause him a problem, either. "In most major cities, just about any restaurant will make just about anything you want," he explains. He orders the same kind of pasta and grilled chicken. When he orders a salad, he doesn't use any dressing except for a wine vinegar or lemon juice.

He Watches Himself All Week and Lets Go on Saturday Night

Burt Staniar seems to be able to balance his frequent dinners out, despite industry functions where preplanned meals are served; but it has taken some work. As chairman and chief executive officer of a major broadcasting company, Burt has business obligations that necessitate many lunches and dinners out. While he is conscious of the food he orders—"I'm much more inclined to have a salad and fish than a burger and fries," he says, and he tends to stay away from heavy sauces and red meats—Saturday night is his dinner without strings attached. "On Saturday night, I would be inclined to order whatever I wanted without regard to nutrition," he confesses.

Twice during the work week, Burt has a business lunch at a nice New York restaurant. He applies common-sense nutrition during these meals. He doesn't eliminate from his diet food that may be high in fat; he just eats less of it, is more aware of how much of it he eats, and eats more slowly so that he can enjoy it longer. During a typical week, Burt may dine out three or four nights, split between in-town and out-of-town business meetings or industry functions. He too may eat out three meals a day when traveling, and he admits that his regimen suffers at banquets or industry functions where the meal is preordered.

Tips on Dining Out: The Real Life Nutrition Plan for Breakfast, Lunch, and Dinner

Many of you may see restaurant menus as mine fields, with danger lurking behind every tempting dish. Can one enjoy the dining experience without asking the kitchen to hold the salt, sugar, sauce, beef, and butter? If you dine out occasionally and eat rich foods in moderation, the answer is yes. A person who is in reasonably good health can periodically indulge in fine dining without restraint.

But if you frequently dine out, you do need to take a little extra care and exercise a bit more control. However, you don't have to abandon fine dining to eat prudently. Dining out while maintaining a nutritious, balanced diet requires planning, knowledge, and some assertiveness.

First, choose a restaurant where you can make nutritious choices such as salads, light soups, vegetables, and fruits. As you learned earlier, dining guides are available that list restaurants preparing foods—regularly or by request—that meet the American Heart Association dietary guidelines. A telephone call to a restaurant also may confirm whether such foods are available.

You need to make careful choices and watch out for pitfalls on menus to maintain healthful eating while dining out. The American Heart Association suggests you look for terms and phrases that indicate low-fat preparation. Feel free to indulge in dishes described as follows:

- "steamed"
- "in its own juice"
- "garden fresh"
- "broiled"
- "roasted"
- "poached"
- "dry boiled" (in lemon juice or wine).

On the other hand, be aware that some low-fat, low-cholesterol preparations are high in salt. If you're watching your sodium intake, avoid items described in any of the following terms:

- "pickled"
- "in cocktail sauce"
- "smoked"

- "in broth"
- "in a tomato base"

Menu descriptions that warn of saturated fat and cholesterol preparation may also indicate high sodium. Avoid foods described with words and phrases like:

- "buttery," "buttered," "in butter sauce"
- "sauteed," "fried," "pan-fried," "crispy," "braised"
- "creamed," "in cream sauce," "in its own gravy," "hollandaise"
- "au gratin," "Parmesan," "in cheese sauce," "escalloped"
- "marinated" (in oil), "stewed," "basted"
- "casserole," "prime," "hash," "pot pie"

If you tend to overeat or you're watching your weight, avoid buffets and all-you-can-eat specials. Don't fill up on crackers, rolls, and pretzels. Instead, have a glass of water as soon as you are seated in order to control your urge to eat, as well as to ensure that you get enough fluids. Eat your meal slowly. If you have dessert, order fresh fruit or sorbet and avoid pastries and whipped-cream desserts. Don't feel you have to eat everything on your plate because you are paying for it or your mother told you it was a sin not to. Restaurant portions are often twice as large as the portions you'd eat at home. To combat this, cut your portion in half and take the uneaten half home; choose appetizers as the main course; order à la carte; or share food with a companion.

The American Heart Association suggests asking the restaurant personnel such questions as the following: Do they or would they

- serve margarine (rather than butter) with the meal?
- serve skim (rather than whole) milk?
- prepare a dish using vegetable oil (corn, soy, sunflower, safflower) or a margarine made with vegetable oil (rather than butter)?
- trim visible fat off meat or skin off poultry?
- limit portion size to 4 to 6 ounces of cooked meat, poultry, or fish?
- leave all butter, gravy, or sauce off an entree or side dish?
- serve fruit (fresh or in a light syrup) for dessert?
- prepare a dish without added salt or monosodium glutamate?
- accommodate special requests if made in advance by telephone or in person?

Restaurants that prepare foods by request offer diners greater control over the amount and type of fat and the amount of salt they consume. If entree descriptions are limited or missing from a restaurant menu, don't hesitate to ask how that food is prepared. For example, is the fish baked in butter, margarine, or olive oil? When ordering, make sure your special requests are noted by the server. Ask that salad dressings be served on the side or, even better, request lemon wedges instead of salad dressing. Similarly, if you order a baked potato, ask that the sour cream or butter be on the side, or eliminate them entirely (Dijon mustard tastes great on a baked potato). For those business breakfasts, toast or English muffins can be ordered dry instead of being soaked in butter, with jelly or honey on the side. Similarly, waffles and pancakes can be ordered to come without a scoop of butter on top. But a better choice is to order your favorite high-fiber cereal.

Often restaurants have food that aren't on the menu (they may be served at another meal) and will bring them out on request. If the menu offers fried fish, ask the chef to lightly season it with herbs and broil or poach it. People who eat in restaurants regularly can't treat each meal out like a celebration and a reason to splurge. Having a chef meet your special request so you get a meal you will enjoy can be some consolation.

In general, simply prepared foods are the best choices for a low-fat meal. Also, choose fresh fish or chicken most frequently. When selecting red meats, order leaner cuts and smaller portions. Avoid processed meats. The selections should be baked, broiled, roasted, steamed, boiled, or poached, with all visible fat trimmed away. Skin should be removed from chicken. With pasta, choose red sauces over white. Ask for your vegetables steamed. Select low-fat dairy products, and ask for milk for your coffee or tea instead of cream or nondairy coffee whiteners.

For a low-sodium intake, avoid salting items at the table; use condiments and steak and soy sauces sparingly; select fresh vegetables instead of canned; and choose "homemade" rather than commercially prepared soups. Choose oil and vinegar over ready-mixed salad dressings; avoid processed meats and cheeses; request lemon slices to season foods; and request that pickles, olives, and potato chips not be served with the entree.

To ensure adequate fiber intake, select a high-fiber cereal for a morning meal; fresh fruit for an appetizer or dessert; steamed fresh vegetables as a side dish, vegetable-grain platters, and whole-grain breads.

The concept of balancing your food intake comes in handy if you're faced with a situation dining out where the choices are few, or your will power is particularly weak. If you evaluate your food intake a day or a week at a time instead of a meal at a time, your overall success at nutritional eating will be more likely and your dining out experience will certainly be more enjoyable.

So let's say you're having a particularly weak moment during a business lunch and you order a rather high-fat meal topped with a rich dessert. Just cut down at dinner than night, or eat "lean" the next day. One high-fat meal will have little, if any, effect on your overall health. It's a constant pattern of overindulgence over time that can cause the problems we discussed in Chapter 2.

Many of you still may feel that a fine restaurant is not the place for dietary dogma. But if you dine out on a regular basis, some moderate substitution is necessary. You can also develop your own set of rules that define your nutritional goals. Such a policy might involve goals of high fiber, low fat, limits on sugar, or a combination of all the above. A general policy for eating, rather than a strict food-avoidance rule, permits more latitude and discretion.

The Dos and Don'ts of Dining Out

	BEST BETS	AVOID
Appetizers	Vegetable juice; bouillon; fresh fruit; seafood cocktail	Deep-fried vegetables; creamed soups; anything cooked in butter
Salads	Any fresh fruits or vegetables with oil and vinegar, lemon juice, or low calorie dressing	Creamy salad dressings; toppings such as cheese, avocados, bacon, or nuts; mayonnaise-based salads
Potatoes/ Rice/Pasta	Mashed, baked, or boiled potatoes; steamed rice; pasta with red sauce	French fried, hash browns, creamed, escalloped potatoes, pasta with white sauce, stuffed pasta
Vegetables	Steamed, stewed, boiled	Creamed, fried, sautéed
Entrees	Roasted, baked, broiled, steamed, poached, grilled, boiled; trim off excess fat	Duck; goose; high-fat sauces; gravy; sautéed, breaded, fried

	BEST BETS	AVOID
Breads	Plain bread or toast; dinner rolls; crackers; plain muffins; pita bread	Sweet rolls; coffee cake; croissants; doughnuts; Danish pastries; biscuits
Desserts	Fresh fruits; frozen yogurt; sorbet; angel food cake; gelatin	Ice cream; custard; pastries; whipped cream
Beverages	Water; fruit juices; low-fat or skim milk	Chocolate milk; milk shakes; soft drinks; alcohol
Italian	Pasta with red clam, meatless marinara, marsala, pesto, or mushroom sauce; pizza with fresh vegetable toppings	Sausages and meatballs; white cheese sauces; garlic bread
Chinese	Stir-fried chicken, seafood, and vegetables; soft noodles; steamed rice and dumplings; fortune cookies	Fried wontons and egg rolls; egg foo yung; fried rice; "crispy" entrees; lobster sauces; soy sauce; MSG
Mexican	Chicken, seafood, and vegetable burritos, enchiladas, and corn tortillas	Guacamole; shredded cheese and sour cream; refried beans; pork and cheese chimichangas; flour tortillas
French	Poached or steamed fish; chicken in wine or other light sauces; niçoise salads; consommé	Pâté; quiche; duck; hollandaise-type sauces; dishes with "beurre" or "crème"; cream-based soups; escargot; French pastries
Greek	Beef shish kebab; pita bread; salads; couscous; tabouli; tzatziki	Lamb; spinach pie; deep-fried falafel
Japanese	Sushi; chicken and fish teriyaki; tofu and vegetables, surimi	Tempura and other deep-fried dishes
Indian	Tandoori chicken; mulligatawny soup; coriander, tamarind, and yogurt-based sauces	Fried breads; coconut milk; curry
Thai/Indonesian	Grilled chicken or shrimp; steamed seafood; tom yom koong soup; Thai fish stew	Sauces or soups with coconut milk
Cajun	Seafood or vegetable gumbo or jambalaya; grilled fish	Andouille and other sausages; fried fish

"Heart Healthy" Restaurants Geared to Address Nutritional Trends

Today's chefs are reinventing the meal.

And so at Eccentric, the restaurant Oprah Winfrey opened in Chicago, there is a seafood bouillabaisse that leaves out the higher-cholesterol items like squid or shrimp, and a tuna steak tossed with four kinds of peppers in a light veal stock.

At Legal Seafoods in Boston, they'll steam your haddock with fresh vegetables in a foil envelope so it cooks in its own juices.

At Chez Eddy in Houston, the grilled red snapper comes with a red pepper sauce, rice, broccoli, snow peas, and carrots. The meal is 25 percent fat and provides only 561 calories and 80 milligrams of cholesterol.

The Four Seasons restaurant in New York is nationally renowned for its fine food but equally noted for its "spa cuisine." Chef Seppi Renggli studied with Columbia University nutritionist Joyce Leung prior to creating his nutritionally balanced meals. With appetizer plus entree, each meal is roughly 700 calories.

At Maxaluna in Boca Raton, Florida, the veal stock is composed primarily of vegetables and herbs flavored with roasted veal bones, which is lighter and easier to digest than cream sauces—not to mention the missing fat and calories.

At Five Feet, a restaurant offering "continental Chinese cuisine" in Laguna Beach, California, sesame and olive oil are predominantly used when cooking, and entrees rarely come with butter or cream sauces. While the entrees change daily, some form of pasta accompanies most meals; fish or meats are grilled, poached, or stir-fried; and distinctive flavor is derived from, for example, ginger, black beans, and garlic, instead of fat.

Dieci, an Italian restaurant in New York, was cited by the New York *Daily News* for its "accommodation to low-cholesterol, low-fat diets." Its owner, Joseph Franco, has been preparing Italian food with an eye toward good nutrition for seven years. Franco was overweight himself, so he began developing recipes for his personal nutrition goals. As a result, he has passed a number of these recipes on to his customers. One example is his preparation of Norwegian salmon. He eliminates the traditional mustard sauce that includes butter and heavy cream and instead grills the salmon and beds it on marinated arugula with balsamic vinegar.

Another restaurateur who drew on his personal experience is Gary Cochran of Beau Jacks Foods and Spirits in Birmingham, Michigan. He recalls that after his father's mild heart attack and subsequent heart surgery, his restaurant learned about the "Eating Away from Home" program of the American Heart Association. Beau Jacks became the first restaurant to bring this AHA program into Michigan. Mr. Cochran, who works with an Oakland County (Michigan) dietitian and the AHA, describes his "Dine to Your Heart's Content" menu as about 15 percent heart healthy. One example of his creative and healthy entrees is the lasagna, layered with fresh zucchini, part-skim mozzarella cheese, fresh basil, fresh garlic, and a meatless marinara sauce.

A late 1990 report by a study group from the Institute of Medicine (noted in the last chapter) called for all restaurants (particularly fast-food) to provide information about the calories, saturated fat, cholesterol, fiber, protein, salt, and vitamins in the standard dishes they prepare. In small restaurants, it might be in a brochure available to a customer upon request. But in larger restaurants and restaurant chains, the report says, the information should be given on wrappers or displayed prominently where the food is bought.

Restaurateurs are beginning to understand their obligations to nutrition-minded patrons. It's a trend that will make good nutrition, like the fabled credit card, something you can't leave home without!

8

The Traveler's Guide to Good Nutrition

Travelers want good food and good nutrition, whether it is at an altitude of thirty thousand feet, in their hotel room or in a hotel dining room, at a spa, in a foreign country, or in an ethnic region of the United States. And fitness buffs don't like giving up their regular morning runs or vigorous weight-room workouts. With more people traveling each day for business and pleasure, this fact has impacted the airline, hotel, and restaurant industries.

As a result, you no longer have to take pot luck when you leave your hometown today. And you can better cope with dietary changes, jet lag, and strange surroundings and still be fresh, in-shape, and alert for meetings, negotiations, or sightseeing. In this chapter, we'll look at ways you can stay fit and maintain good nutrition while on the road.

First You Have to Get There: Eating Right While in the Air

The first travel meal you eat is often on a plane. And fliers love to hate airline food. Just listen to what some of the people we spoke with had to say.

Judy Markey, who travels once a month, calls airline fare "repugnant." While she admits the meat is usually edible, she says "the vegetables are dead."

Jane Hartley, who has flown frequently on business and pleasure trips, says she's dissatisfied with airline food because it is not cooked well, the ingredients are not good, she doesn't like the sauces, and the selections are too limited. Jane singled out Air France as the only carrier that provided food she was happy with. "With most of the airline food," she says, "you can't even tell what you're eating." Jane adds that the food in first class is better, because fresher, untouched foods like fruit, cheese, and cold shrimp are offered, and they are not saturated with sauces.

Barry Nash, who travels regularly on business, says, "I have finally reached the point where I avoid airline food as much as I can. I find it unsatisfactory, and I never feel good after I've eaten it." There is one exception. "If the flight is early enough in the evening, I'm hungry, and it's my only chance to eat other than at 9:30 at night when I get home, I'll eat something on the plane," he admits. Barry says he's tried to specify certain foods through his travel agent but finds it frustrating because he always experiences a breakdown sooner or later. Furthermore, he doesn't feel the special meals are very good, either. "You get a lot better food in business and first class on international flights than you do on domestic American flights," he adds.

Burt Staniar says he picks at the airline food because it is "so awful-tasting." Although he tries to avoid eating airline food, he sometimes eats chicken, he tends to eat the vegetables that are offered, and he never eats the "fake cake."

While airline food continues to have its critics, passengers seem to be eating the food, according to a 1987 survey. Half of the 610 passengers surveyed by Cornell University's School of Hotel Administration found airline food better than it was before deregulation in 1978, while 27 percent said it was the same, and 23 percent said it was worse.

Yet the nation's airlines are spending record amounts on food service in an effort to shed their image as the providers of the airborne equivalent of hospital food. They are hiring well-known chefs to help revamp menus, replacing plastic with silverware and ceramic crockery, and offering more healthful fare.

The nation's ten largest airlines spent $2 billion on food in 1989, an average of $5.05 per passenger, which is 13.3 percent more than in 1988 and 21.7 percent more than in 1987, according to Airline Economics, a consulting concern in Washington. Much of the increase in money spent is due to the airlines' effort to improve food quality. The push for better food reflects the changing airline industry. With only eight American airlines controlling 90 percent of the domestic market, competition is less on fares and more on services—like seat width, frequent-flier programs, and, now, food. The changes are more apparent in the business and first-class sections, for which airlines spend three to four times more for food than they do for coach class.

Particularly in coach sections, the trend in the airline industry is toward lighter fare and more snacks, even though the Cornell survey found that 65 percent of fliers prefer hot meals. Eastern, for example, no longer serves hot meals in coach on flights of less than three hours. So if you're on a short flight, chances are the only airline food you'll be offered is your choice of beverage and a snack.

Irrespective of the food offered, passengers can make good nutritional choices when flying. For example, avoid alcohol in flight. Alcohol aggravates jet lag and has more impact than it does on the ground. Combined with the very low humidity and recirculated cabin air in a pressurized cabin, drinking alcohol in-flight may also lead to dehydration. It's best to avoid coffee, tea, and cola as well, because the caffeine in these beverages also contributes to dehydration. Instead, drink liquids such as water or fruit juices—8 ounces every hour—since doing so helps to combat dehydration. Salted peanuts are best to avoid, due to both sodium and fat content.

Nearly all airlines are offering more healthful alternatives, however. For instance, Continental serves fresh fruit with cereal. American has added mineral water to its beverage carts. United has replaced butter with margarine. And even the ubiquitous peanut does come unsalted.

While airlines admit that they don't focus on nutritional balance when serving snacks, they make sure full-course meals are well balanced. Actually, up to a year's worth of planning goes into the meal you're eating on a flight today.

Most airline food is prepared by large catering organizations like Caterair, Ogden, and Sky Chefs. The Caterair kitchen at Kennedy International Airport turns out as many as twenty thousand meals a day, with assembly-line efficiency. Still, most airlines choose the recipes and specify how the food is to be prepared.

American Airlines runs food surveys and focus groups, has organized a conclave of twelve chefs who meet annually to review the airline's food service, and follows the public's general eating trends. United requires its chefs to dine once a month at restaurants to keep them in touch with what goes on and to improve upon their menu suggestions. The most valued information about airline meals comes from flight attendants. United gets up to seven thousand "Notes to the Chef" from attendants every other month.

Once airlines and caterers get a fix on public taste, menu planning begins. United, which has twenty kitchens, plans most of its own meals. Other airlines, like American, give general guidelines to caterers. But trends on the ground aren't the only consideration in menu planning. Airline food has to survive chilling and reheating and must meet U.S. Department of Agriculture requirements: cold food must be stored below 45 degrees Fahrenheit, warm meals above 140 degrees. Some meals might taste great on the ground but lose their flavor by the time you're airborne and they're placed on your tray table.

Planners also consider menu fatigue—a condition of the frequent traveler facing the same meal flight after flight. American has six different meals for each level of service and rotates the meals monthly at each level. United splits the country into five regions and offers different meals in each. That way, you will get a different meal on a flight from Denver to San Francisco than on one from New York to Miami. Meals with the widest appeal (or that are the least offensive to the most people) are most likely to be selected by carriers.

But with all this planning, if you're thinking about dieting, you may consider your alternatives to standard airline fare. The typical airline lunch or dinner, including the dessert, has about 750 to 800 calories. That's equivalent to a quarter-pound hamburger with french fries. Airlines have slowly been addressing this issue, particularly by serving chicken more often. Unfortunately, most airlines serve the chicken meat that most people don't want. More carriers are buying dark, deboned thigh meat, which costs half as much as white meat. Stockpiles of dark meat have grown in recent years because consumers increasingly prefer white meat. Trans World Airlines is one fan. It includes thigh meat in teriyaki, barbecue, and sweet-and-sour recipes, explaining that the thigh meat "reconstitutes" very well.

If you find the standard airline fare too hard to stomach, you do have alternatives.

First, you can request a "special meal." All major airlines offer free special meals to anyone ordering them a day in advance, no matter where they're seated. Most of the choices are religious (kosher, Hindu, etc.) or dietary (low cholesterol, low sodium, vegetarian, etc.), babies' and children's meals, or fruit or seafood plates, but several carriers even offer entree alternatives such as quiche, crab, and barbecued ribs.

While it is best to order special meals when making reservations, some airlines try to make special accommodations for travelers without a lot of lead time. Delta, which offers fifteen different special meals, will accept requests up to six hours before departure. Similarly, for flights of an hour and a half or longer, United will guarantee a special meal from its sixteen different meal choices if you order twenty-four hours in advance, and the airline attempts to fill requests on shorter notice. American Airlines, which offers an "American Traveler Menu" created with the American Heart Association and the Kenneth Cooper Aerobic Clinic, accepts orders for its heart healthy options six to twelve hours in advance.

Most people don't know about the meals, because the airlines don't advertise them. Obviously, the logistics of trying to serve a lot of special meals on a flight can be difficult, and it costs the airlines more, so most airlines don't want to promote this service. As a result, fewer than 5 percent of all fliers order them.

Still, the ranks of discriminating airline diners are gradually growing. United, for example, served 500,000 more special meals in 1987 than in 1986, about a 1 percent increase. In response to more requests for special meals, TWA expanded its menus. And, according to several airline food suppliers, there have been greater requests for special meals, particularly lighter and less caloric meals.

Secondly, you can BYOB—bring your own bag. Bringing your own wholesome snack or meal is an alternative to standard airline food. We so often pack our picky youngsters foods they like for long trips, but we forget about ourselves. A piece of chicken, fresh fruit, a sandwich of sliced turkey breast and tomatoes on whole wheat bread, or fresh vegetables like carrots and zucchini are satisfying and nourishing. Remember to wrap food well to keep it from drying out, and don't bring foods that require immediate refrigeration.

A final alternative is to just say no. You can avoid calories in airline meals by not eating the dessert, the peanuts, and the salad dressing; or you can just pass on the flight meal and eat before or after you land. Or you can try to fly between meals if your willpower is weak. Ask a reservation agent or travel agent what meals are served on the flight before booking it.

Here are some overall tips to help you avoid discomfort on any flight (the first three are minimal ways to exercise and increase your circulation within the constraints of a plane):

• Take frequent walks up and down the aisles.
• Take occasional deep breaths.
• Frequently loosen and tighten abdominal (stomach) and gluteal (buttocks) muscles.
• Eat lightly during your flight.
• Drink plenty of water before, during, and after your flight.

Hotel Restaurants and Room Service: Accommodations That Make Nutrition Easier

Meal options expand once you check into your hotel. As with airlines, hotels—in their dining rooms, coffee shops, and room-service menus—are offering more selections geared toward good nutrition.

Some five years ago, the Marriott Hotel Division launched a "Good for You" menu program with the sanction of the American Heart Association. As interest and consumer demand has soared, the Hotel Division is putting more chicken and fish, fresh fruit, and other lighter items on its menus. Some of Marriott's resorts—including the Desert Springs in Palm Springs, California, and the Downtown Los Angeles Marriott—have made very innovative menu changes to adhere to their healthy-menu concept.

"Perfect Balance" is the trademark for low-calorie fare offered by Hyatt hotels nationwide. The Hyatt on Capitol Square in Columbus, Ohio, for example, has two special items at breakfast and three at lunch and dinner. The lunch items include stir-fry chicken and shrimp, broiled chicken breast, and broiled fresh fish, all under 330 calories.

Another example of a nutrition-conscious hotel restaurant is the Circular Dining Room at the Hotel Hershey in Hershey, Pennsylvania. The restaurant works with a registered dietitian at the Hershey Medical Center, and at least 50 percent of its menu is nutrition-oriented.

The Desert Garden in Tucson, Arizona, also has specific low-calorie, -fat, and -cholesterol dishes. Nutrition has been one of the hotel's concerns since it opened in 1985, because many of the Tucson visitors are older and more diet-conscious.

While the nature and quality of the dining rooms tend to be reflected in the room-service menus of most hotels, some prepare their "meals on wheels" in separate kitchens. Many experienced travelers watching their diets say this is why they limit their use of room service while on the road. For early-morning meals, however, room service can provide a good, nutritious start for your day. Most large hotels do offer a nutritious breakfast choice. Barry Nash often eats breakfast in his room while traveling on business. He tends to order cereal and fruit, sometimes pancakes and juice, but rarely eggs.

Quick service is one of the most important ingredients to good room-service dining, particularly for more elaborate meals. If you've had a long day and want to dine in the relaxing privacy of your own hotel room, save yourself the disappointment of a cold room-service meal by inquiring about delivery time (30 minutes will usually guarantee the food is fresh from the kitchen and is not being reheated). Also ask if your meal will be prepared in the hotel's restaurant kitchen or in a separate kitchen. If the answer is the latter, or if nothing nutritious or appealing is on the menu, you might opt for a bellhop to quietly pick up a meal from a nearby restaurant.

Pleasure Travel: The Fitness Vacation, with an Emphasis on Nutrition

A new kind of health vacation has emerged in the 1990s as the idea of a restorative, physically challenging getaway has caught on. We're not talking here about spa vacations for the well-to-do. They still exist; but today, with more people in more income brackets concerned about fitness and stress (a subject we'll discuss in the next chapter), pleasure travel has increasingly gravitated toward the "fitness" vacation, where food is always prepared with nutrition in mind, and nutrition and exercise classes are offered.

Today's fitness vacationers are younger, more health conscious, generally success oriented, and often looking for an escape from their harried day-to-day life-styles. Increasingly, they include men as well as women, and sometimes whole families. The prime goal is to reduce stress, eat right, and exercise at a moderate level. Exercise is already a part of these people's daily lives, so they're not looking for a place to help them "get in shape." The word "fitness" is now taken to mean long-term life-style improvement.

A fitness vacation is often a relaxing journey to an exotic setting where guests participate in aerobic workouts, nutrition classes, meditation and yoga, sports training, and more. The ultimate goal is not to lose weight, although many don't mind if that happens, but to gain a more relaxed perspective on life.

According to some estimates, more than 1.2 million Americans are passing on the traditional vacation of sunning, sightseeing, eating, and drinking, opting instead for this healthful alternative. New spas, ranging from the lavish to the rustic, are opening almost monthly. Many hotels and vacation resorts are adding up-to-date facilities and trained staff to their operations. And, wisely, all new programs employ chefs who have broadened their menus and are providing take-home diet advice.

There are 240 different facilities in the United States, Canada, Mexico, and the Caribbean listed in Bernard Burt's guidebook *Fodor's Health & Fitness Vacations* (Fodor's, 1989). And they come in all price ranges, from less than $699 a week to more than $2,000.

Among the newest is Canyon Ranch in Lenox, Massachusetts, the heart of the Berkshire Mountains. A sister center to the acclaimed Canyon Ranch in Tucson, it opened in late 1989 in an historic mansion and includes a 100,000-square-foot fitness center with racquetball, squash, and tennis courts; a running track; a 75-foot swimming pool; and separate spas for men and women with saunas, steam rooms, inhalation rooms, and Jacuzzis. The emphasis is on exercise, nutrition, stress reduction, and permanent lifestyle improvement. The cost for one week is $1,660.

But there is a health vacation for every budget, depending on your particular goals. In Litchfield, Minnesota, you'll find the Birdwing Spa, charging $1,050 for seven nights in a single-room accommodation. Meals, nutrition and fitness counseling, exercise, beauty treatment (including massage, facial, manicure, pedicure, and hair style), and tips are all included in the basic price. *Affordable Spas and Fitness Resorts* (Ventana Press, 1988) is another guide to help the budget- and fitness-conscious.

Other than your checkbook, you need to look at your personal goals. Do you want to lose weight, increase your exercise level, reduce your stress, train for sports activities, or simply be pampered? Do you prefer the mountains to the ocean? Are there special interests that you'd like to develop—gourmet cooking, or yoga? Would you rather be at a place for families or one for singles only?

In his Fodor's book, Bernard Burt classifies the various types of health resorts to help the vacationer find the most appropriate destination to meet his or her needs. Most important is to find the combination of facilities, professional staff, and programming that make you most comfortable. We list those that include nutrition as part of their focus.

- **Life enhancement.** The Hilton Head Health Institute, Hilton Head Island, South Carolina, is this type of program, which generally features a total assessment of the vacationer's condition, with medical tests and personal consultations on nutrition and fitness. These programs aim for long-term physical and psychological benefits, and the size of each participating group is limited to about a dozen men and women.
- **Weight management.** Examples are the Kerr House in Grand Rapids, Ohio, or the Sans Souci Health Resort in Bellbrook, Ohio, which stress learning to lose weight properly and to maintain a healthy balance in body mass. These programs teach proper eating habits, from what to buy in the supermarket to how to prepare meals.

- **Nutrition and diet.** The Bonaventure Resort and Spa in Fort Lauderdale, Florida, is an example of a program that helps develop healthier nutrition habits through lectures and hands-on experience in food preparation. The programs focus on the fundamentals of eating healthy natural foods.
- **Holistic health.** Vigorous or mellow, the programs, like the one at the Feathered-Pipe Ranch in Helena, Montana, stress emotional, intellectual, and spiritual development, combining exercise, nutrition, stress control, and relaxation.
- **Preventive medicine.** The Pritikin Longevity Center in Santa Monica, California, is such a program, taking a scientific approach to health and fitness by combining traditional medical services with advanced prevention concepts and offer participants exposure to medical, fitness, nutritional, and psychology experts.

To further help you find the health vacation of your choice, travel agencies are cropping up that specialize in just this kind of vacation. Spa-Finders Travel Arrangements of New York City offers special discounts at many health spas, fitness resorts, and holistic retreats worldwide. It also offers a free 800 number for booking service (1-800-ALL-SPAS) and a *Spa Finder* catalog for $4.95.

Even cruise vacations no longer have to be limited to an endless procession of formal five-course meals, gala midnight buffets, and minimal sport activities like shuffleboard or Ping-Pong. Today's luxury liners feature fitness facilities and nutrition programs that are equal to anything on land. New health and fitness programs include fresher, lighter, and more healthful foods low in calories, sodium, and cholesterol to complement the floating spas and exercise workouts.

A leader in this trend is Greek-born Chris Tsardoulias, executive food and beverage director for Royal Cruise Line. Working with the American Heart Asssociation, he has created a series of dishes in which fresh herbs replace salt and butter, so you can eat "To Your Heart's Content." Under that title, on menus of the ship the *Royal Odyssey*, you may find light vegetarian lasagne layered with vegetables, cheese, and basil-tomato sauce; scallops dusted with herbs and paprika, then skewered and broiled; and fillets of halibut, salmon, and rock cod poached and served with a tangy lemon coulis. As a further aid to passengers, the Royal Cruise Line distributes a comprehensive nutrition guide providing nutrient analyses, with calorie counts, for each of the new menu items. In addition, the booklet suggests ways to maintain a diet when selecting from standard shipboard menus—substitution techniques like the ones outlined in Chapter 3, such as replacing cream with yogurt and ordering omelets made without egg yolks. Frequent cruise passengers often worry about weight gain, so finding a delicious and healthful alternative is a boon to them or any fitness-conscious traveler.

If working out is your main goal when out of town, Tim Zagat publishes the two-volume *Zagat United States Hotel Survey*, which covers 850 hotels in 38 cities and includes a sports-facilities index. As the fitness industry becomes more sophisticated, hotel facilities are expanding to meet the demand created in local health clubs. Some of the exceptional hotel health centers offer top-of-the-line equipment—for instance, those at the Nikko Chicago Hotel and the Westin Hotel in Washington, D.C. At the Plaza in New York, stationary bicycles were ordered for all eighty of the hotel suites. All the hotels in New York's Morgan Hotel Group (current and planned) are developing fitness programs, from Lifecycles at the Royalton to a five-thousand-square-foot health club at the Barbizon.

Other examples of well-equipped hotel fitness clubs include the Regency Hotel in New York, which is equipped with such state-of-the-art machines as the Versa Climber and Liferower. This facility was designed for both aerobic and strengthening workouts and includes free weights, a massage room, a Jacuzzi, and a steam room. The Rowes Wharf Health Club and Spa at the Boston Harbor Hotel boasts the largest indoor pool in the city. Water aerobic classes are available to guests, as is the exercise room, which includes weight machines, StairMasters, treadmills, rowers, and stationary bikes; the Ritz Carlton Hotel in Laguna Nigel, California has a complete fitness center, daily stretching, firming, and flexing classes, and aerobics, in addition to personalized fitness programs. The most inclusive option is the Personal Best Program. With the help of a computer it offers a risk-factor profile to assess life-style patterns and habits and suggests how poor ones can be changed to improve health.

While hotel workout centers may be attractive for many, some of you may prefer a more solitary exercise routine in the privacy of your own room. The answer is in portable gear such as light free weights or wrist weights, or if your hotel room has a VCR (call ahead to find out), your favorite workout tape.

Nutrition Facts for Foreign Travel

It is best to use common sense when country hopping, because outside the United States, the varieties of exotic foods, the methods of food preparation, and the presence of foreign bacteria can wreak havoc on the American digestive system.

In all, some 850,000 out of 100 million U.S. citizens who travel abroad each year become ill. Don't let your next trip, whether for business or pleasure, become a nightmare. Once you leave the United States, healthy food choices are much more difficult to make.

The cuisine of many European countries is far too high in animal fat, cholesterol, salt, and sugar. Studies on dietary practices in France, for example, show a sharp decline in per capita consumption of grains (an important source of fiber) and an increase in consumption of cholesterol-rich red meat, eggs, and dairy products. Today, fat comprises an unhealthy 45 percent of the total calories in the average French diet. (The U.S. guideline is 30 percent, and the average American diet includes 40 percent fat.) Nutritionists and dietitians in Norway, Great Britain, and Germany are also becoming increasingly concerned about the health-poor eating habits of their citizens. Green vegetables are almost unheard of in the typical Scandinavian diet. And consider the fondness of the British for steak and kidney pie, bangers and mash, fish and chips, scones and clotted cream—or the German predilection for sausages and beer.

Of course, why travel if you can't eat traditional national delicacies? It's almost impossible not to be tempted. But even as you follow the maxim "When in Rome, do as the Romans do," remember that your nutritional needs remain the same no matter where you go. Try to eat meals that provide a balance from the four main food groups: fruits and vegetables; cereals, breads, and whole grains; eggs, meat, fish, and poultry; milk and cheese. Watch the numbers of calories, fats, sugars, and sodium-rich foods. When confronted with an array of exotic dishes, don't overdo it. Try sampling a small taste of everything—as long as it appears to be well cooked and made with wholesome ingredients.

Further, if you're on a special diet, don't hesitate to request the appropriate foods, prepared properly. Many fine restaurants around the world employ chefs who pride themselves in catering to the special health needs of patrons. When you do make a request, it's a good idea to be specific. Don't simply state what you can't eat—clarify what you *can*.

The age-old advice "Don't drink the water" should be taken seriously. According to a special panel of the National Institutes of Health convened to collate health-related information about foreign travel, the only proven, risk-free way to avoid contracting diarrhea is to follow "sensible dietary practices."

During your travels, the safest drinks are bottled, carbonated beverages, beer, wine, and hot coffee and tea. This is particularly true for Mexico and other less-developed countries (you usually don't have to worry about the water in most European countries). As for plain, unbottled water, be sure it's been boiled for at least 10 minutes. And absolutely avoid ice cubes—and even using tap water to brush your teeth.

Especially risky foods include raw vegetables and salads, often washed in the water you need to avoid, and meat or seafood that has not been thoroughly cooked. Other foods to avoid are unpasteurized milk products (use powdered milk instead) and unpeeled fruit. And don't be fooled by some common misconceptions. Mixed drinks are not safe—alcohol does not "burn off" the germs in bad water. Spices do not mitigate the contaminants in food. Seeking out only American food may not be your wisest choice— imported food may not be fresh.

The risk of eating contaminated food may be decreased somewhat if you stick to the beaten path. Most large restaurants and hotels in popular tourist areas are closely monitored by United States travel organizations. As an extra precaution, be sure to ask your travel agent for any news about health problems at restaurants or hotels in the cities you will be visiting. Above all, avoid eating or drinking any wares offered by street vendors.

When you go sightseeing in warm weather, you run the risk of dehydration, heat cramps, heat exhaustion, and even heat stroke. Our total percentage of body water tends to decline as we age. Less body water means a reduction in heat tolerance and the body's ability to regulate internal temperature, especially in women. Physiologists recommend drinking a minimum of three glasses of water a day, preferably four glasses during hot weather or exercise. Remember, water is the best thirst quencher. Whenever a drink contains sugar, salt, fat, or alcohol, absorption into your system will be reduced. If you tire of drinking plain water or just don't like the taste, an herbal tea without sugar or a wedge of lemon in your water are good alternatives. (This is assuming that the water supply is safe or that you are using bottled water.)

One more tip—as is customary with Europeans, pack along a few reliable snacks. Choose favorite convenience foods that travel well, are individually wrapped, and are high in complex carbohydrates. You never know when you're going to arrive somewhere and find all reputable establishments closed. Small packages of whole grain crackers, cheese and cracker snack packs, nuts or seeds, and dried fruits are all healthful travel snacks. If you're going far off the beaten track, individual cans of water-packed tuna and canned fruits packed in their juices are additional items you may want to bring.

The Real Life Nutrition Plan for the Cross-Country Traveler

Most frequent travelers in the United States say they take more trips for pleasure and business within the country rather than abroad. So let's pay particular attention to regional favorites that you will likely come across in your travels.

Distinctive taste differences exist as you go from one region to another. The reason is due as much to the ready availability of the products in each region as to the ethnic backgrounds and preferences of the people who live there.

Few people in the United States today are of native lineage. Most have ancestors who voyaged across oceans to settle here. Along with their tangible belongings, the immigrants brought with them a wealth of food culture. After they arrived in their new country, their food habits had to change slightly, because the familiar foods from the country they came from were not readily available. But a host of new ones were abundant; so they fitted new foods into their old patterns. The result is what we call ethnic foods.

Today we enjoy a great variety of these foods. Ethnic foods happen to do very well in certain regions. In New England, you will find (after pizza parlors) more Oriental restaurants than hamburger havens. Similarly, Oriental restaurants beat out hamburger hangouts in the Middle Atlantic. In the Pacific, hamburger and pizza restaurants tie for first place.

If you ask diners in the various regions what they look for, you come up with a picture of how nutrition-conscious they are. According to research by NPD Research and the National Restaurant Association, New Englanders in general are the most healthful eaters when they dine out because they go for nonfried fish. Lowest on the nutrition list are people in the East South Central states, who order everything fried. (The research eliminated the nationwide favorites french fries, hamburgers, side-dish salads, bread, and pizza, often found in fast-food restaurants.)

The regional favorites were mapped out as follows:

- New England (Connecticut, Massachusetts, Maine, New Hampshire, Rhode Island, Vermont): **Nonfried fish**
- Middle Atlantic (New York, New Jersey, Pennsylvania): **Veal and pasta**
- South Atlantic (Delaware, District of Columbia, Florida, Georgia, Maryland, North and South Carolina, Virginia, West Virginia): **Chicken, fried and nonfried shellfish**
- East North Central (Illinois, Indiana, Michigan, Ohio, Wisconsin): **Beef and dishes made with beef, such as chili**
- East South Central (Alabama, Kentucky, Mississippi, Tennessee): **Fried foods, such as fish, chicken, vegetables**
- West North Central (Iowa, Kansas, Minnesota, Missouri, Nebraska, North and South Dakota): **Mashed potatoes, pan pizza**
- West South Central (Arkansas, Louisiana, Oklahoma, Texas): **Mexican foods such as enchiladas and nachos**
- Mountain (Arizona, Colorado, Idaho, Montana, Nevada, New Mexico, Utah, Wyoming): **Mexican foods such as tacos and burritos**
- Pacific (Alaska, California, Hawaii, Oregon, Washington): **Hispanic and Asian foods, such as burritos, taco salad, Chinese foods.**

We thought it would be helpful to provide nutrition tips for any region of the country where you might find yourself. Judy Stokes, an Atlanta dietitian and food management consultant, has made several recommendations that we felt were right on target:

- If you find yourself in New England, order fish broiled, baked, or grilled, with as little high-fat sauce as possible. Or get it done in polyunsaturated margarine to cut cholesterol.
- If you're traveling to the Middle Atlantic region, you can't really go wrong. Veal is relatively low in cholesterol. Order it made with a little white wine and a sprinkle of Parmesan cheese or with a low-fat tomato sauce. Pasta can be very healthful with vegetables and low-fat cheese. Meat sauces raise the cholesterol.
- Chicken and shellfish tend to be popular items in the South Atlantic region. Watch the frying—it will only provide you with too much fat and too many calories. While shellfish tend to be higher in cholesterol, they are so low in saturated fat content that they are healthful choices—as long as you order them broiled rather than batter-fried.
- If you go with the flow in the East North Central region, you won't be making a good choice. Chili is spicy, high in fat and calories, and a challenge to the digestive tract. It takes longer to digest foods high in fat.
- Similarly, the popularity of fried foods in the East South Central region spells trouble. Nutrition guidelines call for low fat and sodium. Eating fried foods frequently can lead to problems associated with cancer and heart disease.
- The West North Central region favorites should be ordered with care. Mashed potatoes are best without the gravy, and pizza with low-fat mozzarella and vegetables can be a good choice—it's the sausage and pepperoni that should be avoided.
- When traveling in the West South Central region, order chicken enchiladas, not beef. You can find Mexican foods that are low in fat and high in protein, such as beans and corn products. But avoid the refried beans—they contain lard—and do without the high-fat sausage dishes. Go light on the sour cream and sauces, and go easy on the guacamole—it's loaded with fat. Tostadas are a healthful choice if you avoid the fried tortillas and the sour cream.
- In the Mountain states, avoid the fried tortillas and greasy meat.

Look for the leanest beef and the lightest frying oil when ordering tacos and burritos. The cheese, lettuce, tomato, and cornmeal in a taco make it a healthy meal.
• In the Pacific region, stir-fried Chinese vegetables are fine. But
avoid high-sodium soy sauce and fried egg rolls or tempura
dishes. And ask the restaurant to leave out the MSG; it's high in
sodium.

So regardless of where you travel, or whether your trip is for
business or pleasure, or both, you should now know the nutrition
and fitness facts of life while on the road (or air). We bid you bon
voyage—and don't forget to write!

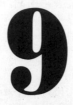

Nutrition and Stress

Bumper-to-bumper traffic, work deadlines, family pressures, overscheduled days that leave no breathing room . . . STRESS. We make our own. We get it from others, sometimes even from our loved ones.

What exactly is stress? According to most experts, stress is the body's response to physiological (surgery, injury), environmental (extreme cold, smoking), or psychological/emotional (job stress, daily hassles, life catastrophes) demands. Most of us think of emotional demands—the pressures of the daily grind—when we talk about stress, the kind that often puts our body in gridlock as our muscles begin to tense. But the broader definition of stress goes well beyond psychological tension and anxiety and encompasses any event that disrupts normal body functioning and affects the appetite. It includes serious injury or illness, such as severe burn or pneumonia; major operations, such as open-heart surgery; pregnancy; and hard physical labor. This chapter will deal with the narrower definition—those stressful events that more consistently affect our daily lives.

Let's look at how stress affects the lives of the people you've come to know in this book.

As a writer, Carole Gerber has a lot of deadlines, and she admits she experiences some career-related stress. She says she tries to manage the stress and not be so harried, but her style is to hold things in, expressing herself less often than she should. When under stress, Carole says, she doesn't eat or she eats less. "I think stress affects everybody's eating habits," she observes. "That's how you can tell fat people from thin people—fat people eat [under stress] and thin people don't." Carole does yoga occasionally when time permits.

Judy Markey, another writer, has even tighter deadlines than Carole, with commitments to a nationally syndicated newspaper column and a Chicago radio show, and she's writing her first novel on the side. But Judy says she handles stress well, and even thrives on having multiple deadlines; she describes herself as a "wired kind of person" who is a "terrible relaxer" and doesn't get harried when she's extremely busy. She is not a retentive personality, nor is she explosive. Stress does affect her eating and sleeping habits, however. She lost five pounds going through her divorce, and stress tends to make her wake up more often.

Jane Hartley handles stress at a middle level, she says, keeping things inside more than letting them out. While she was working in the broadcasting industry at various executive levels over the years, stress affected her eating (she ate more), sleeping (she slept more fitfully), and exercise habits (she exercised less often).

When Barry Nash has a lot to do, he feels harried, but most of the people who work with him describe him as "sanguine." Activity affects his eating habits—he tends to eat less when he is busy doing work that he enjoys. Boredom used to make him eat more. He says there were times in his life when eating was the only thing he looked forward to. He seems to manage his stress with exercise. "I have to make a conscious decision to exercise in the face of stress," Barry explains. "It's real easy to just struggle from waking to sleeping with all the things that press in. But what I'm beginning to understand is the more I exercise, the more stamina I have, the clearer I think, and the more I get done."

Herb Glimcher faces pressure every day and describes himself as fast moving and aggressive in business. But he says he tries to take things in stride, is low-keyed, and doesn't get flustered easily. "I try to control my emotions business-wise," Herb says. "I'm better today than I was ten or fifteen years ago." Stress also doesn't affect his eating habits as much today as it did in the past—then he might have eaten more. His open-heart surgery was the impetus for this change.

Burt Staniar has been in the hot seat for several years. As CEO of a large New York–based broadcasting company answering to a parent company and a board of trustees, he certainly encounters stress. "I know there's a lot of stress in my life," Burt admits, "but I don't feel it. I feel like I'm quite under control." Burt can tell if he feels tension when his sleeping becomes less sound. One way he attempts to manage any stress is through meditation. He read Dr. Herbert Benson's book *The Relaxation Response* (more on this later in the chapter) and tries to meditate a few times a week, although he admits one should do it twice a day. Benson suggests pushing outside thoughts away while meditating, but Burt says, "I find that extremely difficult in my business world because I keep thinking of business things, they keep jumping in, but I keep gently pushing them aside. I think it helps a little bit."

As you see, people react to stresses differently. What is a challenge to one person may be overwhelming to the next. While one thrives on a fast pace, another might feel out of control. During the classic response to stress, your heartbeat and breathing increase, the pupils of your eyes widen, you hear more acutely, and your muscles tighten. These and a number of other changes are part of a primitive physiological reflex that puts the body on guard for danger. Our brains and bodies have been programmed from prehistoric times to release hormones like adrenaline, and even cholesterol, to speed the reaction to danger or stress. Being prepared to flee to safety or attack an enemy was an essential reaction for our ancestors. But fight-or-flight may not be the best response to the psychological wars waged in the workplace or the home.

Unrelieved stress can produce eventual medical problems, which takes quite a financial toll. Consider some of the more common physical symptoms of stress, which often require medical intervention: chest pains, dizziness, heart palpitations, hyperventilation, lower-back pain, stiff neck, stomach upsets, sleep disturbances, drug and alcohol abuse, muscular spasms, fatigue, headaches, and even the flare-up of diseases such as asthma or arthritis. According to some reports, these symptoms and others cost American businesses an estimated $75 billion annually. Other symptoms include anxiety, overeating, irritability, fear, anger, depression, and loss of appetite, all of which may have adverse effects on both nutrition and good health. In general terms, the effect of any stress on your nutritional state depends upon the type of stress, how long it lasts, and how intensely you experience it. But clearly stress has a "nutritional cost" beyond the financial cost, which ranges from the depletion of vitamins and a depressed immune system to an increase in cholesterol and poor eating habits.

While it's almost impossible to eliminate daily pressures or life's misfortunes, there are ways to minimize the effects of stress, whatever its cause. One way is knowing how to manage your stress through your diet, exercise, and relaxation techniques.

Stress and Illness

Modern medicine has been slow to recognize that stress plays a key role in a wide range of illnesses. While research linking stress and illness is not conclusive, some studies point to a wide range of ailments caused by stress, ranging from minor and hardly life-threatening conditions, such as a bad cold, to serious afflictions, such as stroke or cancer.

The notion that life catastrophes can trigger stress-related illness dates back to the 1960s, when psychiatrists Richard Rahe and Thomas Holmes developed a Life Events scale, assigning points to major life changes—100 points for the death of a spouse, 47 points for being fired, etc. The higher your score in a year, the greater your chance of being a hospitable host for a visiting virus.

The greatest emotional stress is often experienced between ages thirty and forty-four, with 60 percent of this age group reporting in one study that they have "moderate" to "a lot of" stress. Divorce, which occurs often within this age range, would be at the very highest range of emotional stress. Loss of a loved one and serious illness are other major emotional stresses.

But everyday annoyances take their toll, too. Things that are especially stressful, according to psychologists, are as diverse as having someone owe you money, filling out forms, waiting in line, keeping a car maintained, and dealing with inconsiderate smokers. According to Delores Curran, author of the book *Stress and the Healthy Family,* some of the most common stresses that families fall victim to are money, children's behavior, spousal relationships, and overscheduled family calendars.

An important factor to keep in mind when connecting stress with illness is the effect of continuing stress. The same stress response that is so helpful in the short term is thought to be harmful in the long run, because our bodies are not meant to stay in a crisis mode. Hormones and chemicals flow into the body in excess and cannot be handled.

Let's look more closely at common physiological responses to extreme or prolonged emotional stress. Adrenaline increases. Metabolism, respiration, and perspiration increase. Digestion slows. The pupils dilate. Blood pressure and the demand for blood flow increase. Stress can also release fatty acids and glucose into the bloodstream, which are converted into fat and cholesterol and deposited on artery walls. A buildup of deposits reduces oxygen to the heart muscles and, in aggravated cases, can cause angina pectoris. At the same time, the immune system becomes depressed, lowering its ability to fight disease. A prolonged stress response could thus influence the progression of infectious diseases by lowering the production of white blood cells.

Stress also releases hormones that can make people susceptible to the formation of blood clots. Those clots can anchor in the arteries and induce a heart attack. Along with cardiovascular problems, stress can also cause muscular, respiratory, skin, sexual, and gastrointestinal disorders. From a purely psychological response to stress, anxiety disorders (such as panic attacks), extreme depression, and suicide could result.

Let's look for a moment at a number of diverse studies correlating stress with a specific personality type, as well as with an enlarged heart, heart lesions, catastrophic heart attacks, high blood pressure, and diminished immunity to colds and upper respiratory diseases.

Studies have shown that type-A personalities (aggressive, more volatile) have a greater incidence of heart disease than type B's (relaxed, less reactive). It is thought that certain individuals are more stress-prone. These "hot reactors" (type A's) have been found to produce the greatest amount of catecholamines (neuro-transmitters that prompt a fight-or-flight readiness of the body).

• Studies by Robert Eliot, director of the Cardiovascular Institute at Swedish Medical Center in Denver, showed that an abundance of stress hormones released into the bloodstream by the brain causes lesions in the heart and changes in blood-vessel walls. (Those considered stress-sensitive in Eliot's studies are people who perceive themselves as never having enough and always losing out to the next guy.)

• Mental stress can cause episodes of potentially serious blood shortage to the heart muscle (termed transient myocardial isch-emias) in some patients who already have diseased coronary arteries, suggested a study reported in the April 21, 1988, issue of the *New England Journal of Medicine*. This finding could help explain the link between stress and many catastrophic heart attacks. Just how mental stress produces the effects on blood flow to the heart is not known, but the brain's production of catecholamines is increased in mental stress, and these substances also make the heart contract more vigorously.

• The April 11, 1990, issue of the *Journal of the American Medical Association* reported on a study that was the first to show a link between stress and high blood pressure. It suggested that chronic job stress—and lack of control over work—can cause high blood pressure and trigger physical changes in the heart, such as enlargement of the heart muscle. Furthermore, the study showed that men with demanding jobs and control over them (such as executives) did not have these effects.

• A study by Arthur Stone, a psychologist at the State University of New York at Stony Brook, discovered that daily stresses increased three to four days before the onset of colds and other upper respiratory diseases in one test group.

• In one study, it was noted that there is a shrinking of the thymus, spleen, and other lymphatic structures involved in the immune system from prolonged stress. There is growing evidence that stressful events may significantly affect the body's resistance to infectious and malignant diseases and that such effects are mediated through the immune system.

Some of the most interesting research into the effects of stress pinpoints how stress can act-as a trigger to raise cholesterol and other lipid levels. Several studies have shown that cholesterol values rise during different types of emotional stress:

- In a Norwegian study, nine female medical students, from twenty-two to thirty years of age, were studied during their most important preclinical exam, a test known to impose considerable mental stress on most students. Blood samples were drawn immediately after the exam, forty-eight hours later, and two months later, during a time when there wasn't academic pressure. All the students had a 20 percent increase in their total cholesterol on the exam day, as compared to either of the other two days.
- Studies of Navy pilots show cholesterol levels are highest among those landing planes on aircraft carriers, though all had similar diets.
- As early as November 1968, the *Journal of the American Medical Association* reported on a two-year longitudinal study, conducted at the University of Michigan, that found that cholesterol levels of men who lost their jobs went up, then dropped later when they found new jobs. The two hundred men were all married and had stable occupational histories.
- A study was conducted in India on sixty-five patients of different age groups who were awaiting surgical procedures. All the patients experienced "statistically significant" rises in their total cholesterol (ranging from 39 to 56.9 percent) just before their operations were performed. The researchers concluded, "These findings support previous reports of the effect of mental tension on serum cholesterol level."
- A study conducted in Helsinki, Finland, found that newborn babies born during the longest periods of labor had elevated triglycerides and diminished HDL ("good") cholesterol.

Stress Calories (or Lack of Calories): The Overeating-or-Undereating Syndrome

Most people react to stress by either over- or undereating. Neither helps alleviate the pressure they're feeling. Overeating only adds another possible stress factor—obesity—to the problems at hand. Usually it's readily available junk food that's at the root of overindulging—a cookie here, a bag of chips there. Nervous munching of notoriously fatty convenience foods will add pounds as well as cause digestive problems. The fat and cholesterol released into the bloodstream during emotional stress only make matters worse. And for those who overeat during busy times, the increase in snacking is often coupled with a decrease in exercise. Furthermore, evidence indicates that the act of eating does not reduce stress, although many people have tendencies to use food as a tension reliever.

Undereating during stress creates a vicious cycle. People under the gun burn energy at a higher rate than normal and also tend to lose and/or inefficiently absorb vital minerals such as copper, necessary for the production of red blood cells; potassium, important to maintaining fluid balance and muscle and nerve activity; magnesium, which is crucial to the functioning of muscles and nerves; zinc, for growth; and calcium, the builder of strong bones and teeth. As we discussed in Chapter 2, calcium is particularly important to women because of osteoporosis, the degenerative bone disease that affects nearly half of all females over the age of forty-five.

The body is best prepared to handle stress if there are adequate stores of all nutrients. Long-term undernutrition can affect the ability to handle stress. A poor nutritional state is in fact itself a stressor.

Foods to Reach for—and to Avoid—When You're Under the Gun

For many, it's natural to reach for food when things begin to get out of control. When you're frazzled, nervous munching on whatever is nearby can have a relaxing effect. But selecting certain foods over others can enhance your energy and help you cope with the stress at hand.

Eat a variety of foods. Stay away from foods high in fat; they take time to digest and linger in your stomach, making you feel sluggish. Complex carbohydrates like fruits and grains can help control the negative impact of stress because they sustain energy and thus discourage mood swings.

Caffeine is another item to avoid. Its effect on the body is similar to the stress reaction—increased heart rate, anxiety, and adrenaline rush. For some, even decaffeinated coffee can have the same effect. And if the pressure you feel is causing sleepless nights, caffeine is likely to prolong the sheep counting.

To thwart the tendency to overeat, choose foods that slow the eating process. Select foods that require utensils to eat rather than hand-to-mouth fare—soup instead of a burger, a baked potato instead of french fries or potato chips. The added motion promotes leisurely eating and gives the stomach more time to feel full.

If stress occurs on the job, it's also advisable to separate mealtime from the office. Eating away from the workplace may give you the break you need from the situation causing your stress.

When stress affects your digestive system and leaves you with a knot in your stomach, try eating several mini-meals or grazing throughout the day. Nutritious, intermittent snacks of fresh fruit and vegetables, a bran muffin, or yogurt give the digestive tract a break. Furthermore, grazing on nutritious foods provides a good alternative for the nervous eater who would normally reach for junk food and the undereater who would normally skip eating altogether.

Here are some additional tips to help you from overeating when stressed:

- Keep low-calorie snacks, like carrot and celery sticks, handy.
- Get in the habit of not finishing everything on your plate. When you go out, ask for a doggie bag.
- If you're going to a party—a stressful situation for many—think ahead about the foods you will eat and what you will drink. Keep your back to the buffet table; taste rather than eat.
- Don't starve yourself all day so you can eat at a party or a special event—your willpower will be gone. Eat small meals throughout the day, and be sure to include some low-fat protein like cottage cheese, low-fat cheese, or skim milk.
- Exercise helps regulate your appetite and relieves pent-up energy. When you feel like eating out of boredom or stress, take a run instead. But more on managing stress through exercise later in this chapter.

Do Certain Foods Affect the Brain?

Links between compounds in the foods people eat and the levels of certain chemicals in their brains are leading some psychiatric researchers to suggest that nutritional supplements might be used as psychiatric drugs. Carbohydrates like those in spaghetti, for instance, can increase the level of a brain chemical that reduces depression. And the amino acid tyrosine can buffer the mental and physical effects of extreme stress.

Although a few foods appear to directly affect moods and functioning (particularly carbohydrates when eaten without any protein), the psychiatrists who use this approach with patients suffering from depression, bulimia, and mania, as well as less serious problems, such as insomnia, say that the general population would not necessarily see mood changes by changing their diets. This approach comes from research that shows in detail just how the foods we eat affect the brain and how a given meal raises or lowers the chemicals called neurotransmitters that transmit signals between brain cells. Within hours after a meal, the levels of certain neurotransmitters vary according to the levels of carbohydrates or proteins that were consumed, according to Dr. Richard Wurtman, a psychiatrist at the Massachusetts Institute of Technology who led research efforts in the late 1980s. Researchers have discovered that a few amino acids (which come from proteins) and certain other substances from food can, once they are digested and enter the blood, readily cross the barrier from the blood to the brain. Most of the research has focused on two, tryptophan and tyrosine.

Tryptophan comes from protein but requires carbohydrates to enter the brain. This substance increases the neurotransmitter serotonin, which lifts some depression and can cause sleepiness. This could explain drowsiness which occurs after one eats a snack of milk and cookies. Tyrosine comes from protein such as that in meat or fish. It increases the neurotransmitters dopamine and norepinephrine, which seem to buffer the effects of stress. Concentrates of tyrosine have been used experimentally, but no studies demonstrate a direct effect from food. One of the uses of nutrients focuses on tyrosine as an antidote to sudden, extreme stress. In fact, researchers at the U.S. Army Research Institute of Environmental Medicine in Natick, Massachusetts, led by psychologist Louis Banderet, tested the effects of tyrosine supplements on soldiers experiencing physical conditions that became progressively harsher. Those who took tyrosine had a significant edge in alertness and response, were in better moods, were less anxious or tense, and felt their thinking to be clearer than the others did. Furthermore, they suffered less from the purely physical rigors of the test—coldness, muscle discomfort, and headaches.

Choline, another substance thought to affect mood, comes from lecithin, such as that found in egg yolks and soy beans. Choline increases the neurotransmitter acetylcholine and, when given in pure form as a supplement, can shorten manic attacks.

But despite the ongoing investigations into the effects of food on stress hormones, it is still unclear how strong a link actually exists. And it should be emphasized that there is no current justification for the use of these amino acids as supplements. Meanwhile, continuing investigations offer one more way to explore the interrelationship between nutrition and stress.

Are Stress-Formula Vitamins the Answer?

The 1980s may have been the decade that held out more solutions to the millions of Americans who suffered from stress than any other. Given the rising interest in nutrition, it was no surprise that the health food industry, among others, responded with "stress formula" vitamin preparations designed, they said, to help the body cope with the heavy demands of a fast-paced world. Though a vitamin supplement may be necessary to ensure recommended levels (RDAs) at times of illness to help the body cope with physiological stress, supplements aren't appropriate for most of us under moderate emotional stress.

Usually included are megadoses of vitamin C, the full complement of B vitamins for converting food into energy (thiamine, riboflavin, niacin, B6, B12, biotin, folic acid, panthothenic acid), and one or more of a number of food factors such as choline, carnitine, and inositol. Such levels definitely are not recommended, even though all of these substances are involved in the formation of neurotransmitters, the chemical messengers that help carry out directives from the brain, and/or in the metabolism, or utilization, of protein, fat, or carbohydrate—fundamental processes that keep us going. These "stress supplements" may contain up to eighty times the recommended daily allowance for B vitamins and up to sixteen times the recommendation for vitamin C. Such megadoses subject the body to still more stress because of the need to excrete the large excesses provided by the supplements.

Advertising accompanying the stress formulas suggests that the need for these nutrients increases as life becomes more hectic. The physiological forms of stress (injury, illness, major operations, pregnancy) are the ones that have been most extensively studied with respect to nutritional requirements. In some cases, a greater intake of nutrients, in the form of either food or supplements, is necessary to enable the body to adapt to the greater strain of the physical problem. It is best to stick with the recommended daily allowances unless advised by your physician.

It is not clear whether the same treatment helps with psychological forms of stress. Much of the research in this area, primarily using experimental animals, has focused on the effects of nutritional deficiencies on the response to stress, not on whether supplemental vitamins improve the ability to function in a stressful environment.

The average American adult usually is able to get adequate amounts of the water-soluble vitamins most commonly found in "stress" preparations from the food he or she eats. It is rare to see nutrient deficiencies like scurvy (lack of vitamin C) or pernicious anemia (deficiency of vitamin B12). Yet some advertising implies that anyone who experiences symptoms such as fatigue and mood changes is not meeting his or her nutrition needs.

Clinical studies have turned up little evidence supporting the benefits of supplemental vitamins on performance under stress. However, studies have shown that large doses of vitamin C may have an antihistamine effect, which helps decrease a cold's severity; no solid evidence indicates that it prevents the cold or flu. Vitamin C has also inhibited some tumors in animal studies, possibly due to immune-boosting effects, although again there's no evidence suggesting it helps people who already have cancer.

Can supplemental vitamins hurt? In general, because these vitamins are water-soluble, any excesses are excreted in the urine. But too much of certain vitamins and minerals can interfere with the absorption of other minerals, and prolonged use of high doses may even have toxic effects. An overdose of any one vitamin throws the body out of kilter, making it work just that much harder to get back on track. In fact, there's clear evidence that megadoses of certain nutrients—ten times the recommended amount or more—may harm immune response. For example, in one study, subjects were given 300 milligrams of zinc per day (twenty times the daily requirement), and their ability to fend off bacteria and viruses decreased. In fact, the ability to fight infection didn't return to normal until six weeks after they stopped megadosing (*American Health,* December 1987).

Large amounts of some of these vitamins can actually add stress through potential side effects: large doses of B6, for example, could possibly cause neurological disorders; too much niacin could lead to hot flushes; and diarrhea could be caused by an excess of vitamin C.

Managing Stress Through Exercise

Besides eating right, regular aerobic exercise is an effective means of dealing with stress. Research has shown that this type of endurance activity triggers the release of endorphins, morphine-like chemicals in the brain, which act as natural tranquilizers. Most regular runners report that after a workout they experience a tremendous sense of relaxation and well-being.

Another chemical theory attempts to explain how aerobic exercise helps the body handle stress. The key to this theory is a series of chemical reactions that take place in the bloodstream when nervous tension, anger, physical activity, or even sexual excitement cause stress. The stress causes acids to be released. These are broken down by the chemical norepinephrine. In large amounts, however, norepinephrine produces a host of ill effects—boosted heart rate, elevated blood pressure, constricted blood vessels, and eye inflammation. But the body works to break the norepinephrine down too, using oxygen to convert it into carbon dioxide and water. If norepinephrine is broken down quickly, its harmful physical effects are minimized. To do that requires a lot of oxygen, though, and fast.

That's where exercise comes in. The arteries of a physically fit person are well developed and can deliver oxygen throughout the body efficiently. Those who aren't physically fit have less-developed arteries, which distribute oxygen more slowly. Only aerobic exercises such as jogging, vigorous walking, racquetball, or swimming—done three or four times a week for at least 20 minutes each time—develop the arteries and provide the oxygen-delivering benefit. Sporadic exercise is too minimal to have an effect on relieving stress or producing fitness and can even be hazardous to an out-of-shape body. Furthermore, exercise can put a lot of stress (physiological) on the body, especially when someone isn't in good condition. The more intense the exercise and the more out of shape the exerciser, the greater the stress.

In response to this stress, the brain interacts with the adrenal glands to release the hormones epinephrine (adrenaline) and cortisol, chemicals that have been linked with depressed immunity in people suffering from grief or other strong emotional distress. When large enough amounts of these hormones surge through the body, they may cause a decrease in the activity of natural killer cells (immune cells responsible for destroying some viruses and tumors), T cells (key for defense against bacteria and viruses), helper cells and B cells (which produce antibodies against specific invaders).

Epinephrine may also stimulate suppressor cells to shut off many or all of the immune system's other cells. In essence, these cells slow down the immune system before it attacks the body's own tissues. When too many of these cells are activated, however, they could head off an attack against bacteria or a virus before it happens. With the immune system thus suppressed, a cancer cell, for example, could potentially run rampant. These explanations are all theory at the present time, but several studies do seem to support them.

A study at Loma Linda University Medical Center in California found that a single bout of exhausting exercise can increase suppressor cells and decrease helper cells in healthy volunteers. Antibodies, the protective proteins created by the immune system in response to foreign invaders, also were found to drop after extreme aerobic exercise.

A study done at the University of Cape Town, South Africa, in 1982 found that ultra-marathoners with the fastest times and the highest weekly training mileage also had the most upper respiratory complaints. A more recent study found low antibody levels in the saliva of cross-country skiers and cyclists after competition.

But do all these studies mean that ordinary aerobic exercise stresses the body? Far from it. In fact, regular and moderate exercise actually cuts down dramatically on the release of such damaging stress hormones as epinephrine and cortisol during a workout. Ideally, one researcher has pointed out, you want exercise to be eustressing, not distressing. Eustress, literally "good stress," means a pleasurable challenge—not a grueling painathon. The best way to experience eustress is to become a conditioned athlete.

Additional Techniques for Managing Stress

Relaxation techniques, maintaining solid and supportive relationships, and being willing to change your schedule or environment to eliminate pressures are all techniques that can help reduce the stress in your life.

One well-known approach comes from Dr. Herbert Benson, a cardiologist and professor at the Harvard Medical School and author of *The Relaxation Response* (1976) and *Beyond the Relaxation Response* (1985). Dr. Benson outlined three steps that lead to reduced blood pressure, heart rate, body metabolism, brain-wave activity, and rate of breathing:

1. Sit comfortably in a quiet environment and concentrate on relaxing all your major muscle groups.
2. Focus for ten to twenty minutes, twice a day, on some word or phrase. Say the word to yourself on each exhalation.
3. Passively push intrusive thoughts from your mind and return to your focus word or phrase.

Another technique for managing stress is based on the theory that it is helpful to be involved in solid, supportive relationships. An investigation done at the departments of medicine and psychiatry at the University of New Mexico School of Medicine supported this theory. The study examined 256 healthy elderly adults who had "satisfying relationships with trusted individuals in whom they could confide" and found them to have lower cholesterol levels and more effective functioning of their immune systems.

Finally, take some control of your life. If you're willing to rearrange your schedule or alter your environment to help reduce your stress, you're halfway there. If you are overburdened at your job, reduce your responsibilities. If you can't seem to get work done at your office, try organizing your time better. Perhaps coming in a bit earlier will enable you to be more productive before your co-workers arrive. Or work during lunch (don't skip your meal, though) when the office is more quiet. Working at home requires similar adjustments in how you organize your time. Establish a routine. If you can't seem to manage the kids, their numerous activities, and the house, get a mother's helper to help shoulder the carpooling. Or reduce the number of after-school commitments your kids are signed up for. You may be overstressing them as well!

So the answer is: never let stress control you. When daily pressures create a knot in your stomach, a tensing of your body, and all the other familiar signs of stress, take stock of your power to manage the stress. Through dietary techniques—eating a variety of foods (particularly complex carbohydrates), avoiding fats and caffeine, and sticking with nutritious snacking when using food to relieve tension—and regular but moderate exercise, along with any other methods that you find helpful, you can minimize the stress before it hurts you.

10

Diet Mania and the Fuss About Weight Control

Americans are among the fattest people in the world. According to the 1988 Surgeon General's Report on Nutrition and Health, more than a quarter of all Americans are overweight, and about 34 million need to lose thirty-five pounds or more for medical reasons. Depending on what definition of obesity you subscribe to, some statistics indicate that almost 40 percent of the U.S. population over thirty years of age is overweight at any one time!

Why the epidemic? As most of you have become aware, you need fewer calories as you get older. What you may not know is that Americans have reduced their physical activity 75 percent since 1900. And we're consuming significantly more fat and calories.

Equally epidemic is the interest in maintaining a lean body, the kind of body we all see in trendy magazines, television shows, and movies. As a result, fad diets and gimmicks promising quick weight loss pose great appeal for those who are uninformed and vulnerable. Consumers are pouring money into the $33 billion diet industry, which is predicted to increase by $20 billion within five years. At any one time, about 65 million Americans are on a weight-loss diet. Some statistics indicate that half the adult women and 30 percent of the adult men in this country are on a diet. Yet many of these dieters are trying to meet the ultra-thin standard often set by the media and the fashion industry. While obesity has its health hazard, so does being too thin. The obsession with food can lead to eating disorders, such as anorexia nervosa and bulimia, which can in themselves be life threatening. Most fad diets are equally dangerous, as is the "yo-yo" dieting behavior of weight gain and weight loss that has become so prevalent.

How fat is too fat, how thin is too thin, and what is the right weight for you? Is it better to be a few pounds over or a few pounds under? What is the best approach to weight control? In this chapter, we will answer these questions, and more, so you can learn how to control your weight as part of a life-style approach to healthy eating.

How Fat Is Too Fat, How Thin Is Too Thin, and What Is the "Ideal" Weight?

"I'm not fat . . . I'm just short for my weight." So goes a popular joke among dieters. It does address a common source of angst for overweight individuals—weight-for-height tables that are treated as the definitive verdict on the "ideal" weight.

Most doctors define overweight and obesity based on the 1983 Metropolitan Life Insurance Company Height and Weight Tables. Theoretically, the tables show what people should weigh to have the longest life. A person who is more than 10 percent over the weight on the tables is overweight, while a person who is about 20 percent over (give or take 5 percent depending on whom you talk to) is considered obese. Similarly, a person who is more than 10 percent below the weight on the tables is underweight.

These weight standards are based upon longevity data for optimal weights between ages twenty-five and fifty-nine. They are not based on any scientific determination of ideal weight; they merely reflect the mortality rates of some four million life insurance policyholders, mostly derived from single weighings of people twenty-five to thirty years old. Their usefulness is mainly for the insurance company, which raised premiums for obese people because people who weighed more tended to die sooner. The insurance tables actually became a standard in the medical profession when Metropolitan Life released its first such tables in 1942 (1943 chart); they gave doctors sound evidence to cite when telling patients that they should drop a few pounds.

While the range of values for a given height and sex differentiates small, medium, and large frame sizes in the 1983 Metropolitan Life tables, frame-size standards are approximate, and in some cases can be misleading. How do you determine your frame size? Several studies have shown that the size of the elbow, the chest, the hip, the wrist, or the knee correlates nicely with overall frame size. Metropolitan chose the elbow.

Elbow sizes are best measured with a caliper, which most health clubs or a doctor's office should have. It is also possible to measure your elbow with a ruler by grasping the two knobby protrusions on either side of the elbow with thumb and index finger. Metropolitan provides a table indicating your body frame based on your elbow measurement. So if you happen to have been born with big elbows, you supposedly have a large frame and are expected to weigh more. The converse is true if you've been dealt small elbows. You can see that this notion of an "ideal" weight is not so black and white—and in fact it has generated a good deal of controversy.

Actually, Metropolitan Life doesn't even use the term "ideal" or "desirable" anymore. The 1943 tables were called "Ideal Weights," and in 1959 the tables were renamed "Desirable Weights." In 1983 Metropolitan merely published its "Height and Weight Tables."

The 1983 version actually listed new weights that were higher than those in the older table. Why? Because heavy people seemed to have a lower mortality in 1983 than in 1959, based on Metropolitan's statistical analysis.

The change in the table highlighted an important truth. There is no definitive way to say exactly what someone should weigh. There are too many variables, ranging from genetic makeup to sociological considerations affecting diet and medical care. Furthermore, take into account that insured people are not representative of the U.S. population—they are generally healthier and wealthier than the average.

But we do need guidelines, and the Metropolitan Life figures have become the best known and most widely used. Still, some experts have challenged their validity, arguing that the Metropolitan standard is right for someone in his or her forties, but too heavy for individuals in their twenties and not heavy enough for

Metropolitan Height and Weight Tables

All weights are in pounds for adults 25 to 59 years old. Men's weights and heights include clothing weighing 5 pounds and shoes with 1-inch heels. Women's weights and heights include clothing weighing 3 pounds and shoes with 1-inch heels.

MEN				**WOMEN**			
Height	Small Frame	Medium Frame	Large Frame	Height	Small Frame	Medium Frame	Large Frame
5-2	128–134	131–141	138–150	4-10	102–111	109–121	118–131
5-3	130–136	133–143	140–153	4-11	103–113	111–123	120–134
5-4	132–138	135–145	142–156	5-0	104–115	113–126	122–137
5-5	134–140	137–148	144–160	5-1	106–118	115–129	125–140
5-6	136–142	139–151	146–164	5-2	108–121	118–132	128–143
5-7	138–145	142–154	149–168	5-3	111–124	121–135	131–147
5-8	140–148	145–157	152–172	5-4	114–127	124–138	134–151
5-9	142–151	148–160	155–176	5-5	117–130	127–141	137–155
5-10	144–154	151–163	158–180	5-6	120–133	130–144	140–159
5-11	146–157	154–166	161–184	5-7	123–136	133–147	143–163
6-0	149–160	157–170	164–188	5-8	126–139	136–150	146–167
6-1	152–164	160–174	168–192	5-9	129–142	139–153	149–170
6-2	155–168	164–178	172–197	5-10	132–145	142–156	152–173
6-3	158–172	167–182	176–202	5-11	135–148	145–159	155–176
6-4	162–176	171–187	181–207	6-0	138–151	148–162	158–179

Source: 1979 Build Study, Society of Actuaries and Association of Life Insurance Medical Directors of America, 1980. © 1983 Metropolitan Life Insurance Company.

the decades after the forties. Dr. Reubin Andres, director of the Gerontology Research Center of the National Institute on Aging, and his colleagues developed a new chart which makes age the primary consideration, rather than height and frame, and separates the weight range for each decade between twenty-five and sixty-five years old.

Comparison of Height-Weight Tables

HEIGHT	METROPOLITAN 1983 WEIGHTS FOR AGES 25–59		GERONTOLOGY RESEARCH CENTER WEIGHT RANGE FOR MEN AND WOMEN BY AGE (YEARS)				
	Men	Women	20–29	30–39	40–49	50–59	60–69
ft-in			lb				
4-10	...	100–131	84–111	92–119	99–127	107–135	115–142
4-11	...	101–134	87–115	95–123	103–131	111–139	119–147
5-0	...	103–137	90–119	98–127	106–135	114–143	123–152
5-1	123–145	105–140	93–123	101–131	110–140	118–148	127–157
5-2	125–148	108–144	96–127	105–136	113–144	122–153	131–163
5-3	127–151	111–148	99–131	108–140	117–149	126–158	135–168
5-4	129–155	114–152	102–135	112–145	121–154	130–163	140–173
5-5	131–159	117–156	106–140	115–149	125–159	134–168	144–179
5-6	133–163	120–160	109–144	119–154	129–164	138–174	148–184
5-7	135–167	123–164	112–148	122–159	133–169	143–179	153–190
5-8	137–171	126–167	116–153	126–163	137–174	147–184	158–196
5-9	139–175	129–170	119–157	130–168	141–179	151–190	162–201
5-10	141–179	132–173	122–162	134–173	145–184	156–195	167–207
5-11	144–183	135–176	126–167	137–178	149–190	160–201	172–213
6-0	147–187	138–179	129–171	141–183	153–195	165–207	177–219
6-1	150–192	...	133–176	145–188	157–200	169–213	182–225
6-2	153–197	...	137–181	149–194	162–206	174–219	187–232
6-3	157–202	...	141–186	153–199	166–212	179–225	192–238
6-4	162–207	...	144–191	157–205	171–218	184–231	197–244

Reprinted with permission of McGraw-Hill Publishing Co.

Values in this table are for height without shoes and weight without clothes.

The weight range is the weight for small frame at the lower limit and large frame at the upper limit.

More important than actual weight, many say, in determining your health is how your weight is distributed. If your body is taking on a pear shape, it's not as bad a sign as if it's taking the shape of an apple. Fat accumulated in the abdominal cavity is more disruptive to one's health than fat layered below the skin on the thighs or buttocks. In fact, studies in Sweden focusing on waist and hip measurements indicate that the risk for cardiovascular disease seems to increase sharply when a man's waist measurement is the same as or bigger than his hip measurement. The same is true for women whose hips are not at least 20 percent larger than their waists.

Overweight and underweight can even be individually diagnosed based on a direct measure of the amount of body fat. This can be done by a skinfold test—also called a "fatfold" test. In one of the skinfold tests, a fold of skin from the back of the arm is measured with a caliper that applies a fixed amount of pressure. The fat attached to the skin is considered to be roughly proportional to total body fat. A fatfold over an inch thick indicates overfatness; under a half-inch reflects underweight.

There are other ways to measure total body fat. One increasingly popular and accurate method today is called bioelectrical impedance. This technique measures the resistance of a low-energy electrical current by the body. The more fat storage a person has, the greater the impedance to the electrical flow.

At this point, you are probably most anxious to understand how to avoid fat accumulation anywhere on your body. Maintaining your weight—not adding fat storage to the places where you tend to add pounds—is based on a balance between the food you eat and the energy you expend. Maintaining a set weight depends on a number of factors: your sex, your age, your body composition, and your metabolism. One pound of weight is equal to 3,500 calories. To lose one pound a week, you need to eat 500 fewer calories each day. Add a moderate amount of exercise and you'll burn off even more calories. Men tend to lose weight twice as fast as women because they have more muscle mass, which burns calories faster than fat tissue.

For both sexes, little things mean a lot over a year. Extra weight can creep up on you. One tablespoon of sugar is only 45 calories. But if you eliminate that tablespoon from your diet every day, you lose 16,425 calories over a year, or more than four and a half pounds. Similarly, if you drink two cups of 2 percent milk every day, you could save 40 calories per cup (80 calories a day) if you switch to skim milk. That adds up to a yearly calorie savings of 29,200, or more than 8 pounds. For those of you who drink several colas each day, the savings are even more significant. One Pepsi has 156.6 calories. If you eliminate one Pepsi every day for a year, you'll save 58,254 calories, or a little over 16½ pounds!

Calorie needs decrease about 5 percent per decade starting at about age forty. As metabolism slows due to aging or lessened physical activity, the intake of food must be adjusted. If the food you eat is not used for energy, it will be stored in your body and you will put on weight. It's as simple as that.

It is important to understand, however, that fat and overweight are not necessarily the same. In fact, it is the ratio of fat to lean muscle that scientists now recognize as a more important indication of disease risk than weight alone. It is recommended that men under age thirty carry no more than 13 percent of their body weight in fat; women, designed by nature to conserve more calories, can carry up to 18 percent. As people age, body weight and percentage of body fat generally increase. So even if we maintain a constant weight through old age, our percentage of body fat will likely increase.

Look at the weight charts we discussed earlier and see how "ideal" your weight is.

The Debate About Weight: Is It Better to Be a Few Pounds Over or a Few Pounds Under?

Does thinness necessarily define beauty and health, or have we been brainwashed by Madison Avenue? We certainly have a national obsession with being thin. In fact, like millions of others, you may be convinced that if you could only lose a few pounds you'd be happier, healthier, and more attractive. Thin is definitely in, and the pressure is on to be slightly on the lean side. But what about your health? Is it good to be underweight? In light of the much publicized dangers of being overweight, you'll be relieved to hear the answer is NO. You *can* be too thin.

Losing a few pounds can lead to being undernourished. There are three population groups who are most at risk by being a few pounds underweight: first, adolescents, who are prone to anorexia nervosa (more on this eating disorder later in the chapter); second, heavy smokers, whose appetites are diminished because their taste buds have been dulled; and third, the elderly, our fastest-growing population segment.

Being underweight, in fact, can be particularly dangerous as you enter the fifty-plus years. In this weight-conscious era of less-is-better, there are some physicians who believe that a weight gain of a few pounds over the years actually may help you live longer, provided you are healthy, and that carrying a bit of extra weight is not a medical risk (see the chart on page 260). Research accumulated over the past ten to fifteen years indicates that gradual, modest weight gain seems to go along with a lower mortality rate. The consensus from various studies has been that people who are about 10 percent above the recommended standard have a longer life span than those who weigh less. In fact, one twelve-year study of 750,000 men and women (who were initially screened to exclude those with any illness) found that those who were 20 percent or more below their standard weight had a higher mortality rate than their heavier counterparts. The explanation of these findings is relatively simple. When you try to maintain a thinner-than-average profile, you have fewer calorie reserves to draw on if you get sick, and you are compounding the built-in nutritional problems that naturally occur with the aging process, such as less efficient absorption of essential nutrients.

So does that mean that an extra few pounds is really not detrimental to your health? Not everyone would agree. According to some medical experts, even 5 to 10 extra pounds increase health risks, including high blood pressure, heart disease, respiratory problems, gall bladder disease, arthritis, and several kinds of cancer. Even the psychological burden of being overweight has been identified as an adverse effect on one's health.

Given the disagreement, what is the healthiest answer when it comes to weight control? Maybe it's to put less emphasis on the scale and more on the quality of your food choices. Your ideal weight may unintentionally result.

Meanwhile, the debate continues.

The Obsession with (or Without) Food, and Its Hazards

It has been said that anyone who weighs more than he should has been eating more than he needs. Put another way, one could say that obesity results from overeating—or that obesity results from underactivity.

But what causes the overeating? And why are some people less active than others? And the questions don't stop there. Can obesity be looked at merely as an obsession with food? If so, is this obsession psychological or physiological? Is a person born to be fat, or is it a condition resulting from early food experiences? Why is obesity more of a problem in developed nations like the United States?

Two studies reported in the *New England Journal of Medicine* (May 24, 1990) provide the strongest evidence to date that heredity is the dominant factor determining whether a person is fat, lean, or in between.

One study confirms what has been long suspected: people can eat identical meals, and some will gain more weight than others. The study showed that one person can put on up to three times as much weight as another while eating the same diet. The researchers, Dr. Claude Bouchard of Laval University in Quebec and his colleagues, isolated 12 pairs of lean young men, identical twins, in a closed section of a dormitory and fed them an extra 1,000 calories a day, six days a week, for a total of 84,000 calories over what they were eating before entering the study. The twins in each pair gained almost exactly the same amount of weight and gained it in the same places on their bodies. But among the various twin pairs there were marked differences in weight gain, with one pair adding more than twenty-nine pounds and another pair adding only nine and a half. This study backed the popular belief that some people can eat all they want and never gain weight, or at least gain very little. Those who gain weight more easily have the biological tendency to very efficiently turn virtually all their extra calories directly into fat.

The second study, conducted by Dr. Albert Stunkard, an obesity researcher at the University of Pennsylvania, and his colleagues, found that identical twins ended up with virtually identical body weights as adults, whether they were reared apart or together. The study indicated that childhood experiences played essentially no role in determining variations in the weights of individual adults. The study concluded that genetic differences accounted for 70 percent of weight variation among men and 66 percent of the variation among women, with environment contributing the rest.

Proponents of the view that obesity is environmentally determined say that factors in our surroundings persuade us to overeat, such as the availability of a multitude of delectable foods. Experiments with "cafeteria rats" support this theory. Ordinary rats fed regular rat chow are of normal weight, but if these same rats are offered free access to a wide variety of highly tempting, palatable foods, they greatly overeat and become obese. As part of this environmental view, some believe that early food experiences can promote the habit of overeating throughout life. As the theory goes, parents who encourage overeating at mealtimes, rapid eating, excessive snacking, and eating to meet needs other than hunger instill this kind of learned, habitual behavior in their children.

In fact, many view overeating in very psychological terms. They see eating as a behavior that is triggered by environmental factors entirely unrelated to food. Repeated connections between food and an emotional state, therefore, create a habit. For example, if a child is given love and affection whenever she eats, she may be conditioned to turn to food whenever love and affection are missing from her life. The same could apply to pain (the child gets hurt and gets a piece of candy), anxiety, loneliness, and boredom, so that eating becomes an inappropriate response to emotions that persists throughout life.

What might explain the fact that the average adult in our society gains about 30 pounds between the ages of twenty and fifty, but people in non-Western societies do not? One answer lies with our heavy dietary intake of fat, accounting for 40 percent of all our calories. In scientific studies, rats permitted to eat as much as they wanted whenever they wanted became significantly fatter when given high-fat food than when given low-fat fare. While scientific evidence on humans is not quite as conclusive, people of the Western world, where the diet is high in fat, are heavier than those in other countries where low-fat food predominates.

Why do high-fat foods seem to lead to greater weight gain? Primarily because fat is a much greater concentrated source of calories than either protein or carbohydrate. Excessive calories from any nutrient ultimately are converted to fat.

This brings us to energy-expenditure activity, which is at the other side of the balancing act necessary to maintain weight (input must equal output). Obese people, under close observation, are often seen to eat less than lean people, but they are sometimes so extraordinarily inactive that they still manage to have a calorie surplus. So while heredity is now accepted as an important factor in the cause of obesity, people can overcome their genetic destiny by eating less, especially less fat, and increasing physical activity.

Regardless of the cause of obesity, the motivation to avoid weight gain has been clearly stated by the medical community. In the mid-1980s, a National Institutes of Health panel said that obesity is as serious a health problem in this country as smoking and high blood pressure. Some of the health risks listed by the panel that related to obesity (weight 20 percent above the Metropolitan ranges) are high blood pressure, high blood cholesterol, adult-onset diabetes, several types of cancer, heart disease, gall bladder disease, menstrual abnormalities, respiratory problems, and arthritis.

Obesity has been singled out, based on strong scientific data, as an "independent risk factor" in heart disease and termed "a physical disease with potentially fatal consequences." It can contribute to premature death in otherwise healthy men. (The same is thought to be applied to women, but the data are not yet conclusive here.) A 20 percent reduction in weight can mean a 40 percent reduction in heart disease. In fact, life-insurance statistics show that being 20 percent above desirable body weight lowers a woman's life expectancy by 10 percent and a man's by 20 percent.

Just look at the hazards of obesity. Beyond heart-related diseases, fat people more often suffer postsurgical complications, gynecological irregularities, and the toxemia of pregnancy. Gaining weight often appears to precipitate diabetes in people susceptible to it. The burden of extra fat strains the skeletal system, impacting arthritis, especially in the knees, hips, and lower spine. The muscles that support the stomach may give way, resulting in abdominal hernias. When the leg muscles are abnormally fatty, they fail to contract efficiently to help blood return from the leg veins to the heart; blood collects in the leg veins, which swell, harden, and become varicose. Gout (a condition characterized by the formation of chalky deposits in the cartilages of the joints due to an excess of uric acid in the blood) is more common; and even the accident rate is greater for the severely obese.

There are particular heart risks for overweight women, a recent controversial study found. The March 29, 1990, *New England Journal of Medicine* reported that even slightly overweight women face increased risk of heart attack—and the risk doubles for those who have gained 20 pounds since age eighteen. The thinnest women—those 6 percent or more below ideal weight—had the fewest heart attacks. The eight-year study of nearly 116,000 healthy middle-aged women suggested that 40 percent of all heart disease in women is due solely to being overweight. The study concluded that obesity is harmful to women largely because it increases blood pressure, raises cholesterol levels, and contributes to diabetes.

Similar studies have linked obesity and heart disease in men. But despite the findings, there is not general agreement about whether it is the weight that causes heart disease or related health problems. And there is much debate among health experts over exactly how dangerous extra weight is.

There is little debate as to the danger of being excessively thin. An extreme underweight condition, anorexia nervosa, is sometimes seen in young women and some young men who strive to look like today's lean models. Anorexia is a result of dieting taken to such an extreme that the self-denial used to control weight becomes a form of starvation. Anorexics become severely undernourished, finally achieving a body weight of 70 pounds or even less. The condition can terminate in death, as was the case with singer Karen Carpenter.

The anorexia sufferer is usually from an educated, middle-class, success-oriented, weight-conscious family that is proud of her achievements. She strives to be successful and chooses weight loss as one means to get there. Anorexics tend to be highly competitive, perfectionists, and very self-critical. Weight loss becomes an obsession that rules an anorexic's life. But no matter how much she loses, she is never satisfied, always seeing herself as too fat even when emaciated.

In a related eating disorder known as bulimia, a person—typically an upper-middle-class teenage girl or young woman—eats huge amounts of food at one time, then vomits to get rid of it. It is not unusual for bulimics to compulsively consume more than 5,000 calories at one time, often in the form of nutritionally undesirable foods like ice cream and potato chips. Along with induced vomiting, the binge may be followed by laxatives or diuretics, enemas, fasting, or an overly strenuous amount of exercise. Bulimics tend to be compulsive, and hypercritical of their bodies. Often they are not really overweight and never have been, but most see themselves as too fat and are terrified of getting fatter. Yet a bulimic is preoccupied with food and typically uses food to cope with stress and anxiety. Bulimia always follows, or is part of, excessively strict weight-loss dieting.

Both anorexics and bulimics are obsessed with staying thin. But bulimics are more difficult to spot because they tend to remain at, or close to, their medical ideal weight and their binge-purge activity is "on the sneak." Anorexics, on the other hand, cannot hide their bizarre eating patterns. They severely restrict the kinds and amounts of foods they consume and typically adopt peculiar rituals, like eating the same food at the same time day after day. Furthermore, anorexics literally waste away, so their condition becomes quite visible. Victims of both diseases become severely undernourished.

The physical consequences of bulimia range from mild to severe. The purges may cause some of the worst problems. Self-induced vomiting can cause mouth sores, swollen salivary glands, rotten teeth, and, eventually, tooth loss. Those who purge lose water and minerals, incurring dehydration and chemical imbalances that can lead to heart problems in predisposed people. The abuse of laxatives or diuretics, as well as the frequent vomiting, can result in muscle spasms in the hands and feet, palpitations, severe gastric disturbances such as ulcers, digestive tract disorders, hernias, mood swings, fatigue, and depression. Excessive exercise can lead to muscular and skeletal injuries. Female victims may stop menstruating.

The physical symptoms of anorexia are truly danger signs, but the anorexic sees them as desirable. As her whole body wastes away, including the muscle tissue, her sexual development ceases and she stops menstruating. Her skin becomes dry and yellow from an accumulation of stored carotene released from body fat. She experiences pain on touch, loses the texture and health of her hair, suffers from severe sleep disturbances and anemia, and has a lowered blood pressure and metabolic rate.

Both anorexia nervosa and bulimia have been defined for the first time in medical history within the past thirty years. Both are known only in developed nations and become more prevalent as wealth increases. The cause of these diseases is unknown, but may come in part from a society whose message to young people, throughout the media, is that the "perfect" woman is a thin one. Anorexia nervosa and bulimia may only be an exaggerated acceptance of the unreasonable expectations of our society. As a result, girls as young as twelve are worried that they are too fat, and they go on diets.

The Who and How of Dieting, from A to Z

America has a weight problem. A majority of overweight people are not dieting, while normal-weight people may be dieting too much. Madison Avenue may be instilling the dieting ethic in the wrong audience, because findings strongly suggest that the typical dieter may not be the typical overweight American.

The facts don't lie. Statistics indicate that dieters are still a minority. At any one time, about 65 million Americans are on a weight-loss diet. Of these, 86 percent diet to lose or maintain weight and the rest diet for medical or other reasons. Most dieters are between the ages of twenty-five and forty-nine, yet statistics show that older people are prone to be overweight but less likely to be on a diet.

Obesity is more prevalent among lower socioeconomic groups, yet these groups are not consumers of the plethora of diet-related products and services (most of them expensive) on the market. Dieting, in fact, has been shown to increase with education. College graduates are 67 percent more likely than the average American to be on a diet.

The nation's obsessive fixation on weight loss has become big business. Weight Watchers International Inc. (the service) alone has more than a million members and in 1990 the company had revenues of $1.6 billion for its service and all of its products. An estimated 20 million Americans spent close to $1 billion on various liquid diet products and programs in 1990. Add to that diet books, diet foods, fat farms, videocassettes, and assorted exercise devices and you have a $33-billion-a-year industry. And Marketdata Enterprises, a research firm in Valley Stream, New York, predicts the market will top $50 billion by 1995.

Dieting has certainly evolved from a cottage industry to a multifaceted megabusiness, with many different strategies to achieve weight loss. The least formalized approach has been around for years—turning to the latest of hundreds of self-help books on the market offering a new "breakthrough" diet for rapid weight loss. Many of these "designer" diets are now well known: the Grapefruit Diet . . . the Immune Power Diet . . . the Banana-Milk diet . . . high protein . . . no protein . . . Atkins . . . Scarsdale . . . Stillman . . . Beverly Hills . . . the Live for Life Diet.

Before you undertake *any* kind of weight reduction program, you must consult your physician. If you want to find a diet book that is practical, safe, and accurate to guide you, here are a few tips. First, make sure the book was written by a credible authority—a registered dietitian or a medical doctor with nutrition credentials from an accredited university. Secondly, stay away from books promising instant success or rapid results. Losing weight the right way takes time—a safe rate of weight loss for most people is a maximum of about two pounds per week.

Generally, you should avoid a diet plan that is very specific, allowing only certain foods and eliminating others. For example, low-carbohydrate and high-protein diets that offer little or no carbohydrates are often high in dietary fat and can raise blood cholesterol. They tend to be monotonous and thus are hard to follow for a long period. A hazard of going on these regimes is that they cause ketosis, a condition that results from the low carbohydrate content, which causes the oxidation of fats to be incomplete. Ketosis can lead to diarrhea, dehydration, sodium depletion, higher blood fats, increased uric acid production, fatigue, and dizziness. Low-carbohydrate and high-protein diets are frequently deficient in vitamins and minerals and often necessitate supplementation. Furthermore, when carbohydrates are restricted to less than 60 grams a day, water and salt loss occurs, not fat loss. When carbohydrates are reintroduced into the diet, the water weight is quickly regained, even if calories are restricted. The Scarsdale, Stillman, and Atkins' Superenergy diets are high in protein and low in carbohydrates Another high-protein diet is the I Love New York Diet.

High-fat diets are fortunately quite out of vogue today. They taste good because fats contain much of food's flavor. Fats also take longer to digest, so people on these diets usually feel full longer. Dr. Robert Atkins advocated a high-fat, low-carbohydrate approach in his *Dr. Atkins' Diet Revolution*. Obviously, this diet contains too much saturated fat and leads to an increase in cholesterol levels.

High-carbohydrate diets can work well, as long as some fat is also included. The Pritikin approach is extremely low in fat, recommending that as little as 5 to 10 percent one's daily calories come from fat. Some fat is good in the diet.

Some popular diets contend that certain foods, such as grapefruit, are capable of "burning off fat." While foods like grapefruit have benefits in the diet, it is unhealthy to rely on any one food for weight, or fat, loss.

There is also no scientific evidence to support "food combining" or the practice of eating certain foods at certain times and avoiding the consumption of certain foods together at the same meal.

A balanced diet is generally the best way to lose weight. So when you're browsing for a diet book, look for one that offers variety, balance, and moderation. Finally, be leery of a book that promises weight loss without exercise or behavior change. Look for a diet that also teaches you how to keep weight off.

Another approach to weight loss that has been around for some time is the drop-in regimen, like Weight Watchers, Nutri/System, Diet Center, and Jenny Craig. These programs, offering a combination of daily or weekly nutritional counseling (generally not by a qualified nutritional professional) and special foods and supplements, have become their own growth industry. Weight Watchers is the oldest of the group, founded in 1963, then purchased by H. J. Heinz Corporation in 1978. On any given week, about one million members attend weekly Weight Watchers meetings in 24 countries. Enrollment is growing, at a 30 percent annual rate. Jenny Craig is also growing rapidly, now operating several hundred centers around the world. These centers do not require a physician's recommendation; they are not medically supervised; and most require that the dieter purchase that company's food products. For some people, these approaches are successful.

Fat farms and "longevity" centers are also not new, although their focus has evolved. The California-based Pritikin Program, for example, was originally aimed at curing ills when it was founded by Nathan Pritikin in 1976. Today, Pritikin dieters eat foods that are low in fat and high in complex carbohydrates and fiber (fruit, vegetables, grains, chicken). During a 7-, 13-, or 26-day program costing from $3,200 to $9,000, they exercise, take classes in "life-style education," and stress weight/diet management. The Kempner Rice Diet Program was originally developed by Dr. Walter Kempner at Duke University in 1939 to treat hypertension. Dieters, under a doctor's supervision, stay in Durham, North Carolina, for about $2,000 a month and eat fruit and rice three times a day. The average length of a stay is about three months. Actually, four nationally known weight-control programs are based in Durham, which the local chamber of commerce dubs "the diet capital of the world."

The very-low-calorie diet (VLCD) is the most recent approach to dieting for the seriously overweight. Fasting programs target the 34 million Americans who, according to the National Institutes of Health, need to lose 35 pounds or more. Designed to provide weight loss for seriously obese individuals, these expensive programs involve lengthy periods when participants are sustained solely by liquid-protein supplements and a steady diet of group therapy and medical checkups. The major programs available today—Optifast, New Direction, Medifast, and HMR (Health Management Resources)—have the following similarities: All include a fasting period of about three months or more (depending on the amount of weight a person has to lose), during which patients consume liquid-protein beverages made of a powder dissolved in noncaloric liquids. Dieters take in 420 to 800 calories daily and typically shed 3 to 10 pounds a week. The "refeeding" stage follows, in which sensible meals (lean meat, salads or vegetables) gradually take the place of liquids. Health complications can occur during this stage if the dieter engages in overeating or "binge" eating, which can lead to dangerous shifts in salt and potassium levels as well as excessive fluid retention. This combination can cause the heart to race, triggering irregular heartbeats. Last, and most important, comes a maintenance phase, in which patients practice eating sensibly on their own. Behavior modification and exercise are important components of each of these programs.

These VLCD programs vary as to the length of the fasting period, whether they allow modifications to the basic plan, and the specific kind of medical supervision provided. But the important point is that they are medically supervised. New Direction is available only through hospitals, ensuring safety and close medical monitoring.

An over-the-counter version of a liquid diet plan has emerged for the many dieters who don't want a health-care professional looking over their shoulders. Slim-Fast survived the industry shake-out in the 1970s and escaped the need for an FDA warning label because it recommends that users also eat one sensible meal each day and thus was not considered a very-low-calorie diet plan. Along with Ultra Slim-Fast (an added-fiber version), it now accounts for 80 percent of the over-the-counter liquid-diet market.

According to the American Medical Association, fasting and very-low-calorie diets should be used only by obese people under close medical supervision, and for good reason. Certain weight-loss plans may raise the risk of the very diseases that weight loss is meant to prevent. Very-low-calorie diets—liquid protein, 300-calorie-per-day formulas, and the like—can raise the risk of heart attack by disrupting the body's electrolyte balance or damaging heart muscle.

Some fad diets are more hazardous to health than obesity itself. Faddish diets allow the greatest chance for the dieter to regain the weight lost and more, which leads to another potentially serious condition. Most experts agree that the "yo-yo syndrome"—the cycle of gaining weight, losing, gaining and losing again—can be more harmful to human beings than being overweight. Several years ago, Dr. Paul Ernsberger, a neurobiologist at Cornell Medical Center in New York, found in a study of lab rats that fattening the rats didn't raise their blood pressure. But fattening them, putting them on a diet, fattening them again, and putting them on another diet—a cycle familiar to human dieters—did. A more recent study, published in the June 27, 1991, *New England Journal of Medicine*, revealed that repeated changes in weight, irrespective of a person's initial weight, are linked to an increased death rate overall and to as much as twice the chance of dying of heart disease.

It is debatable whether the yo-yo effect is a physiological result of constant dieting or a psychological inability to make the necessary life-style changes to maintain a desirable weight. With some chronic dieters, the more they diet, the more their metabolism slows, and the more they have to restrict their intake to lose additional pounds or even maintain their weight loss. A 1990 article in the *New England Journal of Medicine* by Dr. Philip Kern and colleagues at Cedars Sinai Medical Center offered support for the metabolic theory when it reported that people who lose weight start overproducing an enzyme, lipoprotein lipase, that makes it easier to put weight back on. The fact is that more than 95 percent of those who lose weight regain it within one year.

The Best Approach to Weight Control: Eating for Good Health

So is fighting fat futile? Not necessarily, experts would answer. Most agree that at least part of the reason people regain their weight is behavioral, with dieters following fad diets that involve no essential change in life-style. Over the long haul, only one diet works: consuming fewer calories and burning off more. Exercise is a big component and is the key to long-term weight loss. In fact, it is possible to lose weight by increasing exercise even without eating less. So a diet program that does not incorporate physical activity is doomed to failure and virtually guarantees a yo-yo cycle of losing weight and regaining it over and over.

The National Council Against Health Fraud (NCAHF) introduced eleven guidelines for consumers considering joining a diet program. Positive answers indicate possible red flags for that program:

1. Does the diet promise dramatic, rapid weight loss of more than 1 percent of total body weight per week?
2. Does the diet promote a menu extremely low in calories (800 or fewer per day) without requiring medical supervision?
3. Does the diet make clients dependent on special products rather than teaching how to make good choices from the conventional food supply?
4. Does the diet ignore the components of exercise and behavioral modification?
5. Is the diet promoted by salespeople who refer to themselves as "counselors" but may actually be unqualified to give guidance in nutrition and health?
6. Does the diet require large sums of money up front or ask the client to sign a contract for costly, long-term programs? (Good programs operate on a pay-as-you-go basis.)
7. Do diet-program representatives fail to inform the client about

possible health risks associated with the diet and weight loss in general?

8. Does the diet program promote spurious weight-loss aids, like diuretics or body wraps?
9. Does the diet claim cellulite exists on the body independent of fat? (Fat is fat; cellulite is fat, too.)
10. Does the diet claim that using an appetite suppressant or methylcellulose allows a person to lose body fat without restricting caloric intake?
11. Does the diet claim a unique ingredient or component unavailable in other weight-control products?

For most people, the best weight-loss programs call for restricted calories; a balanced—as opposed to single or two-foods—diet; gradual loss of one or two pounds a week (see our "Real Life Diet" at the end of this chapter); regular exercise; and a maintenance plan to prevent backsliding.

Discipline is needed to make modest dietary changes. Eat less butter, avoid fried foods, have more fresh fruits and vegetables, cut back on meat, and consume more pasta and grain. Several hundred calories a day can be eliminated just by cutting out creamy salad dressings, using mustard instead of mayonnaise on sandwiches, and not piling a mound of butter on a baked potato or table rolls.

Here are some additional tips to help you control your weight:

• People gain an average of seven pounds between November and January—be particularly careful during the holiday months.
• Avoid snacking at critical times like before dinner and while cooking, grocery shopping, watching TV, reading, and during boredom.
• Don't skip meals to control your weight. Try eating only half of everything you like.
• Eat slowly and chew longer. You'll eat less, because your brain will have time to recognize that you're no longer hungry.
• Drink a glass of water before eating to make your stomach feel full.

Before going on any weight-loss program, your first step is to establish whether you are prepared to make a lifelong change in your eating behavior and exercise habits. If you make weight loss a priority and you're prepared to make a permanent life-style change, you *can* achieve long-term success in keeping your weight off.

By eating sensibly and making modest changes in your diet, for example, you can cut at least 500 calories a day. By exercising every other day, you can work off perhaps 1,000 calories or more a week. Most people would lose about a pound to a pound and a half each week on such a program. Maintaining your new weight would require a calorie ceiling level and regular exercise several times each week.

In the next chapter, we'll focus on exercise—an important component to any sound weight-loss program, and an important component to all sound approaches to good health!

The Real Life Diet:
ONE WEEK OF MENUS TO GET YOU STARTED

SUNDAY	1,200 Calories	1,500 Calories	2,000 Calories
BRUNCH			
Citrus Compote	½ cup	½ cup	¾ cup
Spanish Omelet with Salsa & Cheese*	1 sv	1 sv	1 sv
Carrot strips (from medium carrot)	½	½	½
Green pepper ring garnish	1 ring	1 ring	1 ring
Corn muffin	1 small	1 small	2 small
Soft margarine	1 tsp	1 tsp	2 tsp
Hot cocoa, made with skim milk	6 oz	8 oz	8 oz
DINNER			
Easy Oven-Barbecued Chicken Thigh*	1 thigh	2 thighs	2 thighs
Company Baked Mashed Potatoes*	⅓ cup	½ cup	¾ cup
Steamed fresh broccoli with	½ cup	½ cup	1 cup
Lemon juice &	½ tsp	½ tsp	1 tsp
Olive oil	1 tsp	1 tsp	2 tsp
Salad on			
Lettuce leaf	1 leaf	1 leaf	1 leaf
Medium tomato, sliced	½	½	1
Cucumber slices	½ cup	½ cup	¾ cup
Reduced-calorie ranch dressing	1 tbsp	1 tbsp	2 tbsp
Whole wheat dinner roll	½ roll	1 roll	1 roll
Soft margarine	½ tsp	1 tsp	1 tsp
Raspberry Angel Dessert*	⅛	⅛	¼
Beverage**			
SNACKS			
Nectarine, medium	½	1	1
Skim milk	½ cup	¾ cup	1 cup
Beverage**			

	1,200 Calories	1,500 Calories	2,000 Calories
NUTRIENT VALUES			
Calories	1,191	1,510	2,003
Carbohydrate (grams)	153	190	267
Protein (grams)	62	84	95
Fat (grams)	38	48	65
Cholesterol (milligrams)	303	355	377
Sodium (milligrams)	1,752	2,276	2,811
Calcium (milligrams)	936	1,141	1,355
Percentage of calories from carbohydrate–protein–fat	51–21–29	50–22–28	53–19–29

*Recipe provided: Spanish Omelet with Salsa & Cheese, p. 287; Easy Oven-Barbecued Chicken Thighs, p. 288; Company Baked Mashed Potatoes, p. 288; Raspberry Angel Dessert, p. 289.
**Beverages may include water, plain and flavored mineral water, seltzer water, sugar-free soft drinks, coffee, and teas.

MONDAY

	1,200 Calories	1,500 Calories	2,000 Calories
BREAKFAST			
Cranberry juice	½ cup	½ cup	¾ cup
Apple-bran muffin	1 small	2 small	2 small
Low-fat cottage cheese with	⅓ cup	½ cup	¾ cup
Pineapple chunks in juice	¼ cup	¼ cup	¼ cup
Skim milk	½ cup	½ cup	1 cup
Beverage**			
LUNCH			
Salad:			
Turkey breast	1 oz	1½ oz	1½ oz
Cheddar cheese	1 tbsp	1 tbsp	1 tbsp
Garbanzo or kidney beans	1 oz	1 oz	1 oz
Lettuce, carrots, broccoli, on-ions, sprouts, tomatoes—			
any raw vegetables	1½ cups	1½ cups	1½ cups
Reduced-calorie salad dressing	2 tbsp	2 tbsp	2 tbsp
Sesame sticks	2 sticks	2 sticks	2 sticks

	1,200 Calories	1,500 Calories	2,000 Calories
Fresh fruit in season (melon)	½ cup	1 cup	1½ cups
Soft-serve ice milk or frozen yogurt	⅓ cup	½ cup	1 cup
Beverage**			

DINNER

	1,200 Calories	1,500 Calories	2,000 Calories
Salmon Patty with Cucumber Sauce*	2½ oz 2 tbsp	4 oz 2 tbsp	4 oz 2 tbsp
Simmered frozen green peas with pepper & Soft margarine	½ cup 1 tsp	½ cup 1 tsp	¾ cup 1½ tsp
Spinach, Orange, and Red Onion Salad with Orange Dressing*	1 sv 2 tbsp	1 sv 2 tbsp	1 sv 2 tbsp
Sliced strawberries	½ cup	1 cup	1½ cups
Beverage**			

SNACKS

	1,200 Calories	1,500 Calories	2,000 Calories
Skim milk	½ cup	½ cup	1 cup
Celery stalk with 1 tbsp peanut butter	1	1	2
Microwaved marshmallow on graham cracker	1 large 1 square	1 large 2 squares	1 large 2 squares

NUTRIENT VALUES

	1,200 Calories	1,500 Calories	2,000 Calories
Calories	1,201	1,509	1,995
Carbohydrate (grams)	171	218	283
Protein (grams)	69	89	117
Fat (grams)	34	42	57
Cholesterol (milligrams)	75	106	123
Sodium (milligrams)	1,822	2,284	2,900
Calcium (milligrams)	801	918	1,459
Percentage of calories from carbohydrate–protein–fat	54–22–24	54–22–24	54–22–24

*Recipe provided: Salmon Patties with Cucumber Sauce, p. 290; Spinach, Orange, and Red Onion Salad with Orange Dressing, p. 291.
**Beverages may include water, plain and flavored mineral water, seltzer water, sugar-free soft drinks, coffee, and teas.

TUESDAY	1,200 Calories	1,500 Calories	2,000 Calories
BREAKFAST			
Orange juice	½ cup	½ cup	½ cup
Oatmeal, with	½ cup	½ cup	1 cup
Vanilla	¼ tsp	¼ tsp	½ tsp
Chopped dates	½ tbsp	½ tbsp	1 tbsp
Brown sugar	1 tsp	1 tsp	2 tsp
Whole wheat English muffin	½ muffin	1 muffin	1 muffin
Soft margarine	1 tsp	2 tsp	2 tsp
Skim milk	½ cup	½ cup	1 cup
Beverage**			
LUNCH			
Sandwich:			
Turkey pastrami	1 oz	1 oz	2 oz
Swiss cheese	1 oz	1 oz	1 oz
Onion slice & lettuce leaf	1 each	1 each	1 each
Spicy brown mustard	1 tsp	1 tsp	1 tsp
Rye bread	2 slices	2 slices	2 slices
Carrot sticks	1 carrot	1 carrot	1 carrot
Fresh pear	1 medium	1 medium	1 medium
Beverage**			
DINNER			
Quick Fettuccine with	½ cup	1 cup	1½ cups
Tomato, Meat, and			
Mushroom Sauce*	½ cup	½ cup	¾ cup
Parmesan cheese	1 tsp	2 tsp	4 tsp
Steamed Italian vegetable			
blend with			
Reduced-calorie Italian	½ cup	1 cup	1 cup
dressing	1 tbsp	2 tbsp	2 tbsp
Garlic bread	1 slice	1 slice	1 slice
Chocolate frozen yogurt	⅓ cup	½ cup	½ cup
SNACKS			
Soft pretzel	½	1	1
Skim milk	½ cup	½ cup	1 cup
Beverage**			

	1,200 Calories	1,500 Calories	2,000 Calories
NUTRIENT VALUES			
Calories	1,212	1,499	1,995
Carbohydrate (grams)	182	230	284
Protein (grams)	52	60	93
Fat (grams)	33	41	57
Cholesterol (milligrams)	75	80	143
Sodium (milligrams)	1,735	2,209	2,838
Calcium (milligrams)	864	965	1,646
Percentage of calories from carbohydrate–protein–fat	59–17–24	60–16–24	56–18–26

*Recipe provided: Quick Fettuccine with Tomato, Meat, and Mushroom Sauce, p. 291.
**Beverages may include water, plain and flavored mineral water, seltzer water, sugar-free soft drinks, coffee and teas.

WEDNESDAY	1,200 Calories	1,500 Calories	2,000 Calories
BREAKFAST			
Fresh orange, cut into wedges	½	½	1
Toaster whole wheat waffles	1	2	2
Reduced-calorie syrup	1 tbsp	2 tbsp	2 tbsp
Fried egg, in pan coated with oil	1	1	1
Skim milk	1 cup	1 cup	1 cup
Beverage**			
LUNCH			
Baked or broiled fish with			
Lemon &	3 oz	3 oz	4 oz
Margarine	1 tsp	1 tsp	1½ tsp
Corn on the cob			
(6-in ear) with	1	1	2
Margarine	1 tsp	1 tsp	2 tsp
Cole slaw	½ cup	½ cup	1 cup
Crisp & juicy red apple			
(from home)	1 medium	1 medium	2 medium
Beverage**			
DINNER			
Boneless pan-grilled pork chop with thyme & pepper	2 oz	3 oz	3 oz

	1,200 Calories	1,500 Calories	2,000 Calories
Quick Barley Pilaf*	⅓ cup	½ cup	1 cup
Steamed pea pods with	½ cup	½ cup	½ cup
Margarine	½ tsp	½ tsp	½ tsp
Fresh Tomato, cut into			
wedges	½	1	1
Yellow cake (low-fat, low-			
cholesterol) topped with	1 oz	1 oz	2 oz
Peach slices	¼ cup	¼ cup	½ cup
Strawberry yogurt	2 tbsp	2 tbsp	4 tbsp
Beverage**			

SNACKS

	1,200	1,500	2,000
Low-fat buttermilk or			
skim milk	¾ cup	1 cup	1 cup
Reduced-salt whole wheat			
crackers	2	4	4

NUTRIENT VALUES

	1,200	1,500	2,000
Calories	1,205	1,494	2,002
Carbohydrate (grams)	160	200	289
Protein (grams)	74	88	105
Fat (grams)	33	40	52
Cholesterol (milligrams)	348	376	406
Sodium (milligrams)	1,202	1,597	1,949
Calcium (milligrams)	789	899	1,032
Percentage of calories from carbohydrate–protein–fat	52–24–24	53–23–24	57–20–23

*Recipe provided: Quick Barley Pilaf, p. 292.
**Beverages may include water, plain and flavored mineral water, seltzer water, sugar-free soft drinks, coffee, and teas.

THURSDAY	1,200 Calories	1,500 Calories	2,000 Calories

BREAKFAST

	1,200	1,500	2,000
Compote:			
Apricots, canned in juice	¼ cup	¼ cup	½ cup
Stewed prunes	¼ cup	¼ cup	½ cup
Reduced-fat Swiss cheese			
melted on a	1 oz	2 oz	2 oz
Garlic bagel half	1	2	2

	1,200 Calories	1,500 Calories	2,000 Calories
Skim milk	1 cup	1 cup	1 cup
Beverage**			

LUNCH

	1,200 Calories	1,500 Calories	2,000 Calories
Pita pocket:			
Water-packed tuna, mixed with	2 oz	3 oz	3 oz
Lemon juice	1 tsp	1½ tsp	1½ tsp
Reduced-calorie mayonnaise	1 tbsp	1½ tbsp	1½ tbsp
Spinach leaves	¼ cup	⅓ cup	⅓ cup
Alfalfa sprouts	1 tbsp	1½ tbsp	1½ tbsp
6-in whole wheat pita bread	½	1	1
Seedless black grapes	15	15	30
Beverage**			

DINNER

	1,200 Calories	1,500 Calories	2,000 Calories
Meat loaf with	2 oz	2 oz	3 oz
seasoned tomato sauce	2 tbsp	2 tbsp	4 tbsp
Onion-Stuffed Baked Potato*	½ sv	½ sv	1 sv
Steamed french-cut green beans with	½ cup	½ cup	1 cup
black pepper (to taste) & margarine	1 tsp	1 tsp	2 tsp
Crunchy carrot coins	½ cup	½ cup	½ cup
Vanilla pudding made with skim milk, topped with	½ cup	½ cup	1 cup
Sliced banana	½ small	½ small	½ small
Pecan pieces	1 tbsp	1 tbsp	1 tbsp
Beverage**			

SNACKS

	1,200 Calories	1,500 Calories	2,000 Calories
Frozen fruit-juice bar	1	1	1

NUTRIENT VALUES

	1,200 Calories	1,500 Calories	2,000 Calories
Calories	1,212	1,495	2,007
Carbohydrate (grams)	175	203	296
Protein (grams)	61	84	98
Fat (grams)	32	40	52
Cholesterol (milligrams)	102	124	161

	1,200 Calories	1,500 Calories	2,000 Calories
Sodium (milligrams)	1,143	1,533	1,920
Calcium (milligrams)	879	1,162	1,403
Percentage of calories from carbohydrate–protein–fat	57–20–23	54–22–24	58–19–23

*Recipe provided: Onion-Stuffed Baked Potato, p. 292.
**Beverages may include water, plain and flavored mineral water, seltzer water, sugar-free soft drinks, coffee, and teas.

FRIDAY

	1,200 Calories	2,000 Calories	

BREAKFAST

	1,200		2,000
Blueberries	¼ cup	¼ cup	½ cup
Frosted shredded wheat biscuits	4	6	8
Skim milk	1 cup	1 cup	1 cup
Whole wheat toast with	1 slice	1 slice	2 slices
Soft margarine	1 tsp	1 tsp	2 tsp
Beverage**			

LUNCH

Sandwich:			
Grilled chicken breast	3 oz	3 oz	3 oz
Lettuce leaf	1 leaf	1 leaf	1 leaf
Tomato slice	1 slice	1 slice	1 slice
Onion slice	1 slice	1 slice	1 slice
Mayonnaise	2 tsp	2 tsp	2 tsp
Whole-grain bun	1	1	1
Fresh orange	1 small	1 small	1 small
Skim milk	1 cup	1 cup	1 cup

DINNER

Vegetable-cheese pizza (12-in) (homemade or take-home)	⅛	¼	½
Mixed green salad	1 cup	1 cup	1 cup
Reduced-calorie Italian dressing	2 tbsp	2 tbsp	2 tbsp

	1,200 Calories	1,500 Calories	2,000 Calories
Black cherry low-fat frozen yogurt on	⅓ cup	½ cup	½ cup
Cantaloupe wedge	¼	¼	¼
Beverage**			

SNACKS

Apple, sliced	½	½	1
Light microwave popcorn	1 cup	2 cup	3 cup

NUTRIENT VALUES

Calories	1,210	1,496	2,005
Carbohydrate (grams)	172	217	290
Protein (grams)	73	88	114
Fat (grams)	30	38	52
Cholesterol (milligrams)	111	130	164
Sodium (milligrams)	1,502	1,946	2,780
Calcium (milligrams)	923	1,044	1,241
Percentage of calories from carbohydrate–protein–fat	55–23–22	55–23–22	56–22–22

**Beverages may include water, plain and flavored mineral water, seltzer water, sugar-free soft drinks, coffee, and teas.

SATURDAY

	1,200 Calories	1,500 Calories	2,000 Calories

BREAKFAST

	1,200 Calories	1,500 Calories	2,000 Calories
Breakfast banana split:			
Banana, split lengthwise	½	½	1
Low-fat cottage cheese	⅓ cup	½ cup	¾ cup
Sliced strawberries	¼ cup	¼ cup	½ cup
Melted low-sugar spread	1 tsp	2 tsp	1 tbsp
Sunflower seeds	1 tsp	1 tsp	2 tsp
Skim milk	1 cup	1 cup	1 cup
Beverage**			

LUNCH

Grilled lean burger:			
Lean meat patty	2 oz	3 oz	3 oz
Tomato & onion slices	1 each	1 each	1 each
Pickle slices	2	2	2

	1,200 Calories	1,500 Calories	2,000 Calories
Lettuce leaf	1	1	1
Sesame-seed whole grain roll	1 small	1 small	1 small
Oven french fries (2½–3-in sticks)	5	10	15
Root beer float:			
Sugar-free root beer	6 oz	8 oz	8 oz
Vanilla low-fat frozen yogurt	⅓ cup	½ cup	½ cup

DINNER

	1,200 Calories	1,500 Calories	2,000 Calories
Cajun grilled red snapper with	2 oz	3 oz	3 oz
Vegetable oil (coat fillet)	1 tsp	1 tsp	1 tsp
Cajun seasoning (sprinkle on)	⅛ tsp	⅛ tsp	⅛ tsp
Curly noodles with	⅓ cup	½ cup	¾ cup
Reduced-calorie buttermilk dressing	2 tsp	3 tsp	4 tsp
Crisp-tender steamed asparagus with	½ cup	½ cup	¾ cup
Garlic-seasoned margarine	½ tsp	½ tsp	1 tsp
Broiled tomato Parmesan half with	1	1	1
Grated Parmesan cheese	1 tsp	1 tsp	1 tsp
Dry bread crumbs	1 tsp	1 tsp	1 tsp
Margarine	½ tsp	½ tsp	½ tsp
Hot Fudge Brownie Pudding Cake*	2¼ × 3″	2¼ × 3″	4½ × 3″
Beverage**			

SNACKS

	1,200 Calories	1,500 Calories	2,000 Calories
Skim milk	½ cup	½ cup	½ cup

NUTRIENT VALUES

	1,200 Calories	1,500 Calories	2,000 Calories
Calories	1,210	1,500	2,009
Carbohydrate (grams)	156	182	275
Protein (grams)	70	94	110
Fat (grams)	38	48	61
Cholesterol (milligrams)	114	167	185

	1,200 Calories	1,500 Calories	2,000 Calories
Sodium (milligrams)	1,273	1,539	1,964
Calcium (milligrams)	802	881	999
Percentage of calories from carbohydrate–protein–fat	50–23–27	48–24–28	53–21–26

*Recipe provided: Hot Fudge Brownie Pudding Cake, p. 293.
**Beverages may include water, plain and flavored mineral water, seltzer water, sugar-free soft drinks, coffee, and teas.

The Real Life Diet Recipes

Spanish Omelet with Salsa and Cheese
(single serving)

Omelet

1 whole egg
2 egg whites
2 tablespoons skim milk
Dash of salt
Dash of pepper
½ teaspoon vegetable oil

Filling

2 tablespoons Spanish tomato sauce
¼ teaspoon Worcestershire sauce
Dash of garlic powder
Dash of red pepper sauce

Topping

1 tablespoon salsa (mild, medium, or hot)
1 tablespoon shredded cheddar cheese

Beat with whisk until combined: egg, egg whites, skim milk, salt, and pepper. Lightly coat skillet with vegetable oil and heat over medium-high heat. Pour egg mixture into skillet. Reduce heat to low and cook without stirring. As eggs set, lift edges and tip pan to allow uncooked egg to flow to bottom of pan. When cooked add sauce, fold in half, and place on plate. Top with salsa and cheese. Makes 1 serving.

Nutrients per serving: 201 calories, 7 grams carbohydrate, 19 grams protein, 11 grams fat, 224 milligrams cholesterol, 535 milligrams sodium.

Easy Oven-Barbecued Chicken Thighs
(4 servings)

4 chicken thighs, skin removed
½ cup barbecue sauce (your favorite)

Marinate chicken in barbecue sauce in refrigerator about 3 hours. Place in lightly oiled baking dish; cover and bake in 350-degree oven for 45 minutes. Remove cover; baste each piece with sauce in dish. Bake uncovered for 10 to 15 minutes.

Nutrients per serving: 133 calories, 4 grams carbohydrate, 14 grams protein, 6 grams fat, 49 milligrams cholesterol, 300 milligrams sodium.

Company Baked Mashed Potatoes
(4 servings)

4 medium potatoes
Boiling water to cover potatoes
1 teaspoon sugar
¼ teaspoon salt
Pepper to taste
Garlic powder to taste
½ cup nonfat yogurt
1 small onion, minced (or 1 teaspoon dried minced onion)
¼ cup (1 ounce) reduced-fat cheddar cheese, grated
1 green onion, chopped

Add potatoes to briskly boiling water. Stir; reduce heat; cover and simmer until potatoes are tender (20 to 30 minutes). Drain. Mash potatoes; add sugar, salt, pepper, garlic powder, nonfat yogurt,

and onions. Whip until fluffy. (Add skim milk if needed to produce desired consistency.)

Pour into lightly greased baking dish. Top with cheese and bake in
350-degree oven for 10 minutes or until heated through and
cheese has melted. Garnish with chopped green onion.

*Nutrients per serving: 108 calories, 21 grams carbohydrate, 4 grams protein, 1
gram fat, 4 milligrams cholesterol, 131 milligrams sodium.*

Raspberry Angel Dessert
(8 servings)

½ angel food cake
1 package (0.3 ounce) sugar-free raspberry-flavored gelatin
1 cup boiling water
10 ounces frozen sweetened raspberries, thawed
8 ounces low-fat, low-sugar raspberry yogurt

Bake or purchase angel food cake; cut in half vertically. Freeze half
for future use unless you wish to double the recipe. Tear cake into
1-inch pieces. Pour boiling water on gelatin in bowl; stir until dissolved. Separate raspberries with fork; save a few berries for garnish; add remainder to gelatin. Refrigerate gelatin mixture until
thickened but not set—about 15 minutes.

Layer half each of the cake pieces, gelatin mixture, and yogurt in
1½-quart serving bowl; repeat. Garnish with reserved raspberries.
Refrigerate until firm—at least 2 hours.

*Nutrients per serving: 159 calories, 35 grams carbohydrate, 5 grams protein, 0.1
gram fat, 0 cholesterol, 137 milligrams sodium.*

Salmon Patties with Cucumber Sauce
(4 servings)

Salmon Patty

1 pound canned salmon
20 unsalted whole wheat crackers
1 small onion, minced
1 tablespoon lemon juice
1 egg
Dash of pepper

Cucumber Sauce

½ cup nonfat yogurt
½ large cucumber, peeled, seeded and chopped
Dash of onion powder
Dash of pepper

Drain juices into small mixing bowl. Remove skin and large bones from salmon. Break into pieces. Add all ingredients to bowl with juices; stir until well mixed. Let set 5 minutes. Shape into patties and cook in nonstick skillet over medium heat until lightly browned and firm.

For cucumber sauce, combine yogurt, cucumber, onion powder and pepper. Serve over salmon patty.

Nutrients per serving: 242 calories, 11 grams carbohydrate, 25 grams protein, 10 grams fat, 53 milligrams cholesterol, 760 milligrams sodium.

Spinach, Orange, and Red Onion Salad with Orange Dressing

(single serving)

Salad

1 cup fresh spinach leaves, washed and drained
¼ cup orange sections or slices
2 slices red onion, separated into rings

Orange Dressing

1 tablespoon orange juice concentrate
1 tablespoon reduced-calorie mayonnaise

Arrange spinach, orange, and onion on salad plate. For dressing, combine orange juice concentrate with the reduced-calorie mayonnaise. Drizzle over salad and serve.

Nutrients per serving: 83 calories, 16 grams carbohydrate, 3 grams protein, 3 grams fat, 2 milligrams cholesterol, 89 milligrams sodium.

Quick Fettuccine with Tomato, Meat, and Mushroom Sauce

(makes 8 cups)

1 pound extra-lean ground beef or turkey
2 medium onions, chopped
2 cups mushrooms, sliced
1 quart salt-to-taste spaghetti sauce
½ teaspoon salt
Herbs and garlic (optional—to taste)
1 pound fettuccine

Brown ground meat in skillet and drain any fat that accumulates. Add onions and mushrooms; cook until softened. Add sauce and salt. Simmer 10–20 minutes, taste, and adjust seasoning with herbs and garlic according to your preferences. While sauce is simmering, cook fettuccine according to package directions. Drain. Serve sauce over fettuccine. Sprinkle with Parmesan or Romano cheese.

Time-saving tip: Freeze leftovers for future quick meals or snacks.

Nutrients per cup of sauce: 218 calories, 13 grams carbohydrate, 13 grams protein, 12 grams fat, 34 milligrams cholesterol, 189 milligrams sodium.

Nutrients per ½ cup sauce over 1 cup fettuccine: 264 calories, 39 grams carbohydrate, 11 grams protein, 7 grams fat, 17 milligrams cholesterol, 96 milligrams sodium.

Quick Barley Pilaf
(makes 2 cups)

1⅓ cups water or unsalted chicken broth
⅔ cup quick pearled barley
2 teaspoons olive oil
½ teaspoon bouillon granules
2 green onions, chopped
¼ cup chopped mushrooms
¼ cup chopped celery

Bring water or broth to a boil. Stir in remaining ingredients. Cover, reduce heat, and simmer 10 to 12 minutes or until tender. Remove from heat. Let stand 5 minutes. Stir and serve.

Nutrients per ½-cup serving: 120 calories, 23 grams carbohydrate, 2 grams protein, 3 grams fat, 0 cholesterol, 122 milligrams sodium.

Onion-Stuffed Baked Potato
(single serving)

6-ounce baking potato
1 small onion, sliced
1 teaspoon oil
½ teaspoon butter/cheese-flavored granules
Dash of mixed-herb seasoning flakes

Scrub potato and cut *almost through* at ¼-inch intervals. Place on lightly oiled square of foil. Coat onion slices with oil and sprinkle with butter/cheese-flavored granules and herbs. Insert slices between cuts into potato. Bring up edges of foil and seal. Bake in

350-degree oven or on hot grill for 40–50 minutes. For half-servings, seal each serving separately.

Nutrients per serving: 243 calories, 46 grams carbohydrate, 4 grams protein, 5 grams fat, 0 cholesterol, 45 milligrams sodium.

Hot Fudge Brownie Pudding Cake
(12 servings, 2¼" × 3" each)

1 cup flour
¾ cup granulated sugar
2 tablespoons cocoa
2 teaspoons baking powder
Dash of salt
½ cup skim milk
2 tablespoons oil
1 teaspoon vanilla
¼ cup walnuts, chopped
¾ cup brown sugar
¼ cup cocoa
1 teaspoon vanilla
1¾ cups hot water

Sift together flour, granulated sugar, 2 tablespoons cocoa, baking powder, and salt. (If in a hurry, just stir together.) Add skim milk, oil, and vanilla to dry ingredients; mix until smooth. Stir in nuts. Grease 9-inch square baking pan or dish or spray with nonstick coating. Spread batter into pan.

Combine brown sugar and ¼ cup cocoa. Sprinkle over batter. Combine vanilla with hot water; pour over entire batter. Bake for 45 minutes or until brownie rises to the top and the pudding is bubbly and thick. Cut into 12 servings. Lift brownie and sauce, inverting onto dessert plates; top with pudding left in pan.

Nutrients per serving: 173 calories, 41 grams carbohydrate, 2 grams protein, 4 grams fat, 0.2 milligrams cholesterol, 88 milligrams sodium.

Dietary analysis and recipes (pages 277–293) provided by Linda J. Bethel, M.S., R.D., L.D., C.D.E., Bethel Nutrition Services, 1526 Nuremberg Blvd., Punta Gorda, Fla. 33983.

11

Working Out and
Eating Right

Whatever your age, the activity most likely to improve your health is exercise. This magical activity, experts say, can give you strength, endurance, and flexibility and at the same time help to control your weight, reduce depression and anxiety, increase self-esteem, and lower your risk of heart disease. And we've been hearing this advice for upwards of twenty years, when our nation first began an "exercise revolution." In fact, according to a recently published survey and analysis by the Federal Centers for Disease Control in Atlanta, lack of exercise is the leading modifiable hazard leading to death from coronary heart disease—a more important factor than an elevated level of cholesterol!

Yet less than 10 percent of Americans over eighteen years old exercise regularly enough for any discernible health effect, while the other 90 percent do little or nothing at all. Even people with special reason to exercise, such as those severely obese or recovering from a heart attack, do not.

Research has clearly demonstrated that you don't need a lot of exercise to be physically fit. Three to five vigorous 20- to 30-minute workouts a week or their equivalent will give you a healthier heart, and a lower risk of serious diseases. A landmark report by researchers at the Institute for Aerobics Research and the Kenneth Cooper Aerobic Clinic in Dallas was the first to show on such a large scale the huge health differences between being sedentary and being even slightly active. Their eight-year study, published in the *Journal of the American Medical Association* in November 1989, of more than ten thousand healthy men and three thousand healthy women showed the risk of dying from heart disease, cancer, and other top killers was much greater for "couch potatoes" than for others who were only slightly more fit. The study was one of the largest to rely on objective measures of fitness (treadmill performances) instead of participants' answers to questions.

The fact is that physically active people seem to feel and look healthier. Studies show they live longer. They appear to have better-regulated appetites. They eat more, but because exercise increases metabolism—the process of converting food into energy—they burn calories faster and don't gain weight.

In this chapter, we'll look more closely at the positive effects of exercise, the kinds of activities that can keep you fit, motivating yourself to stay active, and the foods (and fluids) that should be part of any exercise program.

Given the Choice, Why Should We Exercise?

In a recent report, the Centers for Disease Control in Atlanta indicated that the risk of not enough exercise equals the risk of smoking a pack of cigarettes per day. That is certainly a pretty compelling statement in favor of exercise for anyone concerned about his or her state of health.

It is not known exactly why exercise reduces mortality, but one possibility is that exercise makes the coronary arteries larger and healthier and thus may decrease dangerous clotting. As a result, it seems to help lower blood pressure, which reduces the risk of stroke and heart attack and lowers the "bad" cholesterol. Exercise also can help curb body fat, which is a risk factor for some cancers. Exercise also increases bowel motility, which may be important in avoiding colon cancer.

The benefits of regular exercise have undergone a great deal of scientific scrutiny, and research studies are ongoing. A side study of Dallas's Cooper Clinic's eight-year research project suggested that moderate exercise dramatically boosts the chances of survival for people with high blood pressure. This study measured the fitness levels of 1,831 men, averaging age forty-two, with high blood pressure. Follow-ups after eight years showed that men in the bottom 20 percent on fitness were about three times more likely to have died than men doing the equivalent of a brisk 30-minute walk five days a week, or a 20-minute swim four times weekly.

The 1989 Dallas study overall is so noteworthy because it is one of the few studies to look directly at fitness rather than rely on verbal reports of exercise and is also one of the few large studies that have looked at women's fitness. This particular study has been expanded to include more than forty thousand subjects and is still under way.

An earlier study, in 1986, of seventeen thousand Harvard graduates, also determined that moderate exercise was beneficial, suggesting it could add up to two years to a person's life.

A six-year study carried out in the mid-1980s of 90 women, ages twenty to seventy, at Seattle's Pacific Medical Center showed that vigorous exercise for at least 30 minutes three times a week prevented significant cardiovascular "effects of aging" until age fifty for active women. Over the six years, the active women's percentage of body fat remained stable, while the body fat of the sedentary women edged up from an average of 28 percent to one of 35 percent, raising their coronary risk.

A series of studies by exercise pioneer Dr. Herbert A. deVries, retired director of the Andrus Gerontology Center at the University of Southern California and co-author with Dianne Hales of *Fitness After 50* (Scribners, 1982), focused on the older population and also found compelling benefits of moderate exercise, results that can be applied to all ages. Exercise was found to significantly alter the deterioration of bodily functions that traditionally accompany aging and possibly even reverse many effects of aging. The research demonstrated that disuse accounts for about half the functional decline that usually occurs between thirty and seventy. Studies have shown that just as three weeks of complete bed rest by people middle-aged and older results in losses equal to thirty years of aging, exercise by this same age group can set the clock back by as many as forty-five years.

Dr. deVries has said the best way to get into sports is to "buy a golden retriever and take him for a good, long hike." While you may not want the responsibility of a dog, the advice to take a long hike is excellent. Almost all of the benefits, with respect to preventing coronary problems, come from expending 1,000 calories a week above the normal routine. For most people, that translates into 45 minutes of vigorous activity, five days a week.

In Dr. deVries's studies, peak fitness occurred after eighteen to forty-two weeks of exercise. Demonstrated benefits include an increased work capacity, improved heart and respiratory function, lower blood pressure, increased muscle strength, greater flexibility, quicker reaction times and clearer thinking, better sleep, and less depression. A study conducted at Ohio State University in the late 1980s monitored 90 seniors on a regular exercise program for nine months over a three-year period and found similar results.

Regardless of when in life a person starts to exercise, improvements in function can occur; but the older a person is when beginning exercise, the more critical it is to consult a physician, begin gradually, and do the exercise properly.

Another benefit of exercise, mentioned briefly in Chapter 9 in relation to stress, might be the good feeling you get from the release of endorphins, those pain-reducing, euphoria-inducing brain chemicals. Most likely, longer episodes rather than shorter workouts will yield the release of these hormones.

Perhaps one of the most important benefits of exercise from a dieter's perspective is its effect on metabolic rates. Whereas calorie-reduced dieting may lower one's metabolic rate, as we pointed out in the last chapter, exercise may offset this effect.

Can Exercise Be Overdone?

The best-known prescription for cardiovascular health is 20 to 30 minutes of aerobic exercise three to five times a week (some experts recommend a duration of up to 60 minutes, especially if the workout is less intense), with the heart rate elevated to the "training range." Also called the "target heart rate," this is usually calculated as 60 to 80 percent of what you get when you subtract your age from 220. Your pulse can be taken with your index and middle finger over your wrist or neck for 15 seconds. Multiply the number of beats you count by four to get the total number of beats over one minute. So if you're forty years old, your target heart rate should be 60 to 80 percent of 180, or 108 to 144 beats per minute, while doing aerobic exercise.

But some people who regularly keep fit take that prescription to an extreme. They engage in exercise regimes that last longer than an hour and are performed with religious regularity every day. Pain and injuries are part of their daily lives.

Thirty to sixty minutes of grueling activity is not necessarily the answer to increasing one's fitness level. You don't need to buy into the notion that you have to run in order to be healthy. Daily physical activity with no particular schedule or level of intensity can also lower your risk of heart disease. According to recent studies, such as one from the Institute for Aerobics Research in Dallas, the highest level of fitness found in a well-trained athlete doesn't offer any more protection from heart disease than the fitness level achieved by someone who goes on daily walks or spends time raking leaves, riding a bike, or walking the dog. The optimum amount of weekly activity, as we mentioned in the last section, should cause you to expend approximately 1,000 calories, something you can do by walking rapidly a half-hour each day.

In fact, some researchers are saying that exercise can be overdone, and exercisers can be breaking down, rather than building up, their bodies. The effects can be subtle, such as lowered sex hormones. Women may miss their periods, and men may have a lower sex drive. But when people push their bodies into overdrive for a long time—running more than 50 miles a week, say, or bicycling more than 100 miles a week—the effect can be serious. So instead of getting quicker, you get slower. You lose protein and you break down muscle tissue. Ultimately, the problems show up as painful injuries like shin splints, pulled muscles, and torn tendons. Along with reproductive changes, other symptoms of overtraining in both sexes include loss of appetite or sudden weight loss, increased pulse rate in the morning before exercise, and prolonged insomnia or restless sleep patterns. Exercise limits vary for each individual, so you need to be aware of your own peak performance and don't push beyond it. If you begin to feel dizzy or faint, short of breath, or have pain during exercise, you need to stop.

Obviously, if weight loss is your goal, intense activity such as running and stair climbing burn more calories per minute. And the more time you spend at whatever you are doing, the more calories you use. Furthermore, the longer your workout, the more likely the used-up calories are coming from your fat reserves, though the exact point at which this occurs is unknown.

Aside from its effect on weight loss, how you perform in your exercise is truly meaningless when it comes to fitness. How far, how fast, how long you exercise are not as important as keeping good health practices and participating every day in activities of your choice. Be redefining fitness and exposing the benefits of activity, we may be able to get the 200 million "fitness failures" in this country back on track.

Types of Exercises and Activities and Their Benefits

There are three major types of exercise—endurance, strengthening, and stretching. All are important in maintaining the best all-around fitness, whatever one's age.

Endurance exercises condition the cardiovascular and respiratory systems and allow a person to do more physical work with less effort and less strain on the vital organs. Endurance activities burn the most calories.

The best and safest way for people to burn calories is to engage in activities in which large muscle groups are used (legs, arms, trunk) and which can be sustained continuously for a relatively long period of time (20 minutes to an hour). Heart and breathing rates should increase, and the exerciser should work up a sweat. Continuous, long-term activities such as walking, bicycling, and swimming use body fat as an energy source, so they're good for weight control or weight maintenance. Other endurance activities include using indoor equipment such as a rowing machine or a ski track, jogging, jumping rope, and aerobic dancing.

Swimming is an excellent endurance exercise that burns fat and tones both the upper and lower body muscles. Some 30 million Americans swim for exercise. Long-distance swimming with short rest periods is most effective for endurance, while swimming short distances, but more rapidly, should be done if muscle strengthening is the goal. To work all of the body's major muscle groups, make sure to alternate your strokes. The freestyle (crawl), butterfly, and backstroke will work and strengthen the upper body muscles, while the breaststroke works both the upper and lower muscle groups. The water resistance also creates an excellent cardiovascular workout that is gentle on the joints. And because we breathe more deeply when swimming, one of the greatest benefits is increased lung capacity. Swim a minimum of 20 minutes at least three times a week.

Walking, which also should be done for a minimum of 20 minutes, is a popular endurance exercise because it can be done in any climate, requires no special equipment other than shoes designed for walking, and is easier on the joints than running. According to a poll done in 1989 by the National Sporting Goods Association, walking is the most popular exercise in America, with 65 million devotees. Any exercise with one foot always anchored to the ground has one-fourth the impact of a jumping activity. As endurance improves, you can increase the pace of your walking, swing your arms and twist your trunk to add upper-body exercise, and walk with hand weights for arm strengthening. Because of the arm pumping and the longer step, walking has a higher level of exertion than running at the same rate, according to a recent book on fitness walking called *Walking Medicine* by Gary Yanker and Kathy Burton (McGraw-Hill, 1990).

One doesn't necessarily have to set aside special time to walk, however, if you get your mileage on the job. A study conducted by Scholl, Inc. in 1988 asked 110 New York workers representing twenty occupations to register their mileage by wearing pedometers at work for one week. Hospital nurses charted the highest mileage, 5.3 miles a day; retail salespeople walked 3.5 miles a day; advertising/public-relations executives walked 2.4 miles a day; bankers, 2.0; lawyers, 1.5; housewives, 1.3; and dentists, at the low end, .85 mile a day. The study also found that the less we walk on the job, the more we like to walk at other times.

Biking is a popular sport in many areas of the country for people of all ages. Biking outdoors, however, can be dangerous. Riders can avoid problems by wearing a helmet and bright reflective clothing when biking at night, and fitting the size of the bike to the rider. Chronic pressure injuries can occur from a poorly adjusted or improperly sized seat.

Jogging, tennis, aerobic dancing, rope jumping, and other impact activities may burn up the most calories over the shortest amount of time, but they are hard on feet, ankles, knees, hips, and backs. Consider, for example, that you're hitting the ground while running with two to three times your body weight with every step. Tennis also can be a problem for shoulders, wrists, and elbows. Though some people can do high-impact activities their whole lives and never see signs of wear and tear, others need to steer more toward low-impact exercises as they get older. The key is to listen to your body.

Often people believe they will have the incentive to exercise if they buy equipment for their home, investing a good amount of money in the process. Yet marketing studies show that most home gym equipment goes unused. The most popular cardiovascular equipment for the home includes treadmills, stationary bikes, step climbers, and ski machines. The benefits of treadmills and bicycles are the same as those listed in our earlier discussion on walking, running, and biking, although the stationary bike is safer and often offers a more intense cardiovascular workout than its outdoor counterpart. The step climber simulates the exercise of climbing stairs and provides an aerobic workout designed to burn calories and increase heart and respiratory rates. This machine also helps firm up lower-body, hip, and leg muscles. Ski machines provide the best all-around workout for the time spent exercising, according to many experts.

Strengthening exercises are the second type of exercise needed for fitness. These exercises increase muscle power, which maximizes all muscle movement and helps protect the joints against injury. More than six hundred muscles attach to the bones of the skeleton and are responsible for all your voluntary movement, from winking an eye to flexing a bicep. Strengthening exercises need to be done only two or three times a week to increase muscle strength by 40 to 75 percent over several months. You might alternate the days you do endurance activities and those when you do strengthening exercises. You can begin your strengthening program using lightweight hand and leg weights, building gradually from perhaps 10-ounce weights (equivalent to a can of soup); or work out on weight machines such as Nautilus or Universal. Exercises such as leg lifts, finger presses, and bent-leg sit-ups are resistive exercises that also strengthen the muscles.

Finally, stretching or flexibility exercises keep the joints from stiffening. Research has shown that most joint aches and pains and stiffness, occurring particularly as we age, are the result of disuse, not of arthritis or some age-related tissue deterioration. Flexibility exercises are best done daily, although three sessions a week have provided significant results. The single most important rule in stretching the body's soft tissues (muscles, ligaments, and tendons) is to hold the stretched position for at least a count of ten. Then relax for several counts and repeat the stretch several times, increasing the repetitions at subsequent sessions until you can comfortably do ten repetitions. Bouncing when stretching is harmful because it tightens, not stretches, soft tissues.

Before you begin any new exercise program or activity, you should see your doctor. If you have any specific health concerns, if you have been relatively sedentary in recent years, or if you are taking medication, you should have a medical checkup.

You should start your new exercise program or activity slowly. It may take you several weeks or longer to become comfortable doing an activity for 20 or more minutes. Endurance improves over time. Gradually increase both the duration and the intensity of your exercise, beginning with five minutes of continuous exercise daily. Your doctor can advise you as to how quickly you can step up your exercise. For those with limiting factors, an exercise stress test may well be recommended by your doctor as you increase the intensity of your exercise.

Exercise regularly. To get the most benefit from your exercise, you should exercise at least every other day. This frequency gives your body a chance to adapt properly and to build endurance and flexibility. Several weeks of inactivity can reverse whatever endurance conditioning you developed (although muscular strength may take six to twelve months of inactivity to slip away completely), so try to maintain an exercise schedule that includes continuous activity for a minimum duration of 20 minutes at an intensity level that is working your heart muscle. Obviously, if you have to stop your program due to an illness or other circumstances, resume at a lower level of intensity and work your way back gradually. As the experts advise, it's better to have exercised and stopped than never to have exercised at all—as long as you start back up again.

It is important that you know your limit. You are probably doing too much if you have persistent muscle soreness or become excessively tired. Begin each exercise session with a five- or ten-minute warm-up period. The older you are, the more important it is to prepare your body for intense exercise. And never stop vigorous exercise abruptly. Cool down afterward—that means taking a two-minute walk-jog after running, a brisk walk after vigorous cycling, or just a slower pace of whatever activity you are doing. Flexibility and stretching exercises are always good to begin and end an exercise session.

After a vigorous workout, don't take a hot shower or sauna. The heat opens up blood vessels and can lead to circulatory collapse. Wait at least five minutes before showering and keep the water warm rather than hot.

In sum, exercise builds endurance, muscle strength, and flexibility. It also burns calories. Exercise is like a chain reaction—for movement to occur, the muscles must contract, the heart must beat faster to send nutrients and oxygen to the muscles, and breathing must increase to eliminate carbon dioxide and supply additional oxygen to the heart. All of these activities require calories as fuel.

The American College of Sports Medicine, the nation's leading sports and exercise research organization, sets guidelines for the public as well as professional and amateur athletes regarding healthy and effective ways to stay in shape. In 1990, this organization revised its 1978 position paper detailing physical-fitness recommendations for adults. Serious athletes may want to follow these 1990 guidelines:

- Train three to five days a week.
- Exercise at an intensity level of 60 to 90 percent of maximum heart rate, or 50 to 80 percent of maximum oxygen uptake or maximum heart-rate reserve.
- Exercise at your maximum heart-rate level for 20 to 60 minutes each session. It is also recommended that nonathletes exercise at lower intensities for longer periods to guard against injury.
- Exercise should be rhythmical and aerobic, using large muscle groups. Example: walking, jogging, bicycling, rowing, and stair climbing.
- Resistance training, done with or without weights at moderate intensity to maintain fat-free weight, should not be considered an aerobic exercise. One set of 8 to 12 repetitions of 8 to 10

exercises that condition the major muscle groups should be performed at least two days a week.

The following chart lists the energy expenditure (number of calories used per hour) of a healthy man weighing 175 pounds and a healthy woman weighing 140 pounds doing various activities. If you weigh less, you would use fewer calories; the opposite is true if you weigh more than the designated weight. The calories may vary a bit based on environmental conditions.

To Increase Calorie Expenditure—
BE MORE PHYSICALLY ACTIVE

ACTIVITY	CALORIES EXPENDED PER HOUR	
	Man	*Woman*
Sitting quietly	100	80
Standing quietly	120	95
Light activity:	300	240
Cleaning house		
Office work		
Playing baseball		
Playing golf		
Moderate activity:	460	370
Walking briskly (3.5 mph)		
Gardening		
Cycling (5.5 mph)		
Dancing		
Playing basketball		
Strenuous activity:	730	580
Jogging (9 min./mile)		
Playing football		
Swimming		
Very strenuous activity:	920	740
Running (7 min./mile)		
Racquetball		
Skiing		

Source: Derived from McArdle et al., *Exercise Physiology,* 1986.

Staying Disciplined

Some people find it nearly impossible to exercise, particularly after spending eight stressful hours at the office. For them, exercise is one more chore to cram into an already hectic day. And for those willing to begin an exercise program, it is difficult sticking with it for very long. In fact, studies show that half of those who begin an exercise program drop out within six months. Why?

The predictable routine goes something like this: John Smith has high expectations of losing weight, controlling the stress in his life, and improving his health and appearance. He wants to see major changes quickly and gets easily discouraged. He begins a running program with renewed fervor (having failed in his last attempt). Meanwhile, he fails to notice that he doesn't get winded as often when running for a bus, sleeps better, and has higher energy levels. While these minor improvements occur fairly soon after he begins his running regimen (last year he tried biking, rowing, and tennis), he fails to realize that it takes 10 to 20 weeks of sustained physical activity for marked progress in weight loss and appearance.

Studies show that people who enjoy the emotional and physical rewards of exercise are likely to be self-motivated and optimistic. Most are young adults, the well educated, and the financially well off. Dropouts tend to be the very people who would most benefit from regular exercise: smokers, the overweight, the severely stressed.

To succeed at incorporating exercise into your life, you need to learn to recognize those subtle, meaningful changes that show progress, like getting less winded and having more energy. You also need to know how hard you have to work out to get your particular results (consult with an exercise specialist) and how long it takes to see major changes. Meanwhile, hook up with a supportive person to keep you from being a dropout.

Most important, make exercise a part of your life-style. Walk to work if you can. Use the stairs instead of elevators. Take short walks after sitting at your desk for an hour. Such commonplace activities will help make you trimmer, fitter, and less prone to injury or fatigue during more strenuous activities like tennis and bicycling. Set an achievable goal when you begin your more active life, and pick an activity that you enjoy. Most physical activities—

walking, playing golf, bowling, mowing the lawn—may burn only 250 to 300 calories in an hour. But over a year these daily activities add up to about a 30-pound weight loss, if your food intake remains the same.

When beginning an exercise program, remember the 1989 findings of the Institute for Aerobics Research and the Cooper Clinic. It showed the kind of exercise needed to move from the least fit or most sedentary category to the next least fit—the jump that revealed the greatest health benefit—was the equivalent of a walk of a half-hour to an hour a day at a fast but not uncomfortable pace. That's not such an awesome commitment of time or energy, is it? Your overall health and fitness are well worth it!

Fluids and Nutrition Play Important Roles in Exercise

One would assume that people who maintain fitness through exercise would be well aware of the fuel that keeps them at peak performance and health. Actually, sports nutrition is as complicated as general nutrition, filled with facts and myths that need to be sifted through.

There is little doubt among experts about the value of a diet high in complex carbohydrates, or starchy foods, particularly for endurance athletes whose workouts last an hour or more. Consuming carbohydrates for even moderately intense exercise has also been shown to improve performance and extend endurance. Whole grain breads, plain potatoes, pastas, hot and cold cereals, fruit juices, and fresh fruit are loaded with carbohydrates. High-carbohydrate diets increase the supply of glycogen (a form of carbohydrate stored in the muscle, and its main source of stored energy) and glucose (the main fuel for the muscle) and help protect against glycogen depletion and fatigue during intense training.

The best nutritional preparation for peak performance is simple—a well-balanced, high-carbohydrate diet containing adequate levels of carbohydrate, protein, fat, liquids, vitamins and minerals, in amounts high enough to meet the extra energy demands resulting from exercise. A diet providing 70 percent of total calories from carbohydrates (about 12 percent from protein and the rest from fats), has been shown to be best for people who engage in intense daily activity.

Protein is needed to build, maintain, and repair muscle tissue, and it must be supplied daily. Athletes need more total protein in their diets than sedentary people do, but only because they need more calories overall. The percentage of calories from protein should remain at 12 percent regardless of whether a person is active or sedentary. Diets excessively high in protein are not necessary or desirable. Too much protein can impair athletic performance because it is dehydrating, can set off an attack of gout, and places an undue burden on the kidneys and liver, according to a position paper prepared by the American Dietetic Association. Excess dietary protein is stored as fat, not muscle.

Vitamin and mineral supplements also have the tendency to be needlessly used by athletes. Particularly dangerous are vitamins A and D, which are stored in the body and are highly toxic in megadoses, and vitamin B6, which in large doses can damage the nervous system.

A study at Cornell University indicated that active women may need twice the recommended amount of the B vitamin riboflavin to prevent a deficiency. Because this amount is readily supplied by a normal diet, supplementation has not been found to improve performance.

Iron is the mineral most often in short supply in the diets of carbohydrate-consuming athletes. Caroline Buchanan, a registered dietitian who surveyed the research on nutrient supplements and athletics, advised physically active menstruating women to increase their iron intake by eating iron-enriched breads and cereals, cooking in cast-iron pots, and limiting tea consumption, since the tannins in tea block iron absorption. She also suggested eating foods rich in vitamin C, such as citrus fruits and tomatoes, along with foods rich in iron (meats, fish, and poultry), to enhance iron absorption.

Fluids may play an even more critical role than nutrients in exercise. Water is a key nutrient, particularly during the hot summer months. The dangers of the loss of too much body water as sweat during long, moderately intense exercise (65 to 75 percent maximum capacity and longer than 60 minutes) are well known. The adult body contains 40 or more quarts of water, but the loss of even 1 percent—typical after an hour of exercise—can seriously affect performance. Water helps control your body temperature and cools all the working muscles. Recent research suggests that fluid replacement is also important for short, highly intense exercise (80 to 90 percent maximum capacity and 30 to 45 minutes' duration).

A healthy 154-pound man loses approximately 2½ quarts of water per day, assuming that the air temperature and relative humidity are moderate and the man is relatively inactive. Water losses, through sweating, rise dramatically during exercise. The same man can lose three or more quarts of water per hour while exercising in a warm environment. A moderate perspiration rate of two quarts per hour can result in fluid losses exceeding 4 percent of body weight. Body water losses of 2 percent of body weight will result in some decrease in performance, with 5 percent losses causing a substantial reduction in performance. Losses above 5 percent can lead to life-threatening problems, such as heatstroke.

Because thirst does not accurately reflect water needs, people who exercise need to drink water regularly while working out, whether or not they are thirsty. In fact, your thirst will be satisfied before you drink enough fluid to ensure a hydrated body. Therefore, it is important for the recreational athlete to follow these general guidelines for fluid consumption during exercise:

- Drink 8 ounces of water 10 to 20 minutes before exercise.
- Drink while exercising. A good rule of thumb is to drink 4 ounces of water every 15 to 20 minutes during normal exercise.
- After exercising, drink 8 ounces of water within a half-hour of finishing your workout.
- Drink more fluid if you're exercising in the heat. A good indicator of hydration is the color of urine. Almost clear urine indicates adequate fluid in the body.

The type of fluid you drink is also important. Water, the traditional fluid-replacement drink for exercisers, has one drawback—it only replaces water. While replacing the water lost in sweat is critical, replacing glucose, the muscles' fuel, is important to performance.

Several fluid-replacement and energy drinks have been developed to provide both. However, most of them contain large amounts of the carbohydrate sucrose (table sugar), which makes them less suitable for effective fluid replacement. Normally, just over one quart of water can be emptied from the stomach and absorbed from the intestines in one hour. Drinks that have a lot of sucrose empty from the stomach and are absorbed from the intestine more slowly. Thus, lost body fluid is not replaced as rapidly as it is by drinking plain water. Studies have shown that products sweetened primarily by fructose can cause stomach distress and sometimes impair performance.

Fluid-replacement and energy drinks with carbohydrate in the form of glucose polymers (up to a 10 percent solution), such as Exceed, empty from the stomach as fast as plain water. In addition, since glucose is the form of carbohydrate used by the body as fuel, energy is available to the muscles rapidly. Thus, the exerciser both receives energy and replaces fluid.

Studies support the theory that some athletic drinks are more effective than water in keeping an athlete well hydrated and at peak performance. A research team at Louisiana State University, for example, studied the effects of consuming a fluid-replacement and energy drink on nine highly trained cyclists who performed short (40 to 45 minutes), intense bouts of cycling. Seven of the nine men had improved performance when they drank the fluid-replacement and energy drink, compared with drinking plain water. These cyclists were able to extend their time to exhaustion by approximately 4 minutes. The two who did not have improved performances rode less than 25 minutes. A similar study, done at the University of South Carolina in 1987, showed that athletic drinks with the proper concentration of carbohydrates and electrolytes can help to maintain glucose levels and extend athletic performance while maintaining proper hydration. Cold liquids are absorbed more quickly than warm ones, and they do not cause stomach cramps.

So if you want to get the most from your exercise sessions, practice good nutritional and fluid habits. Eating well-balanced meals and drinking liquids spread throughout the day will ensure that you have adequate energy and hydration for peak performance.

However, for those of you who are involved in intensive athletic events that last more than an hour and a half, a more disciplined and specific nutrition regimen is recommended by exercise physiologists and sports nutritionists. They agree that the most effective way to enhance endurance is to begin eating a high-carbohydrate diet (60–70 percent) three days before the event. At the same time, taper off your training program to rest your muscles and allow them to be saturated with carbohydrates. Choices of exactly what to eat before exercising varies from person to person. Dietitian Nancy Clark, M.S., R.D., author of *Sports Nutrition Guidebook* and consultant to sports teams like the Boston Celtics, to the PGA, and to Wimbledon tennis players, offers the following recommendations when counseling sports enthusiasts. Less intensive exercise performance may also be enhanced by her nutrition advice.

1. Eat high-carbohydrate meals every day to fuel and refuel your muscles so they'll be ready for action. Choose high-starch, low-fat foods—bread, English muffins, bagels, crackers, pasta, and so on. These foods also digest easily and help you maintain a stable blood-sugar level.

2. Eat small servings of low-fat protein foods. Here are some good choices:
   two or three thin slices of turkey or chicken (in a sandwich)
   one or two slices of light (in fat) cheese (in pita bread)
   one spoonful of low-fat cottage cheese (with canned peaches or pineapple)
   one or two poached eggs (on toast)
   one glass of skimmed milk (with cereal and banana).

3. Avoid sugary foods, such as soft drinks, candy, syrup, or even fruit juices, one hour before you exercise. While sugar may give you a temporary boost, you are likely to feel sluggish once you've started your workout and your blood-sugar level drops.

4. Allow enough time for food to digest. High-calorie meals take a long time to leave the stomach. The general rule is to allow three to four hours for a large meal, two to three hours for small meals, and one to two hours for a liquid meal. Allow more digestion time before intense exercise than before a low-level activity.

5. You may want to try liquid meals, because liquids leave the stomach more quickly than solid foods.

6. If you have a tendency to be nervous the day of the event, make sure you eat well the day before, and include a hearty bedtime snack.

7. If you have a favorite food that you believe helps you, make sure you include it in your nutrition plan. Take it to the event

if you so desire. Likewise, stick with familiar foods. Don't experiment with new foods before you exercise—leave that to another day.

8. Drink plenty of fluids to prevent dehydration. For endurance events, drink four to eight glasses the day before the event, two to three glasses two hours before the event, and one or two glasses just before you begin. Fluids can be water, juices, and sports drinks like Exceed, Max, and Gatorade.

   Just as important as what to eat to enhance your event or workout is what to eat when you're finished. Again, priority should be given to fluids first and carbohydrates second. Begin to replenish lost fluids and nutrients one to four hours after your workout.

9. Fluids to include are juices (they supply water, carbohydrates, and electrolytes), water (which is always well tolerated), watery foods (watermelon, grapes, and soups), and high-carbohydrate sports drinks (they supply fluids and carbohydrates). Push the fluids—it may take 48 hours to totally replace your fluid loss from an intensive exercise like a marathon.

10. It is important to eat carbohydrates after you work out. Aim for 300 calories (75 grams) of carbohydrates, as in:

    one cup of orange juice and a bagel
    two cups of cranberry juice
    one 12-ounce can of soft drink and 8 ounces of fruit yogurt
    one bowl of cereal with banana.

We hope this chapter has convinced you of the importance of exercise to your health and has exposed you to the variety of activities that can give you the exercise you need. For those of you who are dedicated athletes, we hope you have learned how to enhance your workout performance. Contrary to popular belief, you don't have to give up your favorite foods, confine your food choices to some inflexible dietary regimen, or deny yourself the pleasure of eating when preparing for an intensive (or a less vigorous) athletic event. To borrow a popular credo, you can "eat to win."

12

A Glimpse of the Future

Life expectancy continues to increase. Part of the reason is better nutrition and healthier life-styles. As we enter the twenty-first century, the middle-age and over-fifty segments of our population will begin to swell. It is estimated that there may be more than 100,000 centenarians in America by the year 2000.

Longer life spans translate into more people vulnerable to diet-related chronic diseases. That means there will also be more people in the twenty-first century who are more willing to make dietary changes to improve the quality of their lives. We see this trend beginning now.

People in the 1990s have started to make life-style changes to improve their health and nutrition. In Chapter 3, we introduced you to the challenge of eating at home and maintaining the traditional family dinner hour. We looked at the influence of the working-mom life-style and the time limitations that have altered what we eat and the way we eat dinner as a family. Chapter 4 examined how the supermarket industry has evolved to meet the needs of the 1990s shopper. Chapter 5 gave you a close look at what products are now available in the average supermarket. In

Chapter 6, we discovered how fast-paced life-styles have allowed fast foods to become such a successful American phenomenon.

The latter half of this book looked at how today's healthy life-style trends have impacted restaurant dining, traveling for business or pleasure, and handling stress. In our last two chapters, we saw how even dieting and exercise seemed to take on a specific personality in the past decade.

Changing life-styles will continue into the twenty-first century. By the year 2001, an estimated 84 percent of all women will be working outside the home. Due to the divorce rate and longer life spans, the number of people who live alone—men and women, young and old—will surpass that of married couples with children. The aging of the population coupled with the changing face of the American household will have a profound effect on eating patterns in the coming decade.

Where will we be, from a nutritional perspective, as we enter the twenty-first century? What nutritional products are on the horizon, and what nutritional breakthroughs might we expect? What will the family dinner hour be like—or our supermarkets, for that matter? Will fast food still be synonymous with McDonald's, or will it take on a new and broader meaning? Will we be dining out and traveling more, or less? And how might tomorrow's restaurants, hotels, and airlines accommodate us? If our daily stresses continue to plague us, will we learn through diet and exercise how to cope better? Will we be fatter or thinner; will we be dieting and exercising more, or less? Or will our future approach to food and diet change so that food will no longer be an obsession and the reckless and faddish diets of the 1990s will be heard of no more?

These are the kinds of intriguing speculations we wish to comment on in this final chapter. Our predictions are based on present trends, research, and development . . . and a little imagination.

The Family Meal in the Year 2001

Mom cooks dinner for the family by assembling ready-to-eat offerings into a meal. She may pull together prepared vegetables she picked up after work from the local farmer's market that specializes in organic produce; frozen cooking bags of beef fajitas (one bag is salt-free for Dad because of his high blood pressure; another is a low-calorie version for her teenage daughter; the third bag is higher in protein and calories for Junior, who wants to "bulk up"; and Mom's own is calcium-fortified, since she is concerned about osteoporosis); a rice pilaf mix; and boxed "homemade" fruit tarts.

With the aid of a double microwave oven (only the telephone gets more use), she can heat the beef and rice, then dish out the salad. (Some 95 percent of Americans have a microwave in 2001, and 50 percent have two or more.) Sitting down to the table only minutes after she began to "cook," Mom has a satisfied sense that she has prepared a nutritious meal that accommodates the health and taste needs of every family member. Microwave warming of store-prepared foods is the preferred method of "cooking" at home. In this twenty-first-century world of culinary illusion, fresh means not "made today" but "controlled atmosphere packaging."

But while "cooking" has taken on a broader meaning for the working mom, there still exist those holdouts who insist on the time to cook regularly and from scratch for family and friends. Cooking like this is an enjoyable hobby rather than a chore. In such a family, you may see an aromatic meat loaf surrounded on its platter by a ring of carrots and potatoes. There's a basket of bread Mom baked this afternoon and a big salad rounding out the meal. A quart of ice cream is waiting in the kitchen freezer for everyone to enjoy. What has changed in this turn-of-the-century scenario is the food itself, because virtually every food item has been scientifically redesigned to improve upon nature. (That's also true for the prepared foods offered by the working mom.) The meat in the meat loaf comes from cattle bred for leanness and raised without artificial hormones and chemicals. (Such meat was already available in the early 1990s.) The carrots and potatoes have been genetically altered to resist pests and diseases so they are pesticide-free. Vegetables actually contain more vitamins and minerals than the traditional varieties. Salad dressing and ice cream can be enjoyed by all family members, regardless of whether Dad or Mom is avoiding fat and cholesterol: both items have been made with a laboratory-derived fat substitute (also already available today). Even the flour used in the bread can be augmented by a specially treated fiber made from straw or citrus pulp. This high-fiber addition to the meal leaves everyone feeling quite satiated.

And here's a third scenario. For truly time-pressed families in the year 2001, it's not uncommon to contract with one of many available services that deliver a healthy, customized gourmet meal literally to your door seven days a week. (Most people sign up only for Monday through Friday, allowing weekend flexibility.) It's a very simple concept. You choose a menu plan—calories and nutrients are always provided, since these services work with registered dietitians—and you designate the time you want delivery. The food is hot and delicious and healthy. It beats carry-out pizza or Chinese food.

Nutritional Products on the Horizon: Supermarkets of the Future

So, you might say, the food products available in the year 2001 have nutritional concerns at the forefront. Mother Nature, over the last decade, has received a lot of help from food scientists in order to alter less desirable foods (from a nutrition standpoint) from the 1990s or create new ones that are deemed healthy.

Take beef and pork, for example. Along with breeding livestock for leanness and raising them without artificial hormones and chemicals, agricultural researchers in 2001 have mastered gene transfer technology and applied it to many commercially important kinds of livestock to alter their composition toward leaner products. Through genetic manipulation, the fatty-acid composition of meat, milk, and eggs can be changed, which means less saturated fat in the diet.

Biotechnology has also developed more healthful products in the fruit and vegetable area. In fact, varieties of carrots and celery may be given superior taste and crunchiness by the use of laboratory tissue culture techniques. And fruits and vegetables are all higher in protein, vitamins, and minerals than their twentieth-century counterparts.

Other biotechnological changes in food plants have produced decaffeinated coffee beans straight from the bush. That means that there is no need to process the beans after they are picked to remove the caffeine. Soybeans are available with a nutritionally complete amino acid profile. The texture and nutrition profile of grains have improved, since we now know how to alter the amount and type of their complex carbohydrates. Even vitamins and minerals are enhanced. It's no surprise that the annual sale of engineered foods reached $100 billion as we entered the twenty-first century.

And that's not all that has changed with our twenty-first-century foods. Companies finally have responded to consumer desire for low-calorie, low-saturated-fat, and low-sodium products and produce synthetic foods, including fat, sugar, and sodium substitutes, that taste great. You can have sour cream, butter spreads, yogurt, ice cream, ice milk, and cheeses with little or no fat—or guilt. Food science has discovered how to remove all the cholesterol from beef tallow, milk fat, and egg yolks, and so previously forbidden beef, eggs, and dairy products are available to those watching their cholesterol.

Actually, much of what is done to foods—in the way they have been altered, produced, packaged, and sold—is determined largely by older Americans, who make up the largest segment of the population in the first decade of the twenty-first century. A further influence comes from the ever-growing Hispanic and Asian populations. Ethnic foods represent a growing portion of the food market, and there are more ethnic hybrid foods as well.

All these new and nutritionally enhanced products are available at the local supermarket, where there are aisles devoted to nothing but microwaveable foods, both frozen and freshly packaged. Frozen foods, however, have declined in popularity, with aseptic packaging and irradiated foods taking their place. Freshly prepared items are specially packaged and kept stable in the refrigeration section, as they are now. The number of canned food items has declined.

The traditional metal and glass containers of 1991 have been replaced by pouches made from layers of laminated, recyclable plastic. Because of the shape and flexibility of these pouches, shorter heating times are needed to preserve foods, and more vitamins are retained. As you may have concluded from our working-mom scenario earlier in this chapter, more foods are packaged in single-serving sizes to accommodate the health and taste needs of every family member.

Food labeling is much clearer to the average consumer than it was at the start of the 1990s. Produce labeling, with complete nutritional information, is now the rule, not the exception.

Health concerns have driven the twenty-first-century supermarkets to stock more fruits and vegetables. On the average, they carry 250 different types of exotic and healthful fruits and vegetables. Biotechnology is able to alter genes so that ripening is delayed and the fruit arrives in the stores at its peak, and produce is more resistant to freezing.

Convenience foods have become increasingly important as our pace of life keeps many on the go, and food companies have become quite creative. Our lunchtime soup and sandwich are packaged together and frozen, waiting to be heated in the microwave. Fat and cholesterol have been greatly reduced in most processed foods, such as potato chips, peanuts, and luncheon meats. Microwaveable high-fiber snack foods like snack pellets produced from a variety of grains and potatoes offer convenient low-fat snacking.

Just as food companies have responded to time limitations with convenience foods, supermarkets have responded by offering home delivery of prepackaged meals as well as delivery of all grocery items. With the push of a few buttons on your home telephone, you're able to enter your supermarket account number and the time you request delivery. After circling the items you wish to purchase from the item list supplied by the supermarket, you can fax your request in a matter of minutes. The convenience of home delivery is offered to consumers at very affordable prices to attract customers, who are increasingly frequenting convenience stores, the supermarkets' biggest competition. Busy life-styles have reduced the number of visits to the supermarket and increased dependence on neighborhood convenience stores as the main supplier of family foods. Major upscale stores even employ highly skilled chefs who create specialty items. Lines of fully prepared entrees appear in local grocery stores.

What "Fast Food" Really Means in the Twenty-first Century

Under the constant pressure of the clock, we embrace anything that promises greater speed and efficiency. In the twenty-first century, we define fast food as something that can be prepared in minutes or even seconds. The microwave has changed our perception of what constitutes "fast" food.

Furthermore, fast-food establishments continued to slow down their service in the 1990s. As people demanded more nutritional items as long ago as the late 1970s, fast-food restaurants responded by broadening their menus, adding items lower in saturated fats, adding salad bars and other customer-driven innovations. Fast-food restaurants got bigger, and slower. The concept of pickup windows was the industry's attempt to speed service up; some restaurants even built double pickup windows. As a result, 50 percent of fast-food business in the 1990s came strictly from pickup service.

So it may come as no surprise to you that a great deal of fast-food restaurants in the year 2001 are pickup only. You can't eat inside even if you want to, and most people in the twenty-first century aren't interested in sit-down restaurant service at fast-food restaurants. Most fast-food restaurants have no seats, are very small, and sit on a small piece of land—obviously, parking spaces aren't needed if no one comes inside to eat.

Another change that you might have expected began in the 1980s, when Domino's Pizza actually started the trend of home delivery followed by other pizza establishments. It proved so successful that other fast-food establishments began carrying the trend into the 1990s. Now, in 2001, many large fast-food chains have one easy-to-remember central number within each city. Your order can be taken at the central location and transmitted by computer to a backroom commercial kitchen (located in inexpensive space like a warehouse) near your home, and your food is delivered within twenty minutes.

Somehow, while they're faster and certainly more convenient than their 1991 counterparts, pickup-only and home-delivery-only fast-food restaurants still aren't as fast as your indispensable microwave. The major fast-food operators also offer items available in the frozen-food sections of all supermarkets so they can be eaten at home after being heated by the microwave in only seconds. Fast-food restaurants, by the way, are now required to label the main nutrients on all their food items.

Notwithstanding the almost universal desire for speed, the fast-food "institutions" haven't disappeared. People still eat at places like McDonald's; but it just doesn't imply "fast" and "convenient" like it used to.

Eating Away from Home in the Year 2001: Dining Out and Traveling in Nutritional Style

While the family meal at home has not disintegrated, as some predicted, the telephone and the television continue to be intrusions on a leisurely meal with the family. As a result, many families eat out to be together. Dining out, in fact, has become a trend: in 2001, only 40 percent of the American food dollar is being spent on home-prepared food.

Nutritionally enhanced products are available at all restaurants; and the talents of chefs and dietitians finally have merged to create a healthful haute cuisine. Restaurants regularly provide calorie and nutrient content of all menu items.

Many restaurants have opened accounts with the businesses in their area. The business enters its account number via telephone, faxes its menu choices, and has the restaurant deliver a hot, nutritious meal—with a waiter to serve it. Obviously, this is not inexpensive, but many businesses feel the convenience and time saved are worth the expense.

Americans are also traveling more than ever. Their palates have become even more sophisticated. Fortunately, advances in the packaging, nutritional enhancement, and taste of foods has led to major improvements in airline food. The once-frequent complaint of travelers about the quality of airline fare has become virtually nonexistent.

An Obsession with Nutrition: Diet Analysis by Computer in the Twenty-first Century

In the twenty-first century, being skinny isn't the goal. People want to be *healthy*, and they have become aware that they can reduce their risk of heart attacks and cancer by eating the proper diet.

Maybe one in five adults and fewer than 15 percent of all teenagers are overweight in 2001. This may be, to a great extent, due to the fact that more than three-quarters of those overweight adopt weight-loss plans combining diet and exercise.

Highly sophisticated nutrition information is readily accessed by the average American right from his or her home computer terminal. Anyone can consult a home health-care monitoring system, connected to the home computer, to ascertain his or her nutrient level. At a finger-prick station, a small blood sample can be taken, and the monitor quickly lists your levels of glucose, potassium, sodium, and other nutrients. It records your cholesterol level and breaks down the HDL, LDL, and triglycerides and compares them to the target numbers appropriate for your age.

Molecular science is even capable of defining an appropriate diet for each individual on the basis of his or her genetic makeup. This, too, can be easily accessed by home computer.

Quite commonplace are a wide variety of diet-analysis software packages. They work quite simply. You enter your sex, height, weight, and level of activity, along with a list of foods you have eaten—generally one day's meals and snacks. The computer figures out your daily nutrition requirements, based on current recommended daily allowances. You're then told what you should be getting in the way of nutrients compared with what you are getting. The computer can calculate the nutrient content of those foods using a data base drawn chiefly from publications of the Agriculture Department. Finally, you're told in no uncertain terms how your diet stacks up against government guidelines.

You can also compute the nutritional value of a recipe. The software program may assign a "gloom rating" to your diet or recipe—a number derived from the fat and cholesterol content of the food or foods, balanced against how many nutrients are in those foods. The larger the number, the less healthy your daily diet or your new recipe.

While people already were using their home computers for recipe analysis in the early 1990s, the practice has become much more common by 2001. You just enter the ingredients into the computer in order to get a nutritional profile of any dish. This way you can make sure the meal you plan will offer a balanced plate of calories, fat, protein, carbohydrates, vitamins, minerals, electrolytes, and the like.

The Home Fitness Center and Family Activities: Reduced Stress as Part of a "Kinder, Gentler" Exercise Regime

The fitness boom has taken a new shape by the year 2001. Everyone has been exposed to exercise. Exercise choices are more personalized and certainly less faddish than they were a decade ago. Baby boomers have aged, and the general population is a much older one. Lower-impact, slower-paced at-home exercise and family activities are quite common. Exercise increasingly emphasizes health over competition.

Physical education in the schools has taken on a much greater emphasis, with more than half the children in grades one through twelve participating in daily physical-education programs. In fact, the majority of children over six participate in some form of moderate exercise with their families at home.

Here are a few more facts about exercise in the year 2001. Some form of moderate exercise—at least 20 minutes at one time, at least three times a week—is the norm for people of all ages. Nearly a third do vigorous exercise. And one in five in the over-sixty-five age group participates in vigorous heart-and-lung-strengthening exercise at least three times a week.

The desire for convenience affects the way we exercise, just as it impacts every other aspect of our more healthful twenty-first-century life-style. Every apartment complex, office park, country club, hospital, and government agency incorporates a fitness facility. Most homes have some form of exercise equipment, from the simplest setup, like a stationary bicycle in the bedroom, to the most sophisticated (and expensive), such as a separate gym room with multiple equipment stations.

Since time is an even more valued commodity than it was in the 1990s, many companies have adopted the four-day work week as a norm. Busier people can spend their leisure time with their families, and family activities are much more physical, whether hiking or biking, doing "team" sports, or working out together in the home gym.

More Predictions for the Twenty-first Century

This is where officials of the Office of Disease Prevention and Health Promotion say we should be by the year 2000:

- More than 90 percent of adults know the alterable risk factors for cardiovascular disease—high blood pressure, high blood cholesterol, smoking, and obesity.
- At least 90 percent of adults have had their blood pressure checked in the last two years and know what it is.
- More than half of all adults know that their cholesterol level should be less than 200.
- Three-quarters of the population know that saturated fat—the kind found in animal products—raises blood cholesterol. They also know what foods are high in fat, saturated fat, sodium, cholesterol, calories, calcium, and fiber.
- At least nine out of ten adults have had their blood cholesterol checked in the last five years.
- Fewer than 15 percent of all adults and no more than 15 percent of young people smoke.
- All tobacco-product packages and advertisements provide information on all major health effects, including addiction, and name all ingredients and the potential harm of secondary smoke.
- At least 85 percent of all teenagers link cigarette smoking with "great risk" to health and "social disapproval."
- No more than 5 percent of adults have more than two alcoholic drinks a day.

Revisiting Our Real People in the Year 2001

Let's make some more predictions, now with the people you got to know throughout this book. These are people much like yourselves, people who don't have perfect nutritional habits and who have varying degrees of nutritional knowledge and commitment. Here are our predictions about their nutritional habits in 2001, as the future offers them new products and technologies.

Carole Gerber will most likely assemble ready-to-eat items into a meal rather than cook from scratch. Her home will have a microwave in the kitchen and a small unit in her home office, near her computer. Her interest in nutrition and her computer ability gained as a freelance writer have made her a natural for computer diet analysis. She will continue to focus special attention on the levels of vitamin C and calcium in her diet.

Judy Markey will also enjoy the ease of assembling her dinner from pre-prepared items. Since she likes to munch rather than lunch, the new microwaveable nutritious snack foods will find themselves in her home. She too will have a miniature microwave unit in her home office. Since her children will be grown, Judy will probably dine out frequently, and the prevalence of healthful haute cuisine will have a positive impact on her overall nutrition awareness and consumption.

Burt Staniar will frequently utilize the restaurant-catered business lunch at his office when he is in town. His three-prong health philosophy regarding fats, exercise, and meditation will continue even more successfully, as his secretary can access any nutrition information for him from her computer terminal outside his office. Particular emphasis will be on his levels of cholesterol and the fats and vitamins in his food. Since he is a believer in taking a day or so off his health program, he won't be as diligent in monitoring his diet during weekends. He will be more diligent with exercise on weekends, particularly since his sons will be grown. He will use his new home-exercise room every Saturday and Sunday both for working out and, since the lights can be dimmed, for meditation.

Jane Hartley will continue to buy her fresh produce at the corner markets in New York, and in 2001 most markets will offer organic produce. Jane and her husband might contract for a carry-in service for three weeknights, while her husband enjoys cooking from scratch one night. One night might be spent dining out with his clients. Weekends in town will also be spent at restaurants, sometimes with their children, who will be old enough to appreciate a fine meal. With healthy choices readily available, Jane and her family can have even more nutritious meals. And she may finally commit to regular exercise by converting one of the rooms in their large New York cooperative apartment into a gym that the whole family can use together.

Barry Nash will find pickup-only fast-food service even more accommodating when he is in a hurry during lunch. Fortunately, fast-food outlets will provide nutritional information, so he will be able to make the healthiest choices possible. Fats in his diet will still be a concern, and for that he will consult his home computer. Traveling won't be as hard on him anymore, since healthy and delicious choices will abound in restaurant and airline food. Desserts will still be his passion, but he will be able to get them sugar-free. With his daughters now teenagers, family-centered exercise and activities will be the rule.

Herb Glimcher, who was ahead of his time with the home treadmill he used daily in the early 1990s, will enhance his home gym with the latest equipment for cardiovascular workouts. He will have a computer located in the kitchen of his home which his wife will also use to monitor their fat and cholesterol intakes. Herb may even have a special software package on Pritikin foods.

So you can see, the nutritional strides to be made over the next decade by food scientists will change the way foods are altered, produced, packaged, and sold, and will have quite an impact on consumers' nutritional habits. As technology advances, so will the entire food industry. In the end, consumers will gain nutritional knowledge and good health.

We hope our predictions have not strayed too far from what we do find on the horizon as we enter the next century.

To your good health!

APPENDIX A

Cookbooks

Here are a wide variety of cookbooks that offer information and recipes emphasizing nutrition, quick preparation, or both. With your newfound knowledge of substitution and low-fat cooking techniques, any of these cookbooks could be a valuable addition to your kitchen.

Cookbooks with a Cholesterol Angle

Eater's Choice: A Food Lover's Guide to Lower Cholesterol by Dr. Ron Goor and Nancy Goor (Houghton Mifflin, 1987)

One of our favorite cookbooks. The first half of the book discusses the relationship between saturated fat, cholesterol, and your risk of heart attack. It equips the reader with the skills to make food choices that lower blood cholesterol. The second half of the book provides more than two hundred delicious recipes, from soup to dessert, that are very low in saturated fat. Each recipe lists the total number of calories per portion, along with the saturated-fat calories. More than half the recipes have a "Q" indicating they are quick and easy to prepare.

Controlling Cholesterol by Dr. Kenneth Cooper (Bantam Books, 1988)

While the vast majority of this book is devoted to the facts surrounding cholesterol—what it is, how it affects your health, how you can control it, and the latest research on the subject—a small section includes recipes for controlling cholesterol which were developed by the nutrition department of the Aerobic Center in Dallas. There are several easy-to-prepare chicken and fish entrees, some quick side dishes, and recipes for vegetables, baked goods, sauces, dressings, and desserts. Each recipe includes values for calories, fat, and cholesterol and indicates the number of ounces in one serving portion. Portions tend to be 3 or 4 ounces.

Some of the more noteworthy offerings are Baked Chicken with Brown Rice and Nut Dressing, Baked Seafood seasoned with Mixed Vegetables, Shrimp Creole, Homemade Meat Sauce, and Spinach Lasagne. The soup recipes, while more involved, are also appealing. The sauces (Barbecue, Lime Ginger, Red Wine and Mushroom, and Teriyaki) are easy and versatile, whether used for fish, poultry, or even, in some cases, beef, and whether as a marinade, as a baste for baking, or simply as a dip.

The New American Diet by Sonja L. Connor and William E. Connor (Simon & Schuster, 1986)

The New American Diet has been devised, based on scientific and medical knowledge, for the prevention of atherosclerosis and coronary heart disease, stroke, hypertension, diabetes, several forms of cancer, and a number of other disorders. The authors also contend that it is ideally suited for gradual weight loss and long-term weight maintenance. The dietary program was based on a five-year study of 233 families to ascertain just how many and what kind of desirable dietary changes typical Americans could comfortably make.

The book is made up of three parts. The first part documents the need for a New American Diet. The second part tells in great detail just what the New American Diet is and what it can do, while emphasizing the need to change food habits gradually if the change is to last. Part three is the cookbook, a collection of nearly 350 recipes, international in scope, low in fat, cholesterol, and salt, and high in complex carbohydrates and fiber.

The authors have also considered ease of preparation when developing the recipes. They have simplified recipes that have many steps and minimized the use of unusual ingredients. Several recipes are labeled "quick" (those taking 30 minutes or less to prepare) and "easy" (recipes that can be tossed together in a few minutes but take an hour or so to cook). The recipes are truly imaginative (Parmesan Yogurt Chicken, Spicy Chicken with Spinach, Fish Almondine with Dilly Sauce).

Low Cholesterol Cuisine by Anne Lindsay (Hearst Books, 1989)

This book offers more than two hundred recipes for imaginative and easy-to-prepare meals that are low in fat, cholesterol, and calories. Each recipe lists an analysis, per serving, of cholesterol, fat, sodium, and calorie content, along with the amount of protein and carbohydrate. The author also indicates what vitamins and minerals the recipe is a good source of. Microwave instructions for many recipes allow cooking preparation in minutes. Several recipes can be prepared one or two days in advance, covered, and refrigerated, such as the Beef and Pasta Casserole for a Crowd (serves 14) and the Vegetable Lasagne (serves 8). We particularly liked the All-Purpose Quick Spaghetti Sauce, the Last-Minute Pasta Casserole, and the imitation "fast food" for the kids, like the Herb-Breaded Chicken and the Frozen Hamburger Patties (makes 20 patties). A few recipes for eating solo are also included.

Grilling

Great Grilling by Hillary Davis (Weidenfeld & Nicolson, 1989)

Beautifully illustrated with more than 100 color photographs, *Great Grilling* begins with a guide to everything you need to know about the wealth of equipment now on the market, from what to fuel the fire with to the different types of grills to what accessories you may need. But the main portion of the book is devoted to more than fifty easy-to-prepare recipes that are much higher in flavor than they are in calories. Our favorite is the Grilled Chicken with Sundried Tomatoes, Garlic, and Fusilli Pasta. You can alternate the grilled chicken with grilled shrimp or grilled scallops.

All the recipes are delicious, and one of the great advantages is that they can be readied for the grill ahead of time. In fact, most of the marinades and sauces can be prepared at least a day in advance and stored in the refrigerator.

Each recipe comes with a complete suggested menu that includes appetizer, side dishes, dessert, and beverage. And each menu is made even simpler with "Perfect Timing" tips designed to make sure the individual dishes are coordinated smoothly. Very occasionally, a recipe will call for heavy cream or use butter, but you should be well versed in the rule of substitution by now!

Fish on the Grill by Barbara Grunes and Phyllis Magida (Contemporary Books, 1986)

Consider these facts: fish is low in calories, high in complete protein, and low in cholesterol; grilling uses as little fat as possible and doesn't take much time. This book should be a must for your kitchen.

Part one of the book provides fish-grilling basics—how to select a grill, how to buy fresh fish, general tips on portions and cooking time. A section called "5-Minute Fish" provides guidelines to create quick and impressive recipes. Do remember, however, that butter can be replaced by margarine or even vegetable or olive oil.

Part two includes recipes that are a bit more exotic and involved to prepare—although no recipe is really time consuming. The fish used in the recipes range from the very delicate, such as sole, to the sturdier varieties like swordfish and halibut. Recipes for a few side dishes to go with the grilled fish, such as hush puppies and cole slaw, are also included. Some of our favorite recipes are Cod with Spanish Almond-Garlic Sauce, Halibut Steaks with Tomato-Basil Sauce, Mackerel with Garlic and Tomatoes, Blackened Red Fish, Individual Red Snappers, Rockfish with Lemon Sauce, and Swordfish Steaks with Barbecue Sauce. Several recipes in this book not only include butter but also use mayonnaise, egg yolks, and even bacon drippings (in the hush puppies)—use substitution if preparing those recipes, and enjoy!

Cookbooks Emphasizing Vegetables

Vegetables: The New Main Course Cookbook by Joe Famularo and
 Louise Imperiale (Barron's, 1985)

The authors contend, for good nutritional reasons, that vegetables should take a more prominent position in the menu, as entree or main dish. They don't suggest avoiding meat altogether but believe it should be played down to accommodate the nutritional principle of moderation. We wholeheartedly agree.

Although most recipes in this book are detailed, many are rather complicated and time consuming, and most use the "real thing"—eggs, cream, butter, cheese, bacon fat—we still wanted to include this cookbook, for several reasons. First, the book offers a chapter on how vegetables can be prepared in all cooking methods—baked or broiled, steamed or boiled, sautéed, or deep fried (a no-no). Secondly, the book includes an alphabetical list of vegetables from artichokes to zucchini that is an ideal reference to help you buy, clean, and prepare vegetables.

Finally, while most of the recipes are not appropriate for the very busy cook, we recommend several recipes whose ingredients can be substituted and are not overwhelmingly difficult to prepare—Vegetable Casserole, Vegetable Lasagne, New Potatoes and Other Vegetables with Yogurt and Cheddar Cheese, Okra and Cornmeal Pudding with Old-Fashioned Spicy Tomato Sauce, and Pizza with Vegetable Topping.

The Enchanted Broccoli Forest by Mollie Katzen (Ten Speed Press,
 1982)

This book is a collection of recipes reflecting many different ethnic cooking styles and containing a fairly wide variety of ingredients. There are recipes for light dishes and hearty ones. Obviously, their common trait is their meatlessness, which can be used for the occasional meatless meal and/or as accompaniment to meat dishes. Each recipe lists the preparation time and/or cooking time—ideal when you're looking for a dish that is quick to prepare—and the number of servings it provides.

The book is organized into six chapters. The soup chapter contains many easy recipes for both hot and cold soups. Our favorites were the Cream of Fresh Green Bean Soup and the Green Gazpacho, both taking only 20 minutes to prepare.

The salad chapter offered many unusual recipes. We particularly like the Chilled Marinated Cauliflower and the Marinated Pasta Salad, both taking 20–30 minutes to prepare and then needing refrigeration for at least an hour. The Eggless Egg Salad is a unique recipe using tofu and only taking 15 minutes to prepare. This chapter also had some wonderful salad dressing recipes, such as Garlic and Herb Vinaigrette, Orange and Sesame, Apple Vinaigrette, and Buttermilk and Cucumber.

The entree chapter was divided into seven subsections. The pasta section offered several quick and tasty sauces. Several tofu recipes were quite interesting—Hot Tofu and Sesame Noodles, Tofu Sukiyaki, and several tofu marinades. Under "Casseroles, Melanges and Other Groupings," we liked the Spinach Kugel and the Potato, Panir and Pea Curry. Recipes in the section on main-dish pastries, egg dishes, and vegetables were much too time consuming to recommend here.

"Light Meals for Nibblers" is a small chapter featuring dips and spreads aimed at the busy and the solo eater. The recipes are imaginative, easy to prepare, and keep for several days. The author contends that if you get into the habit of keeping your house well stocked with fresh vegetables and good bread, a dip is all you need to transform these into a light supper. Favorites include Tofu Guacamole, Tofu-Sesame Dip, Tahini Dip, and Pureed Vegetable Dip.

The remaining two chapters deal with breads and desserts.

Salads for All Seasons by Barbara Gibbons (Macmillan, 1982)

In this innovative cookbook of more than 250 recipes, the definition of salad is greatly expanded. Here, a salad can be anything from breakfast to dessert. Barbara Gibbons, the "Slim Gourmet," offers quick and easy recipes drawing on a wide array of cooking styles and ethnic traditions with foods that are naturally high in fiber and low in calories—in fact, she provides calorie counts for every recipe. And her main contention is that making a meal of salad is the quickest, easiest, least fattening, most nutritious "fast food" available today.

The book is long on shortcuts and short on troublesome techniques and exotic or hard-to-find ingredients. The "Salad Basics" chapter is an invaluable and comprehensive body of information on the different kinds of lettuce, other salad vegetables, spices, herbs and seasonings, salad oils, vinegars, and fruit juices used in dressings, as well as buttermilk, sour cream, and yogurt and the natural thickeners and stabilizers. The chapter "Make-Ahead and Marinated Salads" will have special appeal for the cook who arrives just in time for dinner.

Christopher Idone's Salad Days by Christopher Idone (Random House, 1989)

The more than seventy salad variations, all illustrated with full-color photographs, lean toward the gourmet side of food preparation. Ingredients in many recipes may be hard to find—for example, tamarillos, flageolets, kohlrabi bulbs, and mirin (a Japanese cooking wine). Additional recipes called for dandelion greens, star fruits, jicama, lotus root, enoki mushrooms, eels, kumquats, Jerusalem artichokes, and chicory.

While the author does offer calorie counts for each recipe, nearly a fourth have at least 800 calories per serving. Some recipes called for bacon, heavy cream, mayonnaise, or butter, and there even was a recipe that involved sweetbreads. But, complaints aside, the book's primer on greens, oils, vinegars, and herbs was excellent, the presentation of recipes was exquisite, and we recommend half a dozen recipes: Summer Salad (160 calories per serving), Grilled Vegetable Salad (235), Parsley and Bulgur Salad (bulgur wheat is cracked wheat—393 calories), Ceviche (380 calories per serving), and Wild Mushroom Salad (316 calories per serving). Each recipe includes wine suggestions as well.

Chinese (Stir-Fry) Techniques

Slim Wok Cookery by Ceil Dyer (HP Books, 1986)

While we are promoting balanced nutrition rather than weight loss in this book, here is one book that offers portion-controlled recipes and established calorie counts through a reputable nutritional database. Further, it is the only Oriental, stir-fry, or wok cookbook we found that doesn't include recipes that call for deep frying.

Color photographs clearly illustrate the more than 175 recipes in this book. Entrees are under 375 calories, and desserts are under 200. Recipes are quick to prepare, and care has been taken, as chef Robert Briggs cautioned us in Chapter 3, to cut the oil used in stir-fry to a minimum.

All recipes are quick and nutritious, so favorites can be quite a personal choice. Among ours: for appetizers, Mini Chicken Balls and Chicken Pinwheels; meat, Greek-Style Pitaburgers and Veal Scallopini Piccata; poultry, Chicken with Shiitake Mushrooms, Grilled Chicken Piquant, and Chicken with Vegetable Rice; fish and shellfish, Scampi, Fillet of Sole with Rice and Bean Sprouts, and Sole and Shrimp Imperial. In the "Vegetables" section, Stir-Fried Tomatoes with Capers is our favorite; and there's even a steaming chart giving the exact number of minutes each vegetable requires. In the "Pasta & Rice" and "Dessert" sections, recipes were more involved. The "Basics" section offered a Beef, Chicken and Vegetable Broth and a Quick Tomato Sauce that you might find particularly useful.

Pasta/Italian

Pasta Fresca by Viana La Place and Evan Kleiman (William Morrow and Company, 1988)

The title of this book, as defined by the authors, means pasta that is "fresh, vivid, and uncomplicated." This book looks at pasta and sauces together as complete dishes. In keeping with the authors' philosophy of simplicity, most sauces in the book can be prepared in about the time it takes to boil water for the pasta. Some sauces are as simple as lemon juice, raw tomatoes, and olive oil. Vegetables of all kinds—artichokes, fennel, asparagus, sweet peppers, zucchini—become sauces. More complicated stuffed and baked pastas are included, however.

In terms of the pasta itself, the authors stress that fresh pasta and dried pasta are equally good, but are used for different reasons. In fact, to critics of dried pasta, the authors are quick to point out that today, all over Italy, dried pasta is eaten much more often than fresh because of its flavor, texture, and convenience.

Some favorites include: Spaghetti and Broccoli Soup (it can be thrown together in 15 minutes from start to finish), Penne al Maestro (substitute for the eggs), Penne Pizza Style, Penne with Spicy Tomato Sauce, Linguine Fini from the Pantry, and Linguine with Crabmeat. We loved the entire chapter "Pasta with Raw Sauces," where the only cooking required is boiling the water for the pasta. Vegetables are cooked only by the heat of the pasta. Try the Spaghetti with Tomato-Lemon Sauce, the Thin Linguine with Arugula and Spicy Tomato Sauce, Spaghetti with Goat Cheese and Tomato, Pesto of Sun-dried Tomatoes with Arugula, and Pasta Sautéed with Herbs. The chapters on baked or stuffed pasta and gnocchi are quite appealing but a bit too involved for the everyday meal.

Italian, Fast and Fresh by Julie Dannenbaum (Harper & Row, 1988)

This book's subtitle touts "Delicious Meals to Make in Less Than an Hour." The author stresses that Italian cooking, like Chinese, is based on simple procedures, respect for basic flavors, and good, fresh ingredients. She cautions the reader not to overcook. And she promotes the nutritious quality of Italian food: "Italian food is one of the healthiest diets in the world. It is high in carbohydrates from pasta, and low in cholesterol because relatively little meat is used, high in fiber from greens and dried beans, high in protein from cheese."

However, the reader needs to sift through those recipes that call for butter and cream and high-fat cheeses to get to lower-fat offerings. Some suggestions include: for appetizers, Flounder Fillets Cooked in Oil and Vinegar, Pasta Vinaigrette, Lemon Pasta Salad, and Primavera Salad; vegetables, Italian Green Beans, Potatoes with Peppers, Grilled Plum Tomatoes, and Spinach with Garlic; soups, Chicken Stock (especially flavorful here), Spinach and Chicken Soup, Potato and Scallion Soup, and Celery Rice Soup; pasta, the Large-Quantity Tomato Sauce, Red Clam Sauce, and Zucchini and Linguine (other pasta recipes are higher in fat from butter, cream, or cheese); seafood, Poached Fish Fillets, Sweet and Sour Flounder, and Broiled Scampi; meat and poultry, Veal Steak with Lemon (substitute for the butter), Veal Marsala (again, watch the butter), and Chicken Mario. The sections "Rice, Gnocchi and Polenta," "Pizza, Eggs and Sandwiches," and "Fruits and Desserts" do not fit the busy homemaker's needs; save them for a rainy day.

Gourmet—Simpler, Fast, and Health-Conscious

At Home with the French Classics by Richard Grausman (Workman
  Publishing, 1988)

Good nutrition should not mean staying away from any particular food or ethnic style. Richard Grausman makes that particularly easy for the person who loves French cooking but tries to stay clear of too much butter and cream. He's updated classic French recipes to make them more compatible with today's health and calorie concerns, reducing the amounts of salt, sugar, butter, egg yolks, and cream without altering the essential nature of the dishes.

He goes one step further by providing clear, easy instructions considerate of the time restraints on today's busy home cook. If a step is not imperative, he eliminates it. If a shortcut works, he uses it. When something can be done in advance, he tells you. Finally, he has used ingredients in this book that, for the most part, can be readily found at local supermarkets. He makes the less accessible items optional or gives comparable substitute ingredients.

Certainly, many recipes in this book take longer than possible for an average weeknight dinner when you're getting home at 6:00 or 7:00 p.m. However, quicker recipes are included—you just need to look for them. And even the longer recipes offer useful food ideas.

Note that the author has not eliminated creams, butters, eggs, and the like, only used less of them. In addition, he offers the readers the option to omit even the small amount of such an ingredient he has called for when possible.

The New York Times 60-Minute Gourmet by Pierre Franey (Ballantine Books, 1979)

Readers of *The New York Times* have found Master Chef Pierre Franey's column, "The 60-Minute Gourmet," the answer to their needs for complete recipes for delicious meals in under one hour.

In this book, Franey has organized the best of these recipes for maximum cooking convenience. Each main course is displayed on a double page with appropriate side dishes and garnishes. He saves you the time of meal planning.

What he does not always save you in this, his first solo venture into authoring cookbooks, is the ingredients with saturated fat—the butter, the egg yolks, the heavy cream. But a little substitution can go a long way, and Franey's recipes are truly delightful. This book contains basic broiled fish dishes, broiled meats, a basic recipe for broiled chicken, and the simplest method for preparing a chicken sauté plus variations on that method. The information he gives you with each recipe makes cooking an interesting and fun adventure.

Cooking with Craig Claiborne and Pierre Franey (Ballantine Books, 1983)

Once called the "Rodgers and Hart of food writing," the *New York Times* cooking team of Claiborne and Franey offer six hundred recipes, featuring international gourmet delights and American regional favorites, using more herbs and spices and less salt, butter, and cream. They haven't, however, cut much from their rather rich desserts.

Also, time constraints don't seem to be a particular focus of this book, which make us somewhat reluctant to include it. However, Mr. Claiborne's bout with high blood pressure a few years prior to writing this book led him to abandon salt in the preparation of foods in his kitchen. As a result, he and Chef Franey have tailored the recipes for taste by a discriminating use of herbs and spices. The recipes are more involved than in Franey's *The 60-Minute Gourmet* while they do reflect lighter foods. Finally, the book is laid out by types of foods without offering meal planning ideas for the hurried cook.

Cuisine Rapide by Pierre Franey and Bryan Miller (Times Books, 1989)

The title of Pierre Franey's latest book does not mean "fast food" as Americans think of it. As Franey explains in his introduction, "It conveys a style of home cooking that is efficient, accessible, and refined." All recipes were designed with the demands and limitations of busy home cooks in mind, and virtually all the ingredients are widely available in supermarkets.

Franey's cooking style in this book has changed from his earlier cookbooks to meet today's demand for lighter, purer, more healthful food. In other words, he has decreased the amounts of butter and cream and added more olive oil and vegetable purees.

From hot appetizers to cold soufflés, the more than 250 recipes in this book can be made in under one hour. *Cuisine Rapide* has clear instructions, helpful sidebars, and 65 line drawings illustrating special cooking techniques such as roasting peppers.

The Way to Cook by Julia Child (Alfred A. Knopf, 1989)

In her seventh and latest cookbook, Julia Child acknowledges that attitudes about food have changed since the 1960s when her first book came out. She points to the time constraints on shopping and cooking, and our evolving health consciousness and awareness of what is in our food. "That very awareness is the best of all reasons for learning *The Way to Cook*," Mrs. Child suggests.

Fresh, healthy home cooking is what the author hopes to provide in this book of 800 recipes and 600 photographs. To maximize the book's instructiveness, Mrs. Child has grouped her discussion around method (stewing, braising, etc.) rather than by food type (beef, lamb, chicken).

Furthermore, she has organized her chapters around "master recipes" such as your basic sauté of chicken, preceding many less detailed variations, such as Chicken Provençal, that are easily made once the basics are understood. The major proportion of the master recipes are low in fat or even fat-free. Ms. Child is here very conscious of calories and fat, and she lists the low-calorie and low-fat recipes in the index.

She has included many new ideas of her own, such as all-purpose soup bases, where you start out with onions and chicken stock pureed with cooked rice to make a fat-free cream soup: by adding other items, you can turn it into chicken soup, a cucumber soup, a broccoli soup, and the like. Also included are suggestions for cooking longer recipes, such as stews and braises, in stages to allow you a home-cooked main course in only a few minutes' time.

There is no greater cooking teacher than Julia Child, and she has finally offered the reader an emphasis on lightness, freshness, and simpler preparations.

Microwave Gourmet Healthstyle Cookbook by Barbara Kafka (William Morrow, 1989)

Since the microwave oven has become such a staple in the American kitchen, we wanted to include a cookbook on microwave cookery. This book, with its accent on nutrition, seemed the most appropriate to include.

Featuring more than four hundred recipes and menu plans focusing on weight loss, this book also offers nutritional information on each recipe—calories, cholesterol, fat, sodium, protein, carbohydrates, and the percentage of RDAs. Obviously, between the food processor and the microwave, food preparation and cooking time is minimal. It is worth noting, however, that some well-known chefs are against the use of the microwave for "real cooking." They suggest its best use is for rewarming, defrosting, and sometimes for starting up or finishing off a recipe. Nonetheless, the nutritional information provided throughout this book is accurate and useful. And the author does admit that some cooking methods, such as roasting poultry, just don't work well in the microwave. The chapter on salads and vegetables, particularly the section on vegetable meals, and the chapter discussing basics and sauces, are quite useful.

Mediterranean Light by Martha Rose Shulman (Bantam Books, 1989)

The staples of the Mediterranean cuisine—fish, fresh vegetables and fruit, grains, legumes, pasta, garlic, and olive oil—are the very foods recommended by state-of-the-art research for weight loss, a healthy heart, and protection against cancer. Martha Shulman lowers the oil, butter, and sugar content of dishes with novel techniques such as replacing fatty meats with "meaty" vegetables like wild mushrooms and cooking Parmesan rinds in a dish and removing them before serving. The result is an appealing new way to diet, a contemporary cuisine that is delicious and filling without being rich.

Included are enticing recipes from every corner of the Mediterranean basin, from the familiar foods of France, Italy, and Spain to exotic lesser-known dishes from North Africa, Lebanon, and Yugoslavia. The author also supplies a colorful variety of menus—from high-protein Middle Eastern breakfasts and hearty Provençal midday dinners to light late-night suppers.

Jim Fobel's Diet Feasts by Jim Fobel (Doubleday, 1990)

Many recipes in Mr. Fobel's recent book are quick and easy; they're most appropriate for those who are not on a diet that severely limits fat, cholesterol, and sodium. Butter and cheese are used, but judiciously, in recipes like lasagna, enchiladas, and even shepherd's pie. None of the recipes has more than 350 calories a serving; many have considerably less. Several recipes are extremely low in fat; others are moderate. Every recipe lists the content of calories, fat, cholesterol, sodium, carbohydrates, and protein.

Dietitians' Food Favorites by the American Dietetic Association Foundation (Restaurants & Institutions Magazine/Cahners Publishing Company, 1985)

While not a diet book, *Food Favorites* is a diverse collection of tasty and nutritious recipes that have become personal favorites of members of the American Dietetic Association, the nation's largest professional organization for dietitians and nutritionists. Recipes reflect regional and ethnic influences and family favorites passed down from generation to generation, along with the dietitians' extensive knowledge of foods, food science, and nutrition.

Conceived by the leadership of the American Dietetic Association Foundation, a not-for-profit corporation established to promote health through nutrition, the cookbook addresses information on healthful dietary modifications in the chapters "Nutrition and Food Selection" and "Using the Dietitians' Food Favorites Cookbook." In addition, each recipe provides a nutrient analysis for one portion, and many of the recipes are coded for use by those who wish to lower their intake of fat, cholesterol, and/or sodium or increase the fiber in the diet.

The Good Book of Nutrition by the American Cancer Society (available through your local chapter)

This official American Cancer Society guide to healthful eating is based on the society's dietary guidelines, established to help reduce the risk of cancer through the following nutritional recommendations: cut down on fat; eat more cabbage-family vegetables; add more high-fiber foods; choose foods with vitamins A and C; and cut down on the intake of salt-cured, smoked, nitrate-cured foods. As the book points out, cancer research has shown that diet has been linked to the development of 35 percent of all cancers. *The Good Book of Nutrition* contains more than two hundred pages of recipes, from appetizers to desserts.

Cooking Light magazine, published bimonthly, by Southern Living, Inc., has many nutritious and time-saving ideas.

APPENDIX B

FMI Supermarket Directory: Nutrition & Health Programs 1989

Food Marketing Institute (FMI) is a nonprofit trade association conducting programs in research, education and public affairs on behalf of its 1,600 members—food retailers and wholesalers and their customers in the United States and overseas. FMI's domestic member companies operate approximately 19,000 retail food stores with a combined annual sales volume of $180 billion—more than half of all grocery sales in the United States. FMI's retail membership is composed of large multi-store chains, small regional firms and independent supermarkets. Its international membership includes more than 200 members from over 50 nations.

Company	Program Name and Description
ASSOCIATED GROCERS, INC. P.O. Box 3763 Seattle, WA 98124	NUTRI GUIDE In-store brochures and color-coded shelf tags identify foods for calorie controlled, fat modified or sodium restricted diets.

Company	Program Name and Description
	A slide presentation also is available for community use.
BASHAS' MARKET P.O. Box 488 Chandler, AZ 85244	HEALTH POWER Bimonthly newsletter offers nutrition facts and consumer tips.
BEL AIR MARKETS P.O. Box 13778 Sacramento, CA 95853	"DINE RIGHT" STORE TOURS Two-hour nutrition tours show consumers how to get more nutrition for fewer calories. Registered dietitians conduct the tours developed by Bel Air with Sutter Heart Institute. Healthiest foods by brand name are pointed out; customers receive cookbook recommendations and a deli coupon for a lunch from Bel Air.
BIG BEAR STORES CO. 770 West Goodale Blvd. Columbus, OH 43212	HEART WISE In-store nutrition education program teaches consumers how to shop for "heart healthy" foods, with in-store literature and recipes plus free Heart Wise shopping tours with registered dietitians. This program was a cooperative effort with the Riverside Heart Institute of Ohio.
BI-LO, INC. Drawer 99 Mauldin, SC 29662	CONSUMER TIPS Tips are part of weekly TV spots, newspaper ads and distributed in stores to customers.

Company

Program Name and Description

Bi-LO INFO
Weekly information in newspaper ads, our monthly mailer, *The Sampler,* and in leaflets in the stores.

"WALTER CAMPAIGN"
A produce campaign based on nutrition and information marketing.

BORMAN'S, INC.
Box 33446
Detroit, MI 48232-5446

HEART-SMART
Store posters and weekly ads of healthy foods and preparation tips flagged by the "heart smart" logo in cooperation with Henry Ford Heart & Vascular Institute.

NUTRI GUIDE
In-store brochures and color-coded shelf tags identify foods for calorie-controlled, fat modified or sodium restricted diets.

NUTRI-FACTS
Brochures, recipes and point-of-sale information on red meat, poultry and seafood.

BREAD AND CIRCUS
1163 Walnut Street
Newton Highlands, MA
02161

COOKING CLASSES
A series of six different cooking classes with themes for multifocus programs; classes offered in breadmaking, cajun and oriental cuisine.

Company	Program Name and Description
	"WHOLE THINGS CONSID- ERED" Publication discusses informa- tion and recipes on "organically grown" foods and natural alter- natives to nonfood items such as toothpaste, shampoo, and deodorant.
H. E. BUTT GROCERY CO. P.O. Box 999 San Antonio, TX 78204-0999	NUTRI GUIDE In-store brochures and color- coded shelf tags help consumers identify foods to be used in so- dium restricted, fat modified and calorie controlled diets.
H. E. BUTT GROCERY CO. P.O. Box 999 San Antonio, TX 78204-0999	PHARMACY AND HEALTH IN- FORMATION Handbills and ad tips are avail- able through the pharmacy. Blood pressure testing and diabe- tes information pamphlets are also provided in the store.
BYERLY'S, INC. 1601 W. County Rd. C Roseville, MN 55113	SPECIAL FOODS SHOPPING GUIDES An in-store program, "Special Foods for Special People," offers eight color-coded shopping guides. One recently revised guide gives foods high in potas- sium and iron. Based on USDA data, the guide lists foods with more than 200 mg potassium and 2 mg iron per serving.

Company

Program Name and Description

IN-STORE INFORMATION &
FOOD LISTS
Recipe cards and shelf tags for
fat-modified, sodium-restricted,
gluten-restricted and expanded
food exchanges are in the stores.
Fact sheets on apple varieties
also help consumers with their
shopping and cooking. Other
lists are on food supplements,
lactose-free foods and information to assist renal patients. A
registered dietitian and Byerly's
home economist contribute to
the information. Home economists in the store also help consumers with nutrition, special
diet products, food preparation,
menu planning and party planning. The *ByerlyBag* monthly
newsletter features the column
"Micro Notes," with tips on microwave cooking.

CITY MARKET, INC.
P.O. Box 729
Grand Junction, CO 81502

NUTRI-WISE
Product shelf tags for sodium,
calories, sugar, fat and cholesterol assist customers trying to
moderate their diets. Pamphlets
and recipes in the Nutrition Information Center feature basic
nutrition & fitness information
and recipes. Nutrition articles in
weekly ads cover new products
in shelf tag categories and produce in season. Food manufacturers also offer their pamphlets
in the information center.

Company

Program Name and Description

COMMUNITY PROGRAMS
Consumer and radio programs
with local high school and ele-
mentary school children are developed. "Wogging" 5 days a
week is one program; recipes &
articles are also in ads and *Eaters'*
Almanac. Projects with local
heart, cancer and diabetes asso-
ciations, state beef council and
yearly food and fitness expo also
serve the community.

THE COPPS CORPORATION
2828 Wayne St.
Stevens Point, WI 54481

FOOD FOR LIFE
This nutrition awareness program offers free pamphlets and
recipes. Monthly health and nutrition topics are: "Osteo . . .
What?," "Serving Seniors,"
"Food for Kids" and "Dental
Diet." Information is reviewed
by 13 health professionals. In-
store displays, posters, demonstrations and store tours show
new methods of food preparation and new foods. A monthly
column in Copps' advertising
flyer discusses health and nutrition along with cooking tips.

NUTRI GUIDE SERVICE
Brochures and color-coded shelf
tags in the stores aid shoppers
following physician and dietitian
recommended diets.

Company	Program Name and Description
	NUTRI-CARE MEAT FACTS Brochures and recipes of nutrition information on calories and nutrients in meat are available. **COMMUNITY HEALTH SCREENINGS** Cholesterol and blood pressure screenings offered at the store as well as Lifescan, a computerized health hazard appraisal, helping customers learn more about their health risks.
D'AGOSTINO SUPERMARKETS, INC. 2525 Palmer Avenue New Rochelle, New York 10801	**D'AGS CONSUMER NEWSLETTER** Bimonthly newsletter covers various topics to help customers make wise food choices and care correctly for food. It also advises on how to reduce wasting food through sensible meal preparation. **GOOD FOOD NEWSLETTER** With artwork from children in a Manhattan school district, D'Agostino's created the *Good Food Newsletter*. Distributed to 10,000 families in Manhattan, the newsletter encourages children to eat "power breakfasts" that provide good nutrition. This community project also promotes the breakfast program in the schools and has been translated into Spanish and Chinese.

Company

Program Name and Description

CONSUMER BROCHURES
Various brochures developed
with the Greater New York Dietetic Association are available in
the consumer center each week.
They include "The Vitamin and
Mineral Connection," with
health advice about vitamin and
mineral supplements, and "The
Cholesterol Control."

RECIPE FOR FUN
As an extension of the advertising program, four new recipes
are created weekly for various
departments. Nutrition information is included where possible
on in-store recipe cards.

G&R FELPAUSCH CO.
127 South Michigan Ave.
Hastings, MI 49058

NUTRI-FACTS "RECIPE OF
THE WEEK"
Weekly 3 × 5-inch recipe cards
feature Nutri-Facts recipes. A
distribution survey is conducted
three times a year to determine
dollar value for sales produced
from the cards.

FELPAUSCH CONSUMER
NEWSLETTER
Bimonthly newsletter features
seasonal food topics and nutrition information. It is free of
charge to customers from the
consumer information centers
and service counters.

Company	Program Name and Description

NUTRI GUIDE
In-store brochures, color-coded shelf tags identify foods to be used in sodium-restricted, fat-modified and calorie-controlled diets.

"RAINBOW OF GOODNESS" PROGRAM
Fluorescent colored guides in produce sections provide point-of-service information and nutritious snack ideas. Weekly seafood recipes with nutrient analysis are also available.

FIESTA MART
2300 North Shepard
Houston, TX 77008

NUTRI GUIDE
In-store brochures with color-coded shelf tags help consumers identify foods to be used in sodium-restricted, fat-modified and calorie-controlled diets.

FIRST NATIONAL SUPERMARKET
17000 Rockside Road
Maple Heights, OH 44137

NUTRI-SCAN
A comparative in-store nutritional program includes shelf tags, a consumer brochure and 80-page book. Factors and levels of calories, fat and sodium are illustrated by orange squares for over 800 brand name foods in the book and on shelf tags. The nutritional information is generated from the Nutri-Scan computerized data bank of over 3,000 products.

Company   Program Name and Description

FLEMING COMPANIES, INC.
6301 Waterford Blvd.
Oklahoma City, OK 73118

PEPCLUB
Information program for retailers includes posters, newsletters, and paycheck stuffers in quarterly installments. It also promotes seatbelts; safe summer play for children; nutrition, health and information on health professionals where possible, such as on in-store recipe cards.

SHOP SMART/EAT SMART
This point-of-sale nutrition program for Fleming's associates (retailers) gives consumers color-coded shelf tags for locating foods lower in calories, fat, sodium and cholesterol. This Nutri Care program also includes: a consumer booklet listing hundreds of products by brand in certain nutrition categories; advertising copy, promotional buttons and stickers for in-store use.

THE FOOD EMPORIUM
1400 Food Center Drive
Bronx, NY 10574

FOOD EMPORIUM COOKING SCHOOL
One-session ethnic cooking classes are taught by food authorities and include health-related topics about low-sodium, low-calorie foods.

DEMO KITCHENS
Chefs demonstrate techniques 7 days a week, make recipes avail-

Company

Program Name and Description

able to customers, and offer sampling demonstrations on weekends.

VITAL SIGNS
The Vital Signs program uses shelf tags to highlight nutritional advantages of select foods. The tags indicate sugarfree, fiberrich, low sodium, fat and cholesterol foods. This program advertisement appears on paper bags.

GATEWAY FOODS
1637 St. James St. Box 1957
LaCrosse, WI 54602-1957

CONSUMER SERVICES
Food for Thought consumer newsletter; a video point-of-purchase program; recipe cards; an educator's bulletin; consumer tips for print advertising; a consumer panel resource; and quality assurance response services available.

GIANT EAGLE MARKETS
101 Kappa Dr., Ride Park
Pittsburgh, PA 15238

GIANT EAGLE CONSUMER SERVICES
Celebration—fundraisers for non-profit organizations. Future Shoppers Program—store tours and in-school presentations educate tomorrow's consumers. Other services include consumer panels, nutrition information kiosks, consumer newsletter, customer relations and cooking schools.

NUTRI GUIDE
In-store brochures, color-coded shelf tags help consumers iden-

Company   **Program Name and Description**

tify foods for sodium restricted, fat modified and calorie controlled diets.

GIANT FOOD INC.
Box 1804
Washington, DC 20013

EAT FOR HEALTH
A nutrition program developed with National Cancer Institute provides consumers *Eat for Health* guides useful for finding foods low in fat, calories, cholesterol, sodium, and high in fiber. Shelf tags and p-o-p recipe cards also help shoppers select lean cuts of meat and recommend eating white meat and skinless poultry. Stickers displayed in meat department, consumer newsletters, and healthy preparation tips in new meat and poultry *Eat for Health* guides also assist consumers.

FAT & CHOLESTEROL GUIDE
A 27-page consumer guide, *Fat, Cholesterol & Your Heart,* encourages diets low in fat and cholesterol to reduce risks to heart disease. It focuses on monitoring blood cholesterol. "Heart healthy" recipes and shopping tips are given. The guide coordinates with Giant's in-store shelf labeling that identifies content of fat, cholesterol and fiber in various foods.

Company	Program Name and Description
	CONSUMER GUIDES In-store brochures and booklets feature a variety of topics, such as sodium, calcium, fats and cholesterol; seniors, pregnancy, nutritious lunches; meats, cheese, seafood and poultry.
	SUMMERTIME FOOD SAFETY BULLETIN Giant customers can pick up a bright yellow and blue bulletin about safe food handling of favorite summer foods at checkouts. In a checklist format, it advises on refrigerating and preparing foods and using clean utensils. It also gives handling tips for fresh and frozen meats and dairy products in case of loss of refrigeration due to an electrical storm. USDA's Meat and Poultry Hotline number is also listed.
	TEL MED A call-in service of over 250 recorded messages on health nutrition and medical concerns.
GRAND UNION COMPANY 100 Broadway Elmwood Park, NJ 07407	**FRESH FISH** Brochures on seafood safety, nutrition and cooking tips.
	FINE FOWL Brochure on poultry safety, nutrition complete with cooking tips.

Company

Program Name and Description

SALAD AND VEGETABLE GUIDES
Brochure describes salad and vegetable care; nutrition and cooking tips.

CONSUMER CORNER
Biweekly column in full-color roto features food safety, company policy, nutrition issues. Home economists take consumer calls the toll-free number advertised in the roto.

NUTRITION LIFE LINE
Consumer education helps consumers to reduce fat intake. Videos, recipes, in-store registered dietitians and food sampling offer consumer information on fat in today's diet.

NUTRITIONAL INFORMATION FOR A HEALTHIER YOU
Fact sheets answer questions about food content and possible health risks associated with additives and other ingredients. Recommendations include safe levels of sodium consumption and ways to identify high sodium foods.

HANNAFORD BROS. CO.
P.O. Box 1000
Portland, ME 04104

NUTRI GUIDE
In-store brochures and color-coded shelf tags help consumers identify foods to be used in

Company

Program Name and Description

sodium-restricted, fat-modified and calorie-controlled diets.

NUTRI-FIT
An expanded shelf-tag nutrition awareness program adds calcium and fiber to the color-coded tags. A mini quiz about monitoring fats, sodium and calories is another part of the program. In addition, nutrition information on 37 cuts and species of meat, poultry, and seafood with cooking tips is offered by this point-of-sale program.

HARRIS TEETER, INC.
P.O. Box 33129
Charlotte, NC 28210

HELPIN' OUT IN THE KITCHEN
Pass-out leaflets are available on an information board in produce department. Nutrition, vitamin and low-sodium foods are discussed. Point-of-purchase "channel" cards contain nutrition information and calories for produce.

HEINEN'S
20601 Aurora Rd.
Warrensville Heights, OH
44146

A LA CARTE
The monthly newsletter frequently features health and nutrition articles. Some *A La Carte* recipe cards have nutrient data.

SALUTE
The program developed with University Hospitals of Cleveland in March 1988 promotes the relationship between diet

Company

Program Name and Description

and health. Dietitians give tours on shelf labeling; health screenings; and advice on fat-controlled, nutrition-to-go deli foods.

The *Health Line* monthly newsletter is another component of the Salute health program. Food baskets for diabetics; fitness tips; advice on fat and cholesterol; and special reports for new babies and mothers are also offered.

HYDE PARK COOPERATIVE
1137 Lafayette Dr.
South Elgin, IL 60177

CONSUMER INFORMATION CENTER
Registered dietitians are available to answer consumer questions on food and nutrition. A weekly recipe sheet features ad specials and nutritional analyses of the recipes. A monthly newsletter includes a "Healthy Eating" column and a wide variety of consumer, food and nutrition information.

THERAPEUTIC DIET SERVICE
Special diet shopping lists have been developed for sodium-restricted, fat-modified, calorie-controlled and gluten-restricted diets. Specially modified recipes are available on request.

Company   Program Name and Description

KINGS SUPERMARKETS, INC.
2 Dedrick Place
West Caldwell, NJ 07006

CUSTOMER INFORMATION
LEAFLETS
Topics include: "Fiber: The
Facts"; "Calcium & You"; "Feeling Great on the Fast-Track";
and other selected nutrition information resources. All stores
have a variety of other food-
buying leaflets with appropriate
nutrition information.

THE KROGER CO.
1014 Vine St.
Cincinnati, OH 45202-1119

NUTRI NEWS
A pocket-size brochure contains
nutrition, preparation and storage information with input from
National Land Regional Advertising.

GRILLIN' TIPS
A consumer brochure advises on
selecting and preparing seafood
for the grill. Recipes for grilling
fish steaks, oysters, clams and
mussels are offered in this colorful brochure produced by National Fisheries Institute for
Kroger.

DOROTHY LANE MARKET, INC.
2710 Far Hills Ave.
Dayton, OH 45419

MARKET-REPORT
This bimonthly newsletter includes store news, recipes, product information and seasonal
food information. Food safety
tips are also provided to ensure
proper handling of perishable
foods in various months.

Company

Program Name and Description

CUSTOMER HOTLINE
Resident Home Economists are available to answer customer inquiries on nutrition, food preparation, menu planning, recipes, party planning and use of specialty products.

COOKIN-SCHOOL
Single session cooking classes are offered on a variety of topics, including special diets, ethnic foods and techniques.

LUCKY STORES, INC.
6300 Clark Ave.
P.O. Box BB
Dublin, CA 94568

NUTRI GUIDE
In-store brochures and color-coded shelf tags identify foods to be used in sodium-restricted, fat-modified and calorie-controlled diets.

MARSH SUPERMARKETS, INC.
501 Depot St.
Yorktown, IN 46396-1599

NUTRI GUIDE
In-store brochures and color-coded shelf tags identify foods to be used in sodium-restricted, fat-modified and calorie-controlled diets.

NUTRI-FACTS
Nutritional information about fresh meat and poultry; brochures for each meat group available.

IN-STORE COMPUTER RECIPES
Recipes include nutritional facts.

Company

Program Name and Description

MINYARD FOOD STORES
777 Freeport Parkway
Coppell, TX 75019

SHOPPING GUIDES
Weekly newsletter distributed in
the stores contains nutrition information and recipes.

CONSUMER CENTER
The Center in the front end of
the stores serves as a distribution
location for manufacturers' pamphlets, nutrition information
and recipes.

TOO SMART FOR STRANGERS
VIDEO
On a free-loan basis for customers, a 40-minute Disney produced video teaches children
about safety and self-protection.

NASH-FINCH COMPANY
125 Mt. Vernon Drive So.
Iowa City, IA 52240

AISLES OF NUTRITION
In-store brochures and color-
coded shelf labels concurrently
identify foods reduced in calorie, low-fat and low-sodium
products. Each brochure is
color-coded to match the product shelf tags.

OLSON'S FOODS, INC.
P.O. Box L
Lynnwood, WA 98046

NUTRITION AND HEALTH
PROGRAMS
Meat Nutri-Facts and Nutri
Guide shelf labeling systems are
offered. Joint programs with
area hospitals also conducted for
cholesterol screening, calcium
analysis and blood pressure
screening. Consumer Informa-

Company	Program Name and Description
	tion Centers are available in stores.
P&C FOOD MARKETS, INC. P.O. Box 4965 Syracuse, NY 13221	NUTRI-FACTS Nutritional information about fresh meat and poultry includes graphic displays with nutrition analyses. IN-STORE CONSUMER IN-FORMATION Brochures, recipes and videos available.
PAY LESS SUPER MARKETS, INC. P.O. Box 639 Anderson, IN 46015	NUTRI-FACTS Nutri-Facts program provides accurate information about calories and important nutrients in meat. NUTRI GUIDE Nutri Guide is a shopping service with brochures and color-coded shelf tags for customers on sodium restricted, fat modified and calorie controlled diets.
PORT WEST, INC. P.O. Box 5377 Ketchikan, AK 99901	NUTRI GUIDE A dietary classification service designed to assist people on special diets through color-coded shelf tags and brochures, which identify foods low in calories, saturated fat, cholesterol and sodium. MEAT NUTRI-FACTS A nutritional information program about beef, pork and lamb

Company

Program Name and Description

features displays and pamphlets of accurate nutrient data and nutritionally analyzed recipes.

PRICE CHOPPER SUPERMAR-
   KETS
P.O. Box 1074
Schenectady, NY 12301

IN-STORE CONSUMER INFORMATION
In-store home economists conduct educational programs dealing with food nutrition and/or consumerism. They also assist with diet advice, store tours, party and menu planning. A wide variety of printed material is available throughout the stores.

DIAL-A-DIETITIAN
This hotline is operated by registered dietitians in conjunction with the Hudson Valley Dietetic Association to answer nutrition questions.

BUY LINES
Buy Lines is a monthly publication designed to provide consumers with information on food, products and current consumer issues.

SUPER SAMPLES
Super Samples in-store product demonstration program introduces consumers to new and existing products.

LITE & LEAN
An adaptation of Meat Nutri-Facts.

Company   **Program Name and Description**

C.O.O.K.S. HOTLINE
"Call On Our Cooking Special-
ists" hotline takes consumers'
food related questions, 9 a.m. to
9 p.m., seven days per week.
Home economists and trained
chefs answer inquiries on nutrition, food preparation, recipes
and food safety. The hotline has
been cosponsored with Mc-
Cormick Spices.

SHOPPING HEART SMART
TOURS
Registered dietitians and home
economists conduct aisle-by-aisle
tours twice a month to show
shoppers how to trim fat, limit
cholesterol and sodium, and add
fiber to their diets. Developed
with the local affiliate of the
American Heart Association,
tours are free to Price Chopper
shoppers.

PURITY SUPREME
101 Billerica Ave.
North Billerica, MA 01862

EAT WISE PROGRAM
A. EAT WISE RECIPES assist
consumers with healthful meal
planning, recipes for meat,
dairy, seafood and produce departments every week. Recipes
include calories and amount of
protein, fat, carbohydrate, sodium and cholesterol per serving. The reverse side of the recipe cards tells how to reduce the
calorie, fat and sodium content
in the recipe.

Company

Program Name and Description

B. EAT WISE SHELF LABEL-ING recognizes products containing 2 grams of fat or less per serving and 140 mg sodium or less per serving on the unit pricing tag.

C. EAT WISE NEWS is a monthly leaflet of nutrition, recipes and food buying tips.

QUILLIN'S IGA
1515 West Avenue South
La Crosse, WI 54601

CONSUMER INFORMATION CENTERS
In-store recipe and information centers answer consumer inquiries. A home economist can help with your menu and party planning and will conduct store tours. Home economists and dietitians also do cooking school classes for the public and special groups.

FOCUS ON FIBER AND FAT
A food labeling class at Quillin's Cooking School is designed to help consumers identify food products that are heart healthy. The labels can be found throughout Quillin's stores indicating foods low in saturated fat or high in double fiber.

RALEY'S
500 W. Capital Ave.
W. Sacramento, CA 95605

NUTRI GUIDE
In-store brochures, color-coded shelf tags aid shoppers on special diets toward foods for sodium-restricted, fat-modified and calorie-controlled diets.

Company

Program Name and Description

RANDALL'S FOOD MARKETS, INC.
16000 Barker's Pt. Ste. 200
Houston, TX 77079

NUTRI GUIDE
In-store brochures with color-coded shelf tags help shoppers to locate foods for their fat-modified, sodium-restricted and/or calorie-controlled diets.

ROCHE BROTHERS SUPERMAR-KETS
P.O. Box 355
Needham, MA 02192

NUTRI-FACTS
This program provides accurate information about calories and important nutrients in meat.

CABLE TELEVISION PRO-GRAM
The series focuses on current issues in food, recipes, nutrition as well as entertainment ideas. The nutrition aspect includes new low-fat, -cholesterol, and -sugar products.

IN-STORE DEMONSTRA-TION PROGRAMS
Nutritious recipes and dietary information are introduced from different departments within the store. Additionally, information on new products with low sodium, cholesterol, sugar and fat is available. The information also is offered to community groups.

SAFEWAY STORES
430 Jackson Street
Oakland, CA 94660

"SNAP"—SAFEWAY'S NUTRI-TION AWARENESS PROGRAM
One component of the SNAP is the "Know Your Foods" program using bright yellow shelf

Company	Program Name and Description

tags. Consumers can easily spot foods low in calories, sodium, fat, and cholesterol, and fiber-rich foods from the tags. Useful in planning your shopping, the *Know Your Foods* guide in the stores lists brand-specific foods along with their nutrient values.

FOODS UNLIMITED
Another SNAP component is the bimonthly magazine *Foods Unlimited.* English and Spanish nutrition pamphlets are also available in nutrition awareness centers in each store. Other nutrition information for consumers includes: produce and meat nutrition signs; meat and a seafood recipe program; color-coded nutrition shelf tags; and a section for consumer response to nutrition questions.

SCHNUCK MARKETS, INC.
12921 Enterprise Way
P.O. Box 4400
Bridgeton, MO 63044-0400

NUTRI GUIDE
In-store brochures, color-coded shelf tags help shoppers identify foods for sodium-restricted, fat-modified and calorie-controlled diets.

FOODSTYLES MAGAZINE
Magazine features recipes, cooking ideas and other food-related information in full-color. It offers knowledge that might improve the quality of consumers' grocery shopping.

Company

Program Name and Description

SHAW'S SUPERMARKETS, INC.
P.O. Box 600
East Bridgewater, MA 02333

CHOLESTEROL NEWSLETTER
A newsletter, *Cholesterol: What's the Big Deal?* explains "fat facts" on types of cholesterol and food options. Shaw's store shelves also have been regrouped into the food categories: "Choose," "Go Easy On," and "Decrease" to guide shopping selections.

NUTRI-WISE
In-store shelf tags and brochures include private and national brands, cross-referenced with information about no sugar added, fat content, sodium and calories.

NUTRI-WISE SEAFOOD PROGRAM
Color-coded recipe cards coordinate with in-store color-coded shelf tags and show modified sodium, fat and/or calories on the reverse side.

NUTRI-WISE TOURS
Registered Dietitians are assigned to stores to help shoppers select nutritious foods. The dietitians use Shaw's as their "laboratory" for teaching people how to read labels.

GAZETTE
Consumer service bulletin published every six weeks. Regular features include articles on food,

Company   **Program Name and Description**

food safety, food handling and storage, nutrition and consumer-related topics.

SPARTAN STORES, INC.
850 76th St., SW
Grand Rapids, MI 49518

NUTRI GUIDE
In-store brochures and color-coded shelf tags identify foods to be used in sodium-restricted, fat-modified and calorie-controlled diets.

STOP & SHOP COMPANIES, INC.
P.O. Box 1942
Boston, MA 02105

TODAY'S SHOPPER
The monthly newsletter covers food and nutrition issues and policies and gives shopping tips; it is available free to customers at checkout and at the Consumer Information Center.

FACTS ABOUT FOOD
Point of sale nutrition information program utilizes an extension of the unit price tag to flag products low in calories, fat, sodium, cholesterol or with a P.S. ratio of at least 2:1. *Facts About Food Guide* gives data for branded products; program nutrients are supplied by the manufacturer. Note: program conducted in a 15-store pilot test.

SHOPPING FOR LESS SODIUM WORKSHOP
"Shopping for Less Sodium" program kit includes background information; posters; reading list;

Company

Program Name and Description

discussion guide and gift certificate for food samples—available free to community groups and organizations.

SUNSHINE FOOD MARKETS
P.O. Box 1108
Sioux Falls, SD 57117

DIET RIGHT WITH SUNSHINE
In-store monthly brochure for the calorie-conscious includes eating tips and recipes. Shelf labels also designate foods low in calories.

CHOLESTEROL LEAFLETS
The colorful consumer leaflets help control blood cholesterol through food choices. Developed with Central Plains Clinic, they explain roles of meat groups, snacks, fats, oils, cheese and other dairy products on blood cholesterol and diet.

EATING AND COOKING LIGHT
A series of newsletters called *Eating and Cooking Light,* provided by the Extension Service. Printed by Sunshine, the topics are: "More Calcium," "Less Sodium," "Less Sugar," "Less Fat and Cholesterol," "Dining Out."

NUTRITION AND HEALTH RESOURCES
Local dietitians and extension home economists write a monthly newsletter on nutri-

Company

Program Name and Description

tion. They also give speeches to consumer groups about low calorie snacks, sodium and low cholesterol foods for adults and children.

TESCO STORES LIMITED
Tesco House, Delaware Rd.
Chestnut Herts EN8 9SL
England

HEALTHY EATING
Nutrition information available on all private label foods. Booklets and leaflets explain healthy diet principles and offer healthy eating recipes. The principles also are integral in TESCO's staff catering facilities. A video of the information is sold in the store. Home economists also are available for group talks.

TODDY'S SUPERMARKETS
6000 S. Holly
Englewood, CO 80111

IN-STORE CONSUMER INFORMATION
In-store consultant is available to answer questions on nutrition, food preparation, menu planning, recipes, etc. The cooking school offers classes including ones for children. The county health department teaches children kitchen safety, nutrition and how-to-shop. Classes on special diets and tested recipes with nutrition information are also offered.

**TOM THUMB PAGE FOOD &
  DRUG CTRS.**
14303 Inwood Road
Dallas, TX 75324

NUTRI GUIDE
In-store brochures, color-coded shelf tags help identify foods to be used in sodium-restricted, fat-modified and calorie-controlled diets.

Company

Program Name and Description

NUTRITION TOUR
Leni Reed's Supermarket Savvy
Nutrition Tour is conducted as
two-hour guided tours for consumers. For a nominal fee, customers learn how to determine
percentage of calories from fat,
how to read labels and interpret
the nutrition information provided by the manufacturer.

TWIN COUNTRY GROCERS, INC.
145 Talmadge Road
Edison, NJ 08818

RECIPE & HINTS PROGRAM
Recipes on display are available
every week in meat, dairy, fish
and produce departments. Calorie content, grams of protein, fat
and carbohydrates are listed
along with sodium levels, in all
Foodtown stores. General household hints are also printed up on
3 × 5-inch cards for customers.

VALU FOODS, INC.
4701 O'Donnell Street
Baltimore, MD 21224

NUTRITION HOTLINE &
TOURS
A registered dietitian reponds to
consumer calls about health and
nutrition. The hotline operates
Tuesday, 8:00 a.m. to 12 noon.
To call the Nutrition Hotline,
dial: 301-342-VALU. Find out
about nutrition tours by calling
the hotline.

VICTORY MARKETS INC.
54 East Main St.
Norwich, NY 13815

LOW SALT/NO SODIUM BRO-
CHURES
Numerous brochures and pamphlets are available at the Consumer Information Center and

Company	Program Name and Description
	ideal for use by dietitians and doctors.

THE VONS COMPANIES, INC.
P.O. Box 3338
Los Angeles, CA 90051

NUTRI GUIDE
In-store brochures and color-coded shelf tags help identify foods which can be used in sodium-restricted, fat-modified and calorie-controlled diets.

NUTRI-NOTES
One nutrition topic is covered each month.

NUTRITION CAROUSELS
In addition to *Nutri-Notes,* consumers will find food and nutrition leaflets from companies such as Lipton, Borden, and Gerber. Our nutritionist, Susan Magrann, M.S., R.D., also makes speeches to hospital groups and others.

WAKEFERN FOOD CORPORATION
33 Northfield Avenue
Edison, NJ 08818-7812

KIDS' RECIPE CONTEST
An annual program motivates children, ages 7–15, to show off their culinary skills. In 1989 the winner for the best recipe won a trip to Disney World. Teen television celebrities judged the '89 contest at South Street Seaport where the kid finalists qualified with their Afterschool Appe-teasers (healthy food snacks); Old World/New Wave (traditional ethnic favorites); or Vital Veggies (creative uses of vegetables).

Company

Program Name and Description

WEGMANS FOOD AND PHARMACY
1500 Brooks Avenue
Rochester, NY 14692

LACTOSE INTOLERANCE—
MAKING A SPECIAL DIET EASIER TO SWALLOW
Booklet describes lactose intolerance, how it affects different people; supermarket danger zones and some alternate choices.

SHAKE THE SALT HABIT
Low-salt recipe booklet compiled by Ontario County Cooperative Extension Service and printed by Wegmans to use in combination with "Please Pass the Salt."

GLUTEN SENSITIVITY
Booklet describes sensitivity to gluten.

LEAN MEAT LABELS
Wegmans developed labels to indicate percentages of leanness on their ground beef. Sirloin beef packages now read "90% Lean, Fresh Ground Beef." This labeling responds to consumers selecting meat based on its perceived fat content. Each meat department is equipped with a fat analyzer and leaflets to implement the program.

DRUG LABEL GUIDES
"Read the Label . . . A Guide to Safe Use of Non-Prescription Drugs" contains important information which cannot be found on the label, such as special label

Company

Program Name and Description

alerts, symbol warnings and phone numbers. "Labels in Large Print" booklet features labels of commonly used Wegman's brand non-prescription drugs for senior citizens with sight problems.

EMPLOYEE PROGRAMS (main office only)
Smoking cessation clinics; computerized health assessments; nutrition and weight control workshops; low-impact aerobics; and breast self-examination programs are offered.

SEAFOOD SAVVY BROCHURE
Pocket-size brochure features calories, sodium, cholesterol, fat and Omega-3 fatty acids of numerous fish species.

FOR WOMEN ONLY
A booklet describing calcium and iron concerns.

SWEET SHEET
The leaflet helps customers through the maze of sugars and sweeteners on the market.

FACE THE FATS
Two supplementary booklets:
(1) *Face the Fats—Fats and Cholesterol* guide to the roles of fat and cholesterol in heart disease.

Company **Program Name and Description**

(2) *Face the Fats* hands-on shopping guide developed with Strong Memorial Hospital in Rochester, including a three-month cholesterol screening project.

HAPPY HEART TOURS
In-store tours with a registered dietitian conducted in conjunction with American Heart Association.

Compiled by FMI Consumer Affairs Department.
Since 1989 is the most recent directory produced by FMI at press time, note that programs may have changed or been discontinued, depending on the marketplace.

Index

FOR THE BEST IN PAPERBACKS, LOOK FOR THE 🐧

In every corner of the world, on every subject under the sun, Penguin represents quality and variety—the very best in publishing today.

For complete information about books available from Penguin—including Pelicans, Puffins, Peregrines, and Penguin Classics—and how to order them, write to us at the appropriate address below. Please note that for copyright reasons the selection of books varies from country to country.

In the United Kingdom: For a complete list of books available from Penguin in the U.K., please write to *Dept E.P., Penguin Books Ltd, Harmondsworth, Middlesex, UB7 0DA*.

In the United States: For a complete list of books available from Penguin in the U.S., please write to *Dept BA, Penguin*, Box 120, Bergenfield, New Jersey 07621-0120.

In Canada: For a complete list of books available from Penguin in Canada, please write to *Penguin Books Ltd, 2801 John Street, Markham, Ontario L3R 1B4*.

In Australia: For a complete list of books available from Penguin in Australia, please write to the *Marketing Department, Penguin Books Ltd, P.O. Box 257, Ringwood, Victoria 3134*.

In New Zealand: For a complete list of books available from Penguin in New Zealand, please write to the *Marketing Department, Penguin Books (NZ) Ltd, Private Bag, Takapuna, Auckland 9*.

In India: For a complete list of books available from Penguin, please write to *Penguin Overseas Ltd, 706 Eros Apartments, 56 Nehru Place, New Delhi, 110019*.

In Holland: For a complete list of books available from Penguin in Holland, please write to *Penguin Books Nederland B.V., Postbus 195, NL-1380AD Weesp, Netherlands*.

In Germany: For a complete list of books available from Penguin, please write to *Penguin Books Ltd, Friedrichstrasse 10-12, D-6000 Frankfurt Main 1, Federal Republic of Germany*.

In Spain: For a complete list of books available from Penguin in Spain, please write to *Longman, Penguin España, Calle San Nicolas 15, E-28013 Madrid, Spain*.

In Japan: For a complete list of books available from Penguin in Japan, please write to *Longman Penguin Japan Co Ltd, Yamaguchi Building, 2-12-9 Kanda Jimbocho, Chiyoda-Ku, Tokyo 101, Japan*.